Emotions and Personhood

International Perspectives in Philosophy and Psychiatry

Series editors: Bill (K.W.M.) Fulford, Katherine Morris, John Z. Sadler, and Giovanni Stanghellini

Volumes in the series:

Portrait of the Psychiatrist as a Young Man: The Early Writing and Work of R.D. Laing, 1927–1960
Beveridge

Mind, Meaning, and Mental Disorder 2e
Bolton and Hill

What is Mental Disorder?
Bolton

Delusions and Other Irrational Beliefs
Bortolotti

Postpsychiatry
Bracken and Thomas

Philosophy, Psychoanalysis, and the A-Rational Mind
Brakel

Unconscious Knowing and Other Essays in Psycho-Philosophical Analysis
Brakel

Psychiatry as Cognitive Neuroscience
Broome and Bortolotti (eds.)

Free Will and Responsibility: A Guide for Practitioners
Callender

Reconceiving Schizophrenia
Chung, Fulford, and Graham (eds.)

Darwin and Psychiatry
De Block and Adriaens (eds.)

Nature and Narrative: An Introduction to the New Philosophy of Psychiatry
Fulford, Morris, Sadler, and Stanghellini (eds.)

Oxford Textbook of Philosophy and Psychiatry
Fulford, Thornton, and Graham

The Mind and its Discontents
Gillett

Thinking Through Dementia
Hughes

Dementia: Mind, Meaning, and the Person
Hughes, Louw, and Sabat (eds.)

Talking Cures and Placebo Effects
Jopling

Philosophical Issues in Psychiatry II: Nosology
Kendler and Parnas

Discursive Perspectives in Therapeutic Practice
Lock and Strong (eds.)

Schizophrenia and the Fate of the Self
Lysaker and Lysaker

Responsibility and Psychopathy
Malatesti and McMillan

Body-Subjects and Disordered Minds
Matthews

Rationality and Compulsion: Applying action theory to psychiatry
Nordenfelt

Philosophical Perspectives on Technology and Psychiatry
Phillips (ed.)

The Metaphor of Mental Illness
Pickering

Mapping the Edges and the In-between
Potter

Trauma, Truth, and Reconciliation: Healing Damaged Relationships
Potter (ed.)

The Philosophy of Psychiatry: A Companion
Radden

The Virtuous Psychiatrist
Radden and Sadler

Autonomy and Mental Disorder
Radoilska (ed.)

Feelings of Being
Ratcliffe

Values and Psychiatric Diagnosis
Sadler

Disembodied Spirits and Deanimated Bodies: The Psychopathology of Common Sense
Stanghellini

Emotions and Personhood
Stanghellini and Rosfort

Essential Philosophy of Psychiatry
Thornton

Empirical Ethics in Psychiatry
Widdershoven, McMillan, Hope, and Van der Scheer (eds.)

The Sublime Object of Psychiatry: Schizophrenia in Clinical and Cultural Theory
Woods

Emotions and Personhood
Exploring Fragility—
Making Sense
of Vulnerability

By
Giovanni Stanghellini
and
René Rosfort

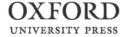

OXFORD
UNIVERSITY PRESS

Great Clarendon Street, Oxford, OX2 6DP,
United Kingdom

Oxford University Press is a department of the University of Oxford.
It furthers the University's objective of excellence in research, scholarship,
and education by publishing worldwide. Oxford is a registered trade mark of
Oxford University Press in the UK and in certain other countries

© Oxford University Press 2013
© Dylan Thomas, *The Poems of Dylan Thomas*,
Copyright © 1939 by New Directions Publishing Corp.
Reprinted by permission of New Directions Publishing Corp. p.263

The moral rights of the authors have been asserted

First Edition published in 2013

All rights reserved. No part of this publication may be reproduced, stored in
a retrieval system, or transmitted, in any form or by any means, without the
prior permission in writing of Oxford University Press, or as expressly permitted
by law, by licence or under terms agreed with the appropriate reprographics
rights organization. Enquiries concerning reproduction outside the scope of the
above should be sent to the Rights Department, Oxford University Press, at the
address above

You must not circulate this work in any other form
and you must impose this same condition on any acquirer

Published in the United States of America by Oxford University Press
198 Madison Avenue, New York, NY 10016, United States of America

British Library Cataloguing in Publication Data
Data available

ISBN 978–0–19–966057–5

Oxford University Press makes no representation, express or implied, that the
drug dosages in this book are correct. Readers must therefore always check
the product information and clinical procedures with the most up-to-date
published product information and data sheets provided by the manufacturers
and the most recent codes of conduct and safety regulations. The authors and
the publishers do not accept responsibility or legal liability for any errors in the
text or for the misuse or misapplication of material in this work. Except where
otherwise stated, drug dosages and recommendations are for the non-pregnant
adult who is not breast-feeding

Links to third party websites are provided by Oxford in good faith and
for information only. Oxford disclaims any responsibility for the materials
contained in any third party website referenced in this work.

To our parents
Ketty e Umberto—Hanne og Birger
The primordial source of our emotions
The inspiration for our becoming the persons that we are

Acknowledgements

This book would not have been possible without the constant encouragement, competent assistance, and financial support of a number of people and institutions.

Giovanni wants to thank all the colleagues and students who generously commented on his lessons and conferences on emotions, vulnerability, and personhood during the years. They have offered an inestimable opportunity for in-depth examination and clarification of these phenomena; allowing these concepts to be communicated and developed.

Among his colleagues, a special thank you goes to Bill Fulford for being an example of profundity conjugated to precision, simplicity, and intelligibility.

Giovanni is also grateful to Arnaldo Ballerini, Massimo Ballerini, Matthew Broome, John Cutting, Thomas Fuchs, Paolo Fusar Poli, Silvio Lenzi, Paul Lysaker, Josef Parnas, John Sadler, Louis Sass, and to the teaching body of the *Scuola di Psicoterapia e Fenomenologia* of Florence. He is especially grateful to Gilberto Di Petta and Mario Rossi Monti, for inspiring conversations.

In writing this book Giovanni remembers his teacher Paolo Rossi, who enlightened his way to philosophy. Paolo was an unforgettable mentor, teaching him the virtue of reason and the value of tolerance.

René would like to thank, first and foremost, the two teachers and friends who initiated, and still nourish, his thinking about philosophy: Jacob Z. Simonsen and Arne Grøn. Without their unflagging support, patience, and keen intellects he would still be roaming around within the narrow limits of his own thoughts. He also wants to express his gratitude to the three institutions that have been involved in the writing of this book: the Faculty of Theology, University of Copenhagen, in particular the Department for Systematic Theology and the Centre for Naturalism and Christian Semantics; the Center for Subjectivity Research, University of Copenhagen; the Department of Philosophy, University of Florence.

René's work has enjoyed essential assistance from the Carlsberg Foundation. Without their generous three-year research grant, this book could not have been realised. He is grateful for their financial support.

Inspiring academic settings and financial support are necessary, but not sufficient conditions for writing about emotions and personhood. René therefore wants to thank the kind and intelligent persons with whom he has discussed some or all of the ideas in this book: Iben Damgaard, Mads Peter Karlsen, Claudia Welz, Lars Sandbeck, Johanne Stubbe Teglbjærg, Carsten Pallesen, Troels Engberg-Pedersen, Niels Henrik Gregersen, Andrea Raballo, Dan Zahavi, Roberta Lanfredini, Borut Škodlar, and K. Brian Söderquist.

Giovanni and René both want to thank our editors at OUP Martin Baum, Charlotte Green, and Sarah Stephenson for their patient and competent assistance in preparing the book.

And last but not least, we express our immense respect and warm gratitude to Fritz Saaby Pedersen, who has read and commented on the whole manuscript. Without his efforts to clarify and amend our English, this book would have been a much more bumpy reading experience.

Finally, Giovanni and René want to express their loving gratitude to their wives for their patient support and indispensable advice during the work on this book. *Grazie*, Paola! *Tak for alt*, Louise!

Copyright Acknowledgements

The authors and publisher are grateful for permission to reproduce extracts from the following material:

"Burnt Norton" from FOUR QUARTETS by T.S.E., copyright 1936 by Harcourt, Inc. and renewed 1964 by T.S. Eliot; "East Coker" from FOUR QUARTETS copyright 1940 by T.S. Eliot and renewed 1968 by Esme Valerie Eliot; "The Dry Salvages from FOUR QUARTETS copyright 1941 by T.S. Eliot and renewed 1969 by Esme Valerie Eliot; "Little Gidding" from FOUR QUARTETS copyright 1942 by T.S. Eliot and renewed 1970 by Esme Valerie Eliot, reprinted by permission of Houghton Mifflin Harcourt Publishing Company and Faber and Faber. All rights reserved.

4.48 Psychosis by Sarah Kane, copyright © 2000 by Methuen Drama, an imprint of Bloomsbury Publishing Plc.

The Poems of Dylan Thomas, by Dylan Thomas, copyright ©1939 by New Directions Publishing Corp. Reprinted by permission of New Directions Publishing Corp.

Contents

Introduction *1*
    How Do You Feel? *3*
    Emotions, Human Beings, and Persons *4*
    The Embodied Nature of Emotions *9*
    Emotions and Psychopathological Vulnerability *11*
    Overview of the Chapters *12*

Part I **Troubled Selfhood**

1 Subjectivity and Naturalism *19*
    Philosophy and Psychopathology in View of Naturalism *19*
    Relaxed Naturalism *23*
    A Phenomenological Alternative *27*
    Hermeneutical Phenomenology *29*
    Why Ricoeur's Theory? *32*
    Reason and Sensibility *40*
    Wounded Thinking *46*

2 A Hermeneutics of 'I Am' *53*
    The Affective Generation of Values *54*
    Fragility of the Heart *57*
    Interpretative Recovery of Selfhood *63*
    Narratives of Time *66*

3 Body and Personhood *71*
    Bodily Ambivalence *72*
    Personhood and the Narrating Self *79*
    Rules and Practices *86*
    The Good Life *88*
    An Ontology of Care *92*
    Becoming a Person through Otherness *93*

Part II **Fragile Personhood**

4 Conceptual Clarity Amidst an Abundance of Feelings *99*
    To Name or Not to Name a Feeling *100*
    Feeling Theories *104*

　　　　Cognitive Theories *107*
　　　　Narrative Theories *110*
　　　　Neuroscientific Investigations of Emotions *115*
　　　　Concepts, Phenomenology, and Ontology *129*
5 Ambivalent Personhood *133*
　　　　Ontological Ambiguity *134*
　　　　The Personal Animal *137*
　　　　Identity and Feelings of Ambivalence *142*
6 Emotions and Personhood *149*
　　　　The Feeling of Emotion *150*
　　　　A Choreography of Emotions *155*
　　　　Moods and Affects *163*
　　　　Intentionality and Temporality *166*
　　　　Narrating Our Emotions *170*
　　　　A Hermeneutics of Care *180*
7 The Feeling Brain *188*
　　　　Considerations on Evolution and Intentionality *189*
　　　　Spinoza, Ricoeur, and Neuroscience on the *Conatus* *192*
　　　　Evolutionary Well-Being *198*
　　　　The Pragmatic Meaning of Life *202*
　　　　Bad Moods, Personhood, and Vulnerability *212*

Part III **Vulnerable Minds**

8 Schizophrenia as a Disorder of Mood *221*
　　　　The Clinical Phenomenology of Schizophrenia *222*
　　　　Delusional Mood, Perplexity, and the End-of-the-World Experience *228*
　　　　The Unfathomed Flatness of Lived Space *230*
　　　　The Objectualisation of Material Things *235*
　　　　The Disintegration of Temporality *236*
　　　　The Source of Vitality *241*
　　　　Disattunement and Disincarnation *246*
　　　　Disembodiment and Appearance of Things *248*
　　　　A Hermeneutics of Schizophrenic Life-Worlds *252*
　　　　Metaphysical Enactment *257*
9 Borderland *261*
　　　　Between Dysphoria and Anger *261*
　　　　Varieties of Bad Moods and Mood Disorders *264*
　　　　Lived Time, Other Persons, and Otherness *272*
　　　　Invalidation Trauma *275*

Temporal Fragmentation and Narrative Identity *277*
Otherness Lost and Found *280*
Indignation, Resignation, and Retaliation *284*
Give Us Our Daily Trauma *287*
A Hermeneutics of Traumatic Existence *290*
A Miscarried Hermeneutics of the *I Am* *292*

10 Emotions, Vulnerability, and a Therapy of Care *296*
The Fragile Dialectic of Selfhood and Otherness *296*
Disintegration of *Logos* and *Pathos* *302*
A Dialectical Conception of Mental Illness *306*
Towards a Therapy of Care *310*

References *319*
Index *333*

Introduction

Emotions and personhood are agreed to be important notions within the field of mental health care. What they are, and how they are related to each other and to the field as a whole, is less evident. To assess this, some conceptual framework seems desirable. This book aims to provide one such framework. It may be considered a contribution to the growing field of philosophy of psychopathology.

The aim of the book is not to arrive at an exhaustive theoretical account of human emotions, or of human personhood for that matter. It investigates the questions of human emotions and their relation to human personhood in the form of the everyday question 'How do you feel?' and tries to clarify the importance of this question in 'normal' life and in psychopathology. Throughout the book, the question will work as the red thread that runs through the various analyses, structuring the different levels of interrogation (ontological, phenomenological, and normative) around one principal concern, namely, to emphasise some of the philosophical and psychopathological implications of that apparently simple question. The following analyses should therefore be read as an attempt to understand human emotions from the combined approach of philosophy and psychopathology with the explicit aim of arriving at a basic conceptual framework for understanding what *emotional* experience means for a human *person*: how does a person experience emotions? What is the relation between the experiential dimension and biological dimension of emotions? What do emotions actually mean for a person's self-understanding? How do emotions figure in a person's relation to the world and other people? How do emotions feature in human vulnerability to mental illness? Do they play a significant role in the fragile balance between mental health and illness? If emotions are significant, how are they so? And how should we develop a therapy centred on the patient's emotional experience?

As we shall argue that emotions and personhood are of vital concern for psychopathology, the principal aim of the book is psychopathological. Still, we make heavy use of various philosophical resources to establish this argument. In fact, the first two parts of the book are spent on establishing a philosophical framework for addressing those issues in psychopathology. In developing this framework, we draw on both the continental tradition (phenomenology and hermeneutics) and the anglophone tradition (mainly philosophy of emotion) in philosophy. This is a difficult ambition to satisfy without disappointing adherents of either tradition. To avoid confusion, then, we should make it clear from the start that the book is unashamedly continental in orientation. One reason for this is the obvious one that we are both trained in this particular tradition, but there is also another reason, which is more methodological. Indeed, our insistence on subjectivity, and our choice of Ricoeur's theory of subjectivity as the theoretical basis of our theory of emotions and personhood, are both central to the psychopathological ambition of the book. The tradition of phenomenological psychopathology to which we hope to make a contribution has developed in constant exchange with the continental rather than the analytical tradition in philosophy. Hence, some of our key notions such as subjectivity, selfhood, embodiment, personhood, mood, experiential and ontological conflict, dialectic, normativity, care, and not least ambiguity and ambivalence, all carry with them a continental flavour known to the reader familiar with the phenomenological tradition in psychopathology. The continental character of these notions is not easily transferred into the vocabulary of analytical philosophy, and they may therefore strike the analytically trained mind as rather quaint.

We have attempted, though, to present our investigations in such a way that a reader educated in analytical philosophy should be encouraged rather than alienated. We also make use of recent and influential neuroscientific explorations of affective consciousness. The conception of personhood and emotions that we promote in the book has as a basic assumption that no warranted account of the relation between emotions and personhood can afford to disregard the biological dimension of emotional experience.

The third, explicitly psychopathological, part of the book uses this framework, combined with insights from traditional and contemporary phenomenological psychopathology, to address the emotional dimension of two central disorders (schizophrenic and borderline disorders). Here we attempt to reaffirm and strengthen the value of the dialectical model of psychopathology by grounding it on the philosophical theory developed in the first two parts of the book. We conceive personhood as the fragile core of an emotional dialectic of selfhood and otherness, and we shall argue that this conception is suitable both to assess the pathogenesis of these disorders and to further the therapeutic effort to help an afflicted person cope with his or her suffering. We believe that this combined use of philosophy and psychopathology is particularly helpful in clinical practice because it provides a philosophically valid framework which is informed and developed with constant attention to the clinical features of mental disorders. On the other hand, we are convinced that the psychopathological profile of the investigations will prove interesting to the philosopher who wants to learn more about the complex relationship between emotions and personhood. In fact, the book is written with the conviction that both philosophy and psychopathology can benefit from mutual collaboration. That this conviction lies at the heart of our endeavours should be evident from the structure of the book, namely, from the fact that the opening of the first chapter explicitly deals with this mutual relationship between philosophy and psychopathology. More specifically, we could say that the first two parts of the book are concerned with issues of *theoretical* psychopathology, that is, the *modus operandi* or background philosophy (including methodological issues) one needs in order to rigorously analyse and treat psychopathological cases, whereas the last part deals with *practical* psychopathology, that is, with the *opus operatum* or the understanding of concrete psychopathological conditions.

In what follows we shall introduce some central issues that both philosophy and psychopathology face when dealing with emotions and personhood. This is meant to serve as an introduction to some of the problems we shall be struggling with throughout the book.

How Do You Feel?

Emotions are, at the same time, some of the most intimate and most intimidating phenomena in a human life. In infancy, we feel before we speak, and as mature adults we often feel that something is right or wrong, appropriate or inappropriate, attractive or disgusting, even though we may not be able to understand and articulate why this is so. The world is opened up by emotions. Emotions play a significant role in our actions and in our thinking about the world. We may, however, also feel caught up in our emotions and sealed off from the world by them. Our relationships with other people are held together by delicate threads of emotion. A peculiar turn of the head or a certain glance from a person we care about can throw us into inexplicable uncertainty and despair. People's attitudes towards one another make up a non-verbal language that is sometimes difficult to translate into sentences and arguments. On the other hand, our spoken words influence, transform, and even create the subtle emotions that bind us together.

It seems glaringly obvious that in order to understand human existence, i.e. both what it *is* to be human and what it is *like* to be human for human persons, we must try to decipher human emotional experience. Nevertheless, emotions have not always been on the forefront of the philosophical and scientific endeavours to understand human nature—not to speak of psychopathological research and mental health care. While literature, music, poetry, drama, paintings, and films have always revolved around the beauty and terror of the human emotions, in academic philosophy they have often, and especially in the twentieth century, been regarded with suspicion or even been intentionally excluded from investigations into human nature. In some philosophical accounts, emotions are considered to stand between us and the world: If we want to understand the world and the place of human beings in this world, then our emotional attitudes in thought and action must be toned down to a minimum or, even better, eliminated altogether. One of the great philosophers of the past century, Bertrand Russell, epitomises this general attitude:

> The emotions are what makes life interesting, and what makes us feel it important. From this point of view, they are the most valuable element in human existence. But when, as in philosophy, we are trying to understand the world, they appear rather as a hindrance. They generate irrational opinions, since emotional associations seldom correspond with collocations in the external world. They cause us to view the universe in the mirror of our moods, as now bright, now dim, according to the state of the mirror.
>
> (Russell 1927, p. 220)

There is, of course, plenty of truth in this. The structures and laws of the physical world, and the intrinsic properties and functions of biological and mental life, must be uncovered by means of a strictly rational and tempered methodology that disregards our individual whims and emotional biases. This is an insight that was already clear to Plato and Aristotle and has been developed and refined over the millennia. However, this warranted methodological approach to the physical world and human nature has always leaked into the general understanding of human ontology: since reason understands and emotions distort, reason must be the hallmark of humanity. Our nature is crowned by reason and rationality, and in order to understand what human beings are we must first and foremost scrutinise the workings of our rational capacities as they stand out in themselves, untainted by the caprices of our flimsy emotions.

Now, it goes without saying that in the history of philosophy, ancient as well as modern, not all philosophers have shared Russell's attitude towards emotions (Dixon 2003, pp. 1–13, 231–51). More importantly, in the last forty years or so, emotions have steadily risen to become a distinguished topic in philosophy, fuelled by the compelling research of empirical sciences such as neuroscience, cognitive science, and evolutionary psychology. Nonetheless, although emotions are being considered very seriously in contemporary philosophy, the nature of emotions and the function of emotional experience in human thought and behaviour are still heavily debated. Several open questions still dominate the research on emotions: what are the emotions? What is the felt aspect of emotional experience and how are feelings related to subjectivity? How do we, as human beings, relate ourselves to and act with regard to our emotions? Even more questions arise if we consider the role of emotions in psychopathology: can mental pathologies be conceptualised as a *dyskrasia*, an unbalanced relationship, between the person and his emotions? How can a rigorous ontology and phenomenology of emotions contribute to improving our understanding of mental pathologies? Can clinical care profit from a theory of emotions and personhood coherent with a rigorous ontology and phenomenology?

Human emotions tend to blur conceptual and disciplinary distinctions. The view of emotions that we shall develop on the following pages understands them as the most embodied of our mental phenomena and the most mental of our bodily sensations. Recent developments in neuroscience and evolutionary biology suggest that the phenomenological dimension of emotions (i.e. our subjective experience of emotions) is difficult, at best, to separate from the ontological dimension (i.e. the biological and the personal nature of emotions). And decisions on how we should act in regard to the ebbs and floods of our emotional experience (i.e. the normative dimension) are inherently connected to our phenomenological and ontological understanding of emotions.

Emotions, Human Beings, and Persons

In trying to answer these questions, we will concentrate on the relation between emotions and personhood. This relation is not at all straightforward or immediately intelligible. To begin with, neither emotions nor personhood have ever enjoyed a very clarified place in the history of Western philosophy. They are both philosophically unstable and hackneyed notions. A few preliminary remarks on emotions, personhood, and their interdependence, are thus in order.

Our theory of emotions is based on the idea that emotions are the basic prerequisite for a person to feel situated in the world, and are thus the *via regia* for the person to understand herself in her existential situatedness. Emotions serve to establish one's feeling involved in the world (*engagement*), one's grasping the meanings of worldly objects (*enactment*), and one's pre-reflective understanding of the actions of other people (*attunement*). As far as the first function of emotions is concerned, emotions make me feel the world as real. Without emotions, the world appears as unreal, devoid of any interest and meaning. Without emotions, things that inhabit my lived space appear as mere *objects*, something that stands in front of me without any relation with my own body. Our emotions enable us to encounter objects in the world as things and persons which matter to us, that is, our experience becomes qualified by our emotional encounter with the world. Things do not show themselves as they are in themselves; rather, as Heidegger famously argued, they appear as equipment (*Zuhandenheit*)—essentially something which exists 'in-order-to'.

Also, emotions provide the motivational background for action (enactment). Enactment means knowledge considered as action-specific, that is, situated and embodied. Emotions situate me in the world and circumscribe my possibilities for action. My body inhabits the world through my feelings and emotions, i.e. it structures my possibilities to use things in view of my vital and existential needs. Emotions thus organise my possibilities to grasp objects as parts of a situation in which I am engaged. We literally *grasp* the meaning of a thing, since this meaning is exactly the specific manipulability of the thing.

Last but not least, emotions provide the background for *attunement*. Attunement between my own emotions and the emotions of other people provides the basis for intersubjectivity. *Attunement* is a pre-reflective, pre-verbal, and tacit bridge linking the emotional lives of other persons with my own. My understanding of the actions of other people is rooted in my capacity to resonate with another person's emotions.

Our theory turns on the argument that the way in which we understand and cope with this emotional engagement with the world is inescapably connected with the way in which we understand personhood. And we go on to argue that emotions and personhood are interdependent to the extent that trying to explain the one without assessing the other will necessarily result in an unsatisfactory account. Central to our theory is the dialectical relationship between moods and affects in the emotional life of a human person. We spend considerable time, in Chapters 5 to 7, to explain the notion of mood and why this phenomenon is important for understanding personhood as fundamental to human emotional life. We understand emotions as kinetic, dynamic forces that drive us in our ongoing interactions with the environment. This definition of 'emotion' focuses on the embodied nature of emotions, but rejects the simple reduction of the body to its physiological mechanism (such as visceral changes mediated by the autonomic nervous system). It obviously also rejects the conceptualisation of emotions as pure 'mental' phenomena. An emotion is not primarily a cognitive phenomenon affecting the mind, but a phenomenon rooted in one's lived body. Also, emotions are characterised by their connection to *motivation* and *movement*. Emotions are functional states which motivate and may produce movements. As functional states that elicit and motivate movement, emotions are *protentional* states in the sense that they project the person into the future, providing a felt readiness for action.

We spend most of Part I establishing a thorough account of human personhood. We do this through a systematic reformulation of Paul Ricoeur's theory of subjectivity. The gist of Ricoeur's theory is that to be a person is not coextensive with being a self. Human selfhood is troubled by an inherent conflictual sense of self due to the continuous eruption of otherness in the heart of the self. A human being is not simply an autonomous self characterised by a sense of voluntary agency and ownership of subjective experience. It is also characterised by a sense of heterogeneous otherness that conditions and disturbs one's voluntary effort to affirm oneself as a self. I am not just a self, but a person among other persons in the world. I discover that my body, the world, and other people condition and challenge my affirmation of myself as a self. I can only become who I am by understanding that I am a person dependent on things I do not have voluntary control of. Otherness is part of what and who I am. Or, to put it differently, I care about being the person that I become through the otherness involved in my body, the world, and other people. Thus, to be a person is *a task of becoming* a person through the appropriation of the dialectical tension of selfhood and otherness. Emotions and feelings are fundamental to this dialectic of selfhood and otherness in my task of becoming a person.

Both emotions and personhood feature as a significant part of everyday human life, often in inescapable connections with one another. We talk about emotions and about being persons (and not things or animals); we live our lives, in thought and action, as human beings with the implicit confidence that we have distinctive human emotions and that being a person is something that characterises every single human being despite any individual peculiarity (personality). Of course, philosophy has not been blind to the ubiquitous use of these notions in everyday life, and several major philosophers during the last century have struggled with the philosophical implications of both emotions and personhood. Few attempts, though, have been made to focus explicitly on the relation between emotions and the notion of personhood. Against the background of Paul Ricoeur's theory of subjectivity, we argue that a satisfactory account of emotions cannot disregard the question of what makes a human being a person, and, on the other hand, that any attempt to understand human personhood needs to take into account the emotional dimension of being a human individual. Indeed, philosophical accounts of either emotion or personhood do normally involve at least an implicit conception of the other. However, in theories of personhood, the complexity of emotions are often only mentioned marginally and not analysed at all. Similarly, theories of emotions hardly ever articulate the idea of human personhood implicit in their accounts.[1] It is often presupposed that human emotions are either more or less similar to the emotions we find in other animals (evolutionarily inspired theories) or significantly different from those of animals (theories that focus on the cognitive or intentional aspect of human emotions).

Another problem stems from the conflation of being a person and being human. Much research on human emotions is carried out on the assumption that if we determine how humans are similar to other animals, and how they differ from them, with regard to anatomy, physiology, and behaviour, then we are in a position to analyse and understand human emotions. We do not agree with this view. Personhood is not tantamount to being human. Although the two notions are deeply related, being a person

---

[1] Admirable exceptions can be found in Fuchs (2000), Goldie (2000), Pugmire (2005), Sartre (1971), Scheler (1966), and Wollheim (1984, 1999).

does not unproblematically coincide with being human. We shall give two preliminary reasons for this distinction and our ensuing focus on personhood.

First, the word 'personhood' captures a dimension that the word 'human' does not, or at least makes this dimension more conspicuous. Whereas considerations on what makes an organism human do not necessarily include the normative dimension of being a human individual, considerations on personhood cannot do otherwise. It is perfectly legitimate to investigate human nature and human emotions without including *normative* questions such as: is this an appropriate reaction? Should I be shameful of my thoughts? Is my desire perverted? What am I guilty of? Why do I not feel anything? Empirical, conceptual or even phenomenological analysis of what it means to be human and have human emotions can, and often should, disregard questions like these, since the aim of such investigations is to explicate and clarify, for example, the conceptual difference between beliefs and desires, the structural nature of human experience, or the function of certain brain areas. With personhood things become more complex. To be a person involves not only the *what I* am (my human characteristics), but also the *how* and *why* I am what I am, in this specific situation or period of my life. A person always evaluates her being this kind of person and is evaluated by the other persons with whom she interacts. In the course of a human life, and particularly in human interaction, the normative dimension is bound to move into the foreground. In other words, personhood captures an important fact about human life, namely 'the pervasiveness of normativity' (Blackburn 1998, p. 53). A recent collection of essays on the nature of personhood opens with a discussion on the relevance and use of the notion of personhood. Instead of maintaining the traditional division of investigations of human nature into analyses of our rational capacities on the one side and of our moral status on the other, the editors argue that:

> [I]t is not a matter of mere stipulation that rational capacities and moral statuses go together. Rather than being an artificial mixture, or a simple confusion, of two distinct phenomena, the composite notion of personhood grasps a real life intertwinement. The ontological and moral facts that intuitively make 'us' special form a holistic unity which is indeed useful to try to conceive as a whole.

(Laitinen and Ikäheimo 2007, p. 9)

Following this lead, we could say that with our focus on the notion of personhood we aim to investigate the 'real life intertwinement' of the phenomenological (experiential) and the ontological (biological as well as personal) dimensions of emotional experience in the normatively structured existence of a human being. It is important, though, to notice that an emphasis on the normative dimension of being a person does not entail any ethical discussion of explicitly moral questions. The present book is not about ethics. The analysis will deal descriptively with the normative aspects of human emotional experience. We do not believe that emotions are essentially ethical in nature, but they do elicit certain thoughts and often prompt a specific kind of behaviour that can only be understood in a normative context. Emotions such as shame, anger or disgust are important elements in what makes us believe that some things are better than others or worth pursuing, and in what makes us desire one person and loathe another. In short, as Ronald de Sousa writes, 'emotions set the agenda for beliefs and desires' (1987, p. 196).[2]

The second reason for our focus on personhood is that the concept of mood plays a central role in our account of human emotions. Humans are meaning-seeking animals and beings that question life and themselves, and moods are, among the phenomena of human subjectivity, the kind of feelings that provoke the most difficult questions: what is this strange feeling? Why do I feel in this way? What do my feelings tell about the person that I am? The concept of mood has not enjoyed much attention in analytic philosophy of emotion in the revival of the last forty years.[3] Moods are often only dealt with in the margins of the analyses of human emotions, or simply dismissed because of their abstruse and subjective nature. Many emotions such as shame, fear, or joy can be analysed in terms of the semantic content of such words and their intentional structure. I feel ashamed *because of* something I have done or because of my nose or because of my smell; likewise I fear people who drive recklessly because their actions behind the wheel contain an element of danger to themselves and others; or I fear an aggressive dog because it can hurt me. I enjoy chocolate because it tastes good and gives me pleasure. Moods, on the contrary, appear to be bereft of any clear semantics or intentional structure. I feel anxious and I cannot explain why; I am euphoric or depressed and I cannot say what makes me so and what this mood means to me. This circumstance has led many philosophers to dismiss moods as insignificant to the fundamental structure and functioning of emotional experience. They are considered superficial subjective states or simply background 'noise' to our otherwise important human emotions. This view is clearly exemplified by the prominent psychologist Paul Ekman:

> Earlier I argued that emotions are necessary for our lives, and we wouldn't want to be rid of them. I am far less convinced that moods are of any use to us. Moods may be an unintended consequence of our emotion structures, not selected by evolution because they are adaptive. Moods narrow our alternatives, distort our thinking, and make it more difficult for us to control what we do, and usually for no reason that makes any sense to us [. . .] If I could, I would forego ever having any mood again and just live with my emotions. I would gladly give up euphoric moods to be rid of irritable and blue moods.
>
> (Ekman 2003, pp. 50–1)

We believe that this attitude is seriously mistaken. First of all, it is a general problem that Ekman ascribes so little significance to the phenomenological dimension of emotions. The fine-grained, and apparently whimsical, tints of our experience of

---

[2] Kurt Schneider distinguishes emotions (*Gefühle*) from bodily sensations (*Empfindungen*) exactly by pointing to the fact that contrary to bodily sensations emotions are always normatively loaded: 'Emotions are characterized by the quality of being either pleasant or unpleasant. This is essential to emotions. Only so far as the above mentioned sensations [unrest, tiredness, appetite, hunger, vitality, tiresomeness, freshness] are qualified as either positive or negative, which is sometimes contained in the meaning of the word (e.g. feeling of sickness [*Übelkeit*]) and sometimes not (e.g. tiredness [*Müdigkeit*]), are they bodily *emotions*, whether they are localised or general vital emotions.' (Schneider 1967, p. 148; our translation)

[3] Goldie (2000), Prinz (2004), and Pugmire (1998, 2005) are admirable exceptions.

the world, other people, and ourselves are considered an insignificant by-product of the impersonal forces of evolution. It may very well be that our subjective experience amounts only to a faint squeak in the deafening evolutionary roar, but an understanding of human experience and action cannot disregard aspects of human nature simply because they appear insignificant on the overwhelming scale of an evolutionary account. Otherwise we end up with a very meagre list of essential human features and a reductive account of human mind, motivation, and behaviour in terms of the functional logic of adaptation, survival, and reproduction. Furthermore, on a more specific level, to decide beforehand what is important and not important with regard to human emotional experience is philosophically, if not scientifically, unwarranted. Strong ontological preconceptions of human nature, such as an evolutionary framework or a radical, post-modern constructivist account, impair the subsequent investigation of human emotions. In other words, we need to leave the question of the personal feeling and meaning of moods open in our approach to emotional experience. Last but not least, moods as the intentionally blurred, non-thematic background of our everyday living are a constitutive part of our experiences and actions. We cannot understand what is it like to be a person without taking into account the phenomenon of moods, that is, the *basso continuo* that disposes for us the way we perceive and behave. No person can understand what he *is* without deciphering his own moods. Moods are probably background 'noise', but not merely so; they are a 'noise' most of us need, and try hard, to make sense of. We could even say that a person is that kind of being that spends much of his life in deciphering his own moods—and as we shall see, especially his bad moods.

The Embodied Nature of Emotions

The embodied nature of our emotions makes them a strong argument for evolutionary explanations of human mind and behaviour. Many of our most common emotions such as fear, anger, and joy can be detected in other primates; although not identical to human emotions, they bear at least a rudimentary similarity. Furthermore, over the last twenty years different branches of neuroscience have identified cross-species mechanisms and reactions on both neurobiological and neuropsychological levels. However, despite these impressive advances in the understanding of the biological dimension of human emotions, emotional experience cannot be disregarded. Biological accounts do not provide a complete picture. We cannot focus on the embodied aspect of human emotions in isolation from the experiential dimension without creating an 'explanatory gap' between what I feel (e.g. emptiness) and what I am told that I actually feel (e.g. a low dopamine activity). Such kind of reasoning is similar to the neglect of consciousness, currently found in influential approaches to the human mind, that opens 'a gap between subpersonal, computational cognition and subjective mental phenomenon' (Thompson 2007, p. 6).

The persistent philosophical challenge, and the concrete psychopathological problem, is to be found in the relationship between the subpersonal level of biological mechanisms and the personal level of experience. On the other hand, given the progressive insight into the neurophysiological mechanisms of the mind, we think it mandatory for any contemporary attempt at understanding human emotional experience to take into account what (neuro)science has to say about human nature. In virtue of the embodied nature of our emotions, the subpersonal, physiological functions of our bodily constitution constantly irrupt into our experiential life by shaping the way we perceive and understand the world, other people, and ourselves. On the personal level, however, our feelings of anxiety are related to the conflictual structure of human existence, and our experience of anguish and guilt are related to our limited understanding of what human existence is and how to cope with it. In short, emotions serve to emphasise the problematic relationship between the phenomenological (how we experience ourselves and the world) and ontological (our condition and place in the world) dimensions of human existence. We cannot understand the nature of human emotions without exploring both these dimensions. If we return to the opening quote from Russell, we could say that the universe as represented 'in the mirror of our mood' is as important for an understanding of human existence as the emotionally stripped understanding of the universe promoted by the natural sciences, since both dimensions of our being humans disclose important aspects of our being the kind of sentient and reflective creatures that we are.

Finally, the question 'how do you feel?' reveals that both the phenomenological and ontological aspects of the question are always embedded in the normative character of human existence. Our emotions and feelings reveal that our experience of the world and our existence in the world matters to us. Our thoughts and actions spring from a normative source and are orientated towards some normative aim. This is the case even for small and seemingly transient features of our daily life such as feeling hunger or thirst, discomfort or ease in a situation, being afraid to speak in front of a colleague, enjoying the laughter of other people or being annoyed by it, craving for an ice cream, avoiding confrontation with somebody, longing for a moment of tranquil solitude, and so forth. We are often not aware of this normative background inherent in the way we go through the humdrum of everyday life. A significant part of our behaviour seems to take place without any distinct feature of emotions, deliberation or choice. It happens, though, that the pervasive nature of normativity comes to the foreground of our lives in the form of distinct emotions and serious choices. I may be hurt by a sharp remark made by my wife, resent my colleague's behaviour, feel attracted by my friend's wife, feel comfort in the presence of a certain person, fear the reactions of my father, or decide whether to lower my face or respond to the insults of my boss. My life is, on various levels and with different degrees of intensity, permeated by the glows of pleasure and stabs of pain. We believe that our moods are an important key to understanding this, often impalpable, normative background of human existence, and we will therefore spend considerable time on these phenomena in the following analyses.

The way we experience the world through the uneven 'mirror of our moods' matters to us as individual persons and, as a consequence of our ensuing behaviour, to the persons around us; in short, our existence as persons is held together in a normative web of heterogeneous values, biological as well as personal. One of the guiding ideas of this book is that emotional experience discloses, and to a certain degree is a co-constituent of, this fundamental normative feature of human personhood. Thus, the following analyses of emotions and personhood will argue that a better understanding of these notions and their mutual relationship will provide a philosophically enriched foundation for psychopathology.

Emotions and Psychopathological Vulnerability

The last part of the book uses the philosophical framework illustrated here to address two central psychopathological conditions: schizophrenia and borderline personality disorders. We have chosen these two psychopathological conditions because each of them illustrates one fundamental aspect of human emotional experience, of the relationship between emotions and selfhood, and of the entanglement of emotions and rationality.

We argue that at work in persons with schizophrenia is not a special kind of bad mood, like sadness or anger, rather a profound alteration of the possibility to be affected. We interpret schizophrenia as a disorder of mood which consists, first and foremost, in switching off a dispositive which discloses—to use Ricoeur's (1987, p. 103 [119]) words—our primordial *in esse*, that is, our basic sense of belonging to the world and our effort to exist. This is the basic drive through which factual reality is given, happens to us, affects us, and motivates us to act. We discuss the nature of this *Ur-emotion* in the light of Ricoeur's concept of *originating affirmation*, but also of Spinoza's *conatus* and Scheler's *Lebensdrang*. This *Ur-emotion* plays a founding role in the constitution of selfhood and in the relation between an embodied self and the world. It provides the latent awareness of our own self and of reality that makes us attune with the external world in a contextually relevant manner without distorting our overall goals, values, and identity. This basic emotion, or basic drive, is jeopardised in persons with schizophrenia, as explained by classical authors in clinical phenomenology such as Minkowski and Blankenburg. When this happens, a hyper-rational form of existence arises whereby body, self, others, and environment are experienced as devitalised and objectified, and the source of one's volitions and actions is experienced as an anonymous mechanism, external to one's own body and self. The analysis of the schizophrenic condition, and more particularly of early stages of schizophrenia, sheds light on the fragile entanglement of emotions and rationality, as well as the role of emotions as the centre of the three main dimensions of experience we met with above: the experience of one's self and of the most primitive form of self-awareness (engagement), object-experience and meaning-bestowing (enactment), and the experience of other people, i.e. inter-subjectivity, the emotion-based pre-conceptual and pre-reflective indwelling or attunement to the world.

In persons with borderline disorder we are faced with the same problem, but with a radically different outcome. At issue is the relation, or better the proportion, between emotional experience and rationality. By experiencing our emotions, we discover *otherness* in ourselves. We usually represent this otherness as an interior part of ourselves that is also exterior—in the sense that it is experienced as an often unknown and troubling feature of our own identity. By means of linguistic representation, we objectify this otherness in ourselves. By doing so, we use our emotions as a manageable source of spontaneity. Rather than menacing our autonomy, through the mediation of language emotions kindle the dialectic of narrative identity. Through the symbolic mediation of language, we appropriate this otherness and turn it into a part of our narrative identity. This capacity for linguistic and narrative appropriation of emotions is lacking in persons with borderline disorder. They are overwhelmed by their emotions, which they feel as an amorphous, untamed presence, a spring of disordered and desperate vitality, or—with Bin Kimura (2000)—an unmanageable *infinite interiority*. The borderline condition thus enlightens the fragile dialectic between emotions and identity.

Overview of the Chapters

The book is divided into three parts: Part I (Chapters 1–3) deals with the problem of subjectivity and selfhood in the light of the question of naturalism. We spend considerable time to establish a hermeneutical theory of subjectivity by gathering together and reformulating aspects of the philosophy of Paul Ricoeur. Part II (Chapters 4–7) turns to dealing explicitly with the relation between emotions and personhood. Against the backdrop of the hermeneutical theory presented in Part I, we look at contemporary theories of emotion and the notion of personhood in order to argue for a philosophically sound way to explain what emotions are, what they mean to us, how they affect our life, and how we make sense of them and cope with them in our life. Part III (Chapters 8–10) is concerned explicitly with emotions and personhood in psychopathology. We aim to show how the hermeneutical framework established in the first two parts can help us to assess the importance of emotions and personhood and to explain why both these notions are central to our understanding of mental disorder and our therapeutic approach to it. We argue that emotional fragility makes vulnerability to mental disorders an inherent part of what it means to be a person.

Chapter 1 provides a preliminary outline of the themes that we deal with throughout the book. We consider the question of naturalism to be a fundamental issue in both philosophy and psychopathology. One way to articulate this question is to look at the nature and relevance of human subjectivity. Continental philosophy and phenomenological psychopathology have a long tradition of research in the notions of subjectivity and selfhood. The same cannot be said to be the case in the Anglophone traditions of philosophy and psychiatry. On the other hand, the latter tradition has dealt more carefully with the challenges and prospects of naturalism. We argue that both subjectivity and naturalism can benefit from a focused analysis on the relation between these two notions with regard to emotions and personhood. We then go on to explain why we have chosen the hermeneutical philosophy of Paul Ricoeur as the theoretical engine for our further explorations, and end the chapter with a discussion of the notion of rationality with regard to traditional distinction between reason and sensibility in human experience. Human rationality, we argue, is an emotional rationality embedded in a complex web of heterogeneous concern, values, and norms.

Chapters 2 and 3 are dedicated to a systematic reformulation of some central aspects of Ricoeur's theory of subjectivity. Chapter 2 deals with the reasons for Ricoeur's shift from his early, more strictly phenomenological approach to his particular version of a hermeneutical phenomenology. We argue that this hermeneutical turn is the result of his lifelong interest in the emotional dimension of experience and the ontological questions that arise from this focus on emotionality.

Chapter 3, the last chapter of Part I, deals explicitly with the nature of Ricoeur's hermeneutic theory. Two major issues are at stake in his analyses, namely, body and personhood. We aim to show how these issues inform and shape his theory of personal identity. The ambivalence of the notion of the body (a biological object as well as a personal organ) provides the theoretical foundation for Ricoeur's proposal of an ontology of care. To understand what it means to be a person, we must try to understand how a person's concerns and values are both embedded in our biological constitution and developed by that person's ongoing interaction with the world, other people, and herself. Selfhood and otherness, experienced primarily but not explicitly in the form of the voluntary and involuntary aspects of being a person, are fundamental in the constitution of human personhood.

In Chapter 4 we spend considerable time on various contemporary theories of emotion. We open a path into this debate about emotions by a preliminary discussion of the difficult issue of getting a conceptual handle on our emotional feelings, which we consider to be a central issue in philosophy of emotion. We then introduce and briefly discuss three major philosophical theories of emotion (the feeling, cognitive and narrative theories) and take a close look at two influential neuroscientific theories. This chapter should equip the reader with the necessary background material for understanding our own account of the intimate relationship between emotions and personhood. Emotions are the most embodied of our mental phenomena, and yet some of the most personal ones as well. To make sense of this complex constitution requires, so we argue, an understanding of personhood.

Chapter 5 then looks at two influential theories of personhood and personal identity. Through the discussion of the biological theory of Eric T. Olson and the constitution view of Lynn R. Baker, we argue that personhood is inherently ambivalent in virtue of its complex ontology. Human beings are personal animals. This means that to explain what it is to be a person involves an approach that appreciates both the biological and the phenomenological aspect of human nature. We propose an approach that focuses on the intimate relation between identity and feeling. We argue that personal identity is constituted not only by who we reflectively consider ourselves to be or which kind of person we are in the eyes of other people, but also by the pre-reflective and sometimes cognitively impenetrable feelings involved in being the person that each of us is.

Chapter 6 provides the theoretical core of our argument. We here try to provide an access to emotional feelings that are frequently left out of philosophical theories of emotion. We approach the emotional dimension of human personhood with the tools of both phenomenology and hermeneutics. We start out with a description of the flow of our emotional experience and of the way it structures the life-world the person lives in, which we then attempt to articulate by sorting the various feelings involved in our emotional experience into two broad phenomenological categories, moods (emotions bereft of any clear semantics or intentional structure) and affects (emotions which have a precise semantic content and intentional structure). This initial distinction enables us to get a conceptual grip on the intentional and temporal structures of our feelings, which allows us to appreciate subjective aspects of our emotional experience that are important for how a person lives with his or her emotion, but are all too often disregarded. Once we have got a hold on the pre-reflective, experiential feature of our emotions, we argue (inspired by Peter Goldie) that narrative structures are fundamental to how a person understands and copes with his or her emotional experience. Whereas cognitive theories focus on the propositional and intentional features of emotion, and feeling theories on the physiological changes in 'the bodily landscape', a hermeneutical approach concentrates on how a person relates to and makes sense of emotional experience. Narratives are central, although not exclusively so, to this interpretive endeavour, because they enable us to articulate the relationship between emotions and personhood by emphasising what our feelings mean to our identity as persons. Such a hermeneutical approach, so our argument goes, is able to provide us with a language for our emotions that exploits the ambivalent nature of human personhood to make sense of our more feeble, cognitively impenetrable, and sometimes ineffable feelings.

In Chapter 7, the final chapter of Part II, we look at the normative aspect of emotions. Whereas the previous chapter dealt with the experiential features of emotional experience and the way we as persons understand and cope with our emotions, this chapter will explore the relation between ontological conceptions of emotion and normativity. In a discussion with the theories of Jesse Prinz and Matthew Ratcliffe, we argue that neither a strict evolutionary nor a strict phenomenological explanation is able to account for the normative aspect of emotional experience. Instead, we focus on the fragile nature of human well-being and argue that moods, and bad moods in particular, may help us understand the normative complexity involved in being a person. We end the chapter with some remarks on the question of emotional vulnerability, which serve as an introduction to the more explicit explorations into the psychopathology of emotions in the third part of the book.

We open the third, and explicitly psychopathological, part of the book with a detailed analysis, in Chapter 8, of the transformations of the life-world in the early stages of schizophrenia. The dramatic transformation of the life-world of persons with schizophrenia involves changes in the spatial, material, and temporal structure of experience and has serious consequences for how such persons live their life as embodied persons, how they understand the existence of other people, and how they interpret their experiences and thus bestow meaning on their life. We argue that moods are fundamental for our access to and understanding of these psychopathological changes. Drawing on classical (including the so-called delusional mood, perplexity, and Josef Conrad's *das Trema*) as well as contemporary psychopathological accounts (especially the construction of schizophrenia as a disembodied type of existence), we suggest that the basic vulnerability to schizophrenia can be considered as a disorder of mood, and especially as the switching off of a dispositive which discloses our primordial *in esse*, that is, our basic sense of belonging to the world. In line with the hermeneutical approach developed in the first two parts of the book, we opt for a dialectical model of the pathogenesis of full-blown schizophrenic symptoms, arguing that these symptoms are the result of the dialectic between the schizophrenic person and his own vulnerability. We focus especially on schizophrenic 'ontological' delusions, interpreting them as a disturbance of the dialectic relation of selfhood and otherness at the heart of being a person.

Chapter 9 first provides a glossary for the varieties of bad moods involved in the borderline condition, and briefly illustrates their place in the spectrum of mood disorders. Then we go on to discuss the borderline condition as a disordered fabric of the self, that is, a disorder of the linguistic and narrative integration of otherness in one's own identity. Borderline persons often experience their own self as dim and fuzzy, are deprived of a sense of identity, and unable to be steadily involved in a given life project or social role. At times they may complain of being insulted by the hypocrisy and insincerity of others, or claim that they are badly treated because of their care for authenticity. They may see others as caliginous, cloudy, and their faces as expressionless; and a moment later they may perceive them as dangerously ambivalent, equivocal, suspect, tenebrous, with evil intent. The main purpose of this chapter is to provide a fine-grained and nuanced description of these rapid, abrupt and dramatic emotional swings and of the changes of the life-world accompanying them. We will interpret these typical changes in the existence of borderline persons as fluctuations between clearly normative emotions and the more diffuse and confusing background of bad moods. A special focus will be on the dialectic between dysphoria and anger, since these emotions, characterising the borderline person's existence, engender very different kinds of existential orientation and enactment, that is, the actualisation of very different configurations of the life-world.

We conclude the book with Chapter 10. Here we develop our conception of human vulnerability to mental illness as the result of severe disturbance, or outright collapse, of the fragile dialectic between selfhood and otherness, involving the brittle entanglement of emotions and rationality. We argue that the uncanny metamorphoses of the life-worlds described in Chapters 8 and 9 are brought about by an extreme disproportion of emotions and rationality, and that the end-products (such as ontological delusions in persons with schizophrenia and ontic ones in persons with borderline disorder) of mental illness are the result of a miscarried hermeneutics of basic emotion-driven experiences. With the fixation in a pathological life-world, the dialectic of selfhood and otherness constitutive of human personhood collapses. This understanding of the vulnerability to mental illness contains a rudimentary framework for engaging with this fragility by means of hermeneutical therapy. A phenomenologically grounded clinical hermeneutics can accompany and help persons affected by mental illnesses in their complicated task of making sense of and communicating their experiences. The aim of such a therapy is to re-establish the dialectic of selfhood and otherness that will help the suffering person to become who she or he is.

Part I
Troubled Selfhood

Chapter 1

Subjectivity and Naturalism

We need a substantial theory of subjectivity when dealing with mental illness. An insistence on human subjectivity does not exclude or pose any obstacle to a scientific investigation of human nature. On the contrary, a better grasp of the subjective dimension of human nature may help clarify how the scientific image of human nature relates to, and is able to influence and possibly alter the way in which human beings understand themselves as individual persons. Without careful attention to subjectivity our explanations of mental illness run the risk of becoming overly reductive in their otherwise laudable effort to meet prevailing scientific standards. This difficult relationship between objective scientific knowledge and subjective experience and self-understanding is at the heart of any philosophy of psychopathology and provides a necessary prelude to our account of emotions and personhood.

This chapter begins with a preliminary look at the relation between philosophy and psychopathology in the light of the thriving attempts to naturalise every aspect of human nature. We argue for a theoretical framework that does not seek to dispose of human subjectivity or reduce it to something that it is not. Recent years have shown that analytical philosophy and continental phenomenology and hermeneutics could gain from a mutual dialogue; in fact, the gap between the two traditions is not as large or deep as it has been. Much has been done to promote such a dialogue in philosophy (e.g. Gallagher 2005; Gallagher and Zahavi 2008; Thompson 2007; Varela et al. 1991; Zahavi 2005), and we argue that the same should be done in the philosophy of psychopathology. The following section introduces our hermeneutical approach to emotions and personhood, and explains why we have chosen Paul Ricoeur's theory of subjectivity as the basis for our approach to human selfhood, and not those of Husserl or Heidegger, as is common in psychopathology. This leads us to a brief introduction to Ricoeur's conception of experience. We will look at his Kantian reading of Husserlian phenomenology, which directs his prevailing interest in ontology that eventually leads him to develop a hermeneutical version of phenomenology. At the end of the chapter, we shall try to explain how Ricoeur's conception of experience bears on the question of naturalism by looking at how it affects our understanding of rationality.

Philosophy and Psychopathology in View of Naturalism

The relationship between philosophy and psychopathology is not simple or obvious. Both disciplines are characterised by strong internal disagreement as to their own constitutive methodological, epistemological, and even metaphysical principles. These internal struggles naturally affect any endeavour to establish a philosophy of psychopathology. One issue that is particularly critical to both disciplines, and their mutual relationship, is the question of naturalism. A very rough outline of how the two disciplines are situated within the broader landscape of contemporary scientific knowledge will help to appreciate the acute character of this problem.

Over the last fifty years the explanatory success of relatively new scientific disciplines such as cognitive science, sociobiology, evolutionary psychology, and neuroscience has rekindled old dreams about a completely naturalised explanation of human nature and behaviour. Such naturalistic ambitions can be traced back to the scientific revolution in the sixteenth century, when the study of nature began to slip from the hands of natural philosophers and theologians into those of technicians, explorers, and physicians. This development accelerated after Darwin in the second half of the nineteenth century, and a major part of twentieth century philosophy can be viewed as attempts to cope with the growing influence from the natural sciences. Two prominent thinkers exemplify the intense debate in the last century, and their statements still serve as a background to contemporary discussions of naturalism. In 1929 Martin Heidegger launched a polemical attack on the scientific enthusiasm blooming in his time:

> No time has known so much and such a variety about human beings [*Menschen*] as is the case today. No time has been able to present its knowledge of human beings so urgently and in so captivating a manner as is the case today. No time has previously been able to offer this knowledge as quickly and easily as today. But also, no time has known less about what a human being is than today. In no other time has the human being become as questionable [*so fragwürdig*] as in ours.
>
> (Heidegger 1990, p. 209; translation slightly modified)[1]

Heidegger's words leave little doubt about his view on the relevance and the detriments, rather than benefits, of the dazzling scientific development of his time. The natural sciences can perhaps inform us of all sorts of interesting details about human nature, but they can never solve the general problems involved in being human. In fact, their discoveries tend to blur and confuse our understanding of ourselves.

Some forty years later, the influential palaeontologist George G. Simpson wrote, in a no less polemical tone, against the philosopher who dreams metaphysically (i.e. uncoupled from scientific methods and the theory of evolution):

> The question 'What is Man?' is probably the most profound that can be asked by man. It has always been central to any system of philosophy or of theology. We know that it was being asked by the most learned humans 2000 years ago, and it is just possible that it was being asked

---

[1] The works of Kant, Heidegger, and Husserl are quoted from the standard English translations. Where we find it necessary we sometimes modify these translations. The page numbers are those of the standard German text, such as they are reproduced in the English translations that we use. Other non-English writers than those mentioned are quoted from existing English translations, if available. To facilitate the consultation of the original texts we have added the page number of the original in square brackets after the reference to the English translation. We have stated when a translation is modified and when it is entirely our own.

by the most brilliant australopithecines 2 million years ago. The point I want to make now is that all attempts to answer that question before 1859 [the publication of Darwin's *On the Origin of Species*] are worthless and that we will be better off if we ignore them completely.

(Simpson 1966, p. 472)

Although Simpson tends to give some kind of credit to '[t]he other, older approaches through metaphysics, theology, art, and other nonbiological, nonscientific fields', he considers such approaches 'merely fictional fantasies or falsities' (p. 473) if they do not acknowledge that explanations of human nature must be carried out in strict continuity with what is revealed in the natural sciences.

This conviction of an abiding necessity for all investigations of human nature to be grounded in natural sciences such as physics and biology has become even more persistent today with the impressive advances of neuroscience and evolutionary psychology. Often the naturalistic framework is conceived as a panacea for the old philosophical problems about consciousness, mind, and self. If only we apply truly scientific methods to such problems, they will reveal themselves for what they really are, namely, inane products of abstruse metaphysical thinking.[2] There is no doubt that both philosophy and psychopathology are deeply influenced by the vaulting ambitions of contemporary naturalism. There is, however, a clear difference as to how the challenges of naturalism are understood and dealt with in the two disciplines.

Philosophy, being the reflective discipline it is, has the theoretical liberty to engage in complex and detailed discussions about the appeal, content, and scope of naturalism. In fact, the last two decades have witnessed a surge in the philosophical debate about naturalism, in particular with regard to such issues as whether or not philosophical methods should be continuous with those of the natural sciences, the significance of scientific truths, the questionable unity of scientific methods, and the ideology behind naturalistic assumptions (e.g. de Caro and McArthur 2004, 2010; Dupré 1993, 2001; Kitcher 1992, 2001). Most philosophers, strict naturalists, more liberal naturalists, and anti-naturalists alike, clearly understand their work as essentially different from that of a scientist. Indeed, philosophy as a discipline, for the most

---

[2] A recent contribution to this view on philosophy is Paul Thagard's book *The Brain and the Meaning of Life* (2010). Thagard attempts to demolish the persistent idea that there are aspects of the meaning of life which are out of the reach of the neurosciences and the endeavours of other empirical sciences. Of love, for instance, he writes in a manner characteristic of his overall argument: 'A full account of the brain mechanisms underlying love should be able to accommodate all of its manifestations, from romance to friendship to compassion. Evidence does not yet suffice to guide construction of a comprehensive theory, but enough is known to suggest what some of the neural mechanisms might be' (p. 156). We may not, for the time being, be able to unite in one comprehensive theory all the separate arguments for a definitive turn to the empirical sciences in our approach to the meaning of life. As science progresses, though, and our technologies and theories become more and more sophisticated, we will eventually be able to rid ourselves of the worn-out cloak of metaphysical philosophy and step up to the challenges of life in the bright and shining armour of the natural sciences. As alluring as this may sound, one could, and (in our opinion) one should, question the soundness of this kind of 'argument-in-the-light-of-future-research-results'.

part at least, does not aspire to be part of the natural sciences, but rather a reflection on the methodological, conceptual, logical, and metaphysical foundation of the different scientific disciplines.

The scenario is more complex in psychopathology. Psychiatry has long striven to become an accepted discipline of the natural sciences as a sub-area of bio-medicine. Many psychiatrists are therefore prone to be suspicious of other methods than those of the natural sciences, even at the risk of losing the subjective aspect of mental disorders. In an illuminating critique of the de-humanising effects of the DSM (Diagnostic and Statistical Manual of Mental Disorders), Nancy C. Andreasen stresses the functionalistic attitude in much present-day psychiatry to the point of concluding that '[r]esearch in psychopathology is a dying (or dead) enterprise' (2007, p. 111). This has left psychopathology in a difficult position. To survive as a discipline it must accommodate the scientific aspirations of psychiatry in general. On the other hand, it cannot lose sight of the phenomenological dimension that constitutes its *raison d'être*. Thus, it seems that psychopathology is compelled to reflect on its own philosophical, or at least conceptual, framework. This is poignantly formulated by three prominent scholars who have struggled patiently with the problematic status of contemporary psychopathology:

> [M]ental-health professionals dealing with such terms as 'reality', 'psychosis', or 'social cognition' are forced to engage, inadvertently or not, in philosophical thinking. They have the choice between a tacit, unacknowledged, and distorting philosophy and a philosophy which critically discloses and discusses its own presuppositions.
>
> (Parnas et al. 2008, p. 578)

It is obvious that simply to spurn the naturalistic framework with Heideggerian indifference and superior ridicule, or else uncritically to wrap one's theories in the mantle of science, are not viable ways of dealing with mental illness. We believe that the philosophical problem of naturalism that is most obviously relevant to psychopathology revolves around the complex relation between the subjective (or personal) and the sub-personal (be that computational or neurophysiological) dimension of human consciousness—that is, a particularly concrete version of the traditional mind-body problem in philosophy. This problem presents itself in psychopathology with an acute exigency not felt in philosophy. Whereas various models of explanatory reductionism abound and flourish in contemporary philosophy, it is more difficult, not to say impossible, to dismiss the subjective dimension of human experience and action as irrelevant or illusory when dealing with mental illness. Although it might be revealed one day that our subjective experiences (such as perceptions, feelings, thoughts, and dreams) possess no causal efficacy in the great chain of being and are thus mere illusory epiphenomena with no ontological status in the natural world, this fact would not change the clinician's need for understanding the peculiar subjective dimension of human nature. Our joys and sufferings are subjective and personal, and any methodological approach and conceptual framework in psychopathology must work out its theories in close connection with that subjective point of view. Or, to put it differently, subjectivity is a kind of 'objectivity' that psychopathology has to deal with. Philosophical problems of human nature in relation to psychopathology are always bound to a specific aim, namely, a better understanding of the subjective experience of the patient.[3]

Relaxed Naturalism

Tim Thornton has recently dealt with the question of naturalism and the problems of reductive tendencies in contemporary psychiatry. He discusses the theoretical and practical problems involved in reductive naturalistic accounts of value, meaning, and fact, and explaining how philosophy is of help to psychopathology he insists on the special character of philosophy of psychiatry:

> Philosophy of psychiatry or, more broadly, philosophy of mental health is primarily a philosophy of and *for* mental health care. It is at its best when it responds to questions and examines the conceptual underpinnings of developing thought in this area.
>
> (Thornton 2007, p. 236; emphasis added)

Inspired by the influential contemporary philosopher John McDowell, Thornton opts for a reconciliatory view on the question of naturalism that he calls an 'anti-reductionist or relaxed version of naturalism' (p. 236; see also McDowell 1994, pp. 89–91). This particular sort of naturalism does not deny that the natural sciences can contribute with important insights to our understanding of human nature and human values, but it argues that it would be wrong to think that these scientifically observable features of reality exhaust the notion of nature. Nature is broader than what the scientist can tell us about it. To understand how human persons suffer and rejoice, we need to understand, Thornton argues, that '[i]n addition to the hard bio-medical facts, the demands of both values and meanings can be seen to be real features of the world' (p. 236). Thornton's rather brief account of this relaxed solution can perhaps be made clearer by turning for a moment to his source of inspiration.

In his book *Mind and World* (1994), John McDowell has argued convincingly against the attempt to align scientific understanding of nature with nature itself. He insists that human understanding is governed by a rational spontaneity that cannot be properly described nor understood by the methods of the natural sciences, or by philosophical arguments in continuity with such methods:

> If we identify nature with what natural science aims to make comprehensible, we threaten, at least, to empty it of meaning. By way of compensation, so to speak, we see it as the home of a perhaps inexhaustible supply of intelligibility of the other kind, the kind we find in a phenomenon when we see it as governed by natural law [. . .] Now if we conceive the natural as the realm of law, demarcating it by the way its proper mode of intelligibility contrasts with the intelligibility that belongs to inhabitants of the space of reasons, we put at risk the

---

[3] For excellent introductions to various philosophical aspects of the problem of naturalism in contemporary psychiatry, see Fulford et al. (2006; in particular, Chapters 12, 13, and 21 to 25) and Thornton (2007). The collections of essays in Radden (2004) and in Kendler and Parnas (2008) are also highly recommendable, although more specialised in their choice of issues.

very idea that spontaneity might characterize the workings of our sensibility as such. The faculty of spontaneity is the understanding, our capacity to recognize and bring into being the kind of intelligibility that is proper to meaning.

(McDowell 1994, pp. 70–1)

McDowell is here developing arguments that form part of Wilfrid Sellars's famous refutation of 'the Myth of the Given' (Sellars 1963b, pp. 161–70). On the naturalist reading of the world, we have, on the one side, a (pre-)given world constituted by complex processes of merely causal relations, and, on the other side, human beings who, more or less accurately, try to understand this given world and themselves by discovering the laws that govern these causal relations. In this picture, we passively receive sensory input from the world that we try to interpret in the most accurate way according to the physical constitution of nature. And the more accurate our interpretations are, the better we understand the laws that govern human meaning and values. McDowell, as Sellars before him, argues that this is a distorting picture of both nature and human meaning. The multitude of meanings that constitute and hold together human life finds no intelligible place in nature as it is discovered and explained by natural science. Human experiences of meaning are characterised by a mixture of a *sui generis* spontaneity and receptive sensibility, which is particularly human in the sense that they are governed by *reasons* and not merely by *causal* relations. Human beings are peculiar creatures endowed with unique (*sui generis*) rational capacities (spontaneity) besides their five senses (receptive sensibility).

McDowell is not arguing against the legitimacy of natural science as such or the use of scientific methodology to explore nature. Neither is he opting for a supernatural conception of nature or a dualistic conception of human beings. He simply argues that the workings of nature, including the beings in it, transcend the laws of nature that are discovered and exploited in the natural sciences:

> [W]hat became available at the time of the modern scientific revolution is a clear-cut understanding of the realm of law, and we can refuse to equate that with a new clarity *about nature*. This makes room for us to insist that spontaneity is *sui generis*, in comparison with the realm of law, without falling into the supernaturalism of rampant platonism [. . .] To see exercises of spontaneity as natural, we do not need to integrate spontaneity-related concepts into the structure of the realm of law; we need to stress their role in capturing patterns in ways of living.

(McDowell 1994, p. 78)

McDowell claims that although he criticises the way philosophers restrict their understanding of nature to that which is disclosed by the natural sciences, his proposed alternative does not slide into what he calls 'the supernaturalism of rampant platonism'. In McDowell's view, nature is more than it is claimed to be in 'bald naturalism' in the sense that it allows for rationality as well as causality, but it is still a nature uninfected by any talk of supernatural entities or processes. Nature is not restrained to the workings of causality. Nature also includes human beings who are endowed with a capacity for understanding and producing behaviour which cannot be fully explained by causal laws. Human meaning is constituted not only by the realm of causal law, but also with what McDowell calls, borrowing Sellars's famous notion (1963b, p. 169), 'the space of reasons'. If our understanding of nature is to have any meaning of all, and in particular a meaning which can allow for human beings 'capturing patterns in ways of living', then nature must be governed by some kind of intelligible processes and relations, which are, in the case of McDowell, both rational and causal. McDowell's critique of strict or bald naturalism is convincing. He manages to show that this restricted kind of naturalism is not able to account for human experience of meaning and value. Human thinking about human life cannot be reduced to the general biophysical laws that make possible and govern such thinking on a sub-personal level.

Following this lead, Thornton recommends that psychiatry adopts a relaxed naturalistic attitude, so that 'nature should not be equated just with the realm of law, but should also be taken to include the space of reasons' which, in turn, involves acknowledging 'that there is more to nature than can be described within the natural sciences' (Thornton 2007, p. 235).

Although we sympathise with this relaxed or more liberal approach to the question of naturalism, where norms and personal judgements about reality are conceived to be just as important as the scientist's stripped notion of objectivity, we cannot help finding some disturbing truth in David Papineau's objection to the *sui generis* character of human rationality (Papineau 1999). McDowell introduces a fundamental difference between humans and other animals, because whereas '[d]umb animals are natural beings and no more' (McDowell 1994, p. 70), humans are rational creatures whose experience and behaviour are inherently constituted and guided by rational norms. This distinction sits very uncomfortable with even the most liberal understanding of naturalism. One of the basic convictions of post-Darwinian naturalism, and natural science in general, is that the differences found throughout in nature are of evolutionary degree, and not of irreducible, *sui generis* kinds. Papineau, for one, is not convinced by McDowell's attempt to steer a relaxed middle course between naturalism and non-naturalism. In fact, he characterises McDowell's project as an exercise in non-naturalism that does nothing to help us understand why human behaviour is so different from that of other animals:

> In the end there seems to be little alternative for the non-naturalist except to hold that the norms of judgement are primitive and not to be further explained. This seems unsatisfactory. Even if we can't reduce judgemental norms to other kinds of facts, it is surely desirable that we should have some kind of understanding of the peculiar force that judgemental norms are supposed to exert on us.
>
> (Papineau 1999, p. 28)[4]

---

[4] Hilary Putnam, who in his later works is greatly inspired by McDowell, also remains rather puzzled by McDowell's sharp distinction between human beings and other animals (Putnam 1999, pp. 48, 192). In the same vein, Simon Blackburn does not understand how McDowell can reject 'mythical' Platonism and still maintain that human beings are endowed with a special 'normative-sensitive' perception (Blackburn 1998, pp. 92–7). Hans Fink, on the other hand, has argued that McDowell's naturalism is incoherent on the semantic level, since it confuses what is included and what is excluded in the notion of nature (Fink 2006). Finally, Donald Davidson maintains that McDowell's proposal simply dismisses the mind-body problem by removing the body and the external world from the equation and thus only amounts to an updated form of mentalism (Davidson 1999).

What bothers Papineau is the cognitive bias involved in this solution. Relaxed naturalism works with what a naturalist would claim is an unwarranted bifurcation of the natural world, that is, two seemingly independent ways of explaining and understanding nature: on the one side, the objective and disenchanted world of the scientist (the realm of law) and, on the other, the partially enchanted human world filled with particularly human values, contrasting points of view, and personal meaning (the space of reason). Since maintaining such a bifurcation when it comes to explaining human nature would be a recoil into dualism, relaxed naturalists such as McDowell and Thornton choose to privilege the rational monotony of 'the space of reason' by ferreting out the a-rational 'realm of law'.[5] Humans are rational and cognitive creatures and should therefore be investigated in terms of reasons, and not causality. Although McDowell claims to respect the causal dimension of human nature, he still argues that 'reasons might *be* causes' (McDowell 1994, p. 71). By conflating anonymous, a-rational causation with human reasons, that is, making primarily rational and cognitive norms constitutive of human experience, thought, and behaviour, we risk losing sight of the complexity of human nature. Humans are indeed rational creatures, but as we all know rationality is extremely precarious. Much of our behaviour is outright irrational, and if we downplay, or neglect in any way, the a-rational, causal dimension of human thought and behaviour, we miss perhaps the most important reason for this precariousness, namely, that besides being rational creatures we are also biological creatures governed by the same biophysical laws as other animals. As Papineau points out, rational norms of behaviour is an ideal that we, most of the time at least, strive to follow, but the fact remains that:

> [H]umans normally reason badly, but can set themselves to do better. We can suppose that humans normally get their beliefs from 'quick and dirty' processes, which no doubt worked well enough in our evolutionary history, but all too often lead us astray in the modern world [...] On the other hand, this is only part of the story. For humans can also deliberately set themselves to use reliable methods instead of the 'quick and dirty' tricks. Even if humans don't always follow norms that offer reliable routes to the truth, they are perfectly capable of this, and characteristically set themselves to do so when it matters.
>
> (Papineau 1999, p. 33)

We agree with Papineau that a convincing argument for a more relaxed naturalism needs to explain *why* and *how* subjective norms, judgements, and values matter to human beings whose existence is indeed influenced and to a certain degree conditioned by their biological nature. Only with such an explanation in place can we hope to understand why we humans reason so badly. As we will see in the next two chapters, Ricoeur offers a theory that explains exactly this complexity of subjective values and biology. We shall also explain in more detail what we mean by the precarious character of our rationality in the last section of this chapter. But for now suffice it to notice that one of the principal risks entailed by relaxed naturalism is that our endeavours to avoid

---

[5] More recent attempts to establish more liberal or relaxed versions of naturalism inspired by McDowell's account can be found in de Caro and MacArthur (2004, 2010).

the overt reductionism of a stricter form of naturalism may tip the philosophical seesaw back to some version of common sense or pragmatic rationalism (McDowell 1994, p. 44). This strategy overemphasises the cognitive aspect of human nature on the cost of the non-cognitive or affective aspects (Bernstein 1995, Blackburn 2006). One hard-won insight of the discussions of philosophical naturalism, which cannot be eclipsed in our understanding of mental illness, is that many aspects of human experience and behaviour are not rationally or cognitively transparent. Mental disorders, in particular, teach us that human rationality is disturbingly precarious, and that rational explanations alone are not always useful for making sense of such disorders. Moreover, we learn from clinical practice that the subjective experience of mental suffering reveals a constant struggle to cope with the brute and meaningless forces at work in mental disorders—and that both this struggle and these forces are hardly reducible to rational explanations. One of the consequences of dismissing or toning down the significance of the a-rational factors in human experience and behaviour is that we thereby tend to neglect the importance of the cognitively impenetrable aspect of our feelings and emotions. One way to avoid the temptation of reducing the non-cognitive or affective aspects of human experience and behaviour to cognitive dispositions is to turn to phenomenology.

A Phenomenological Alternative

Now, one of the many merits of Thornton's book is that it addresses the question of naturalism from within the contemporary discussions in analytical philosophy of mind, since the previously predominant continental tradition in psychopathology has often neglected the question altogether. However, this emphasis on analytical philosophy of mind also casts an oblivious shadow over recent developments in phenomenology and hermeneutics that might serve as valuable contributions to the question of naturalism. Much phenomenology today has abandoned its previous predilections for the complex text-exegetical analysis of Husserl and other classical phenomenologists, and has instead begun to take an active part in the discussions of naturalism.[6]

Contrary to current approaches in analytical philosophy of mind, the phenomenological approach does not start out with two separate, and seemingly irreducible, aspects of human nature—the objective and the subjective—which are then to be reconciled in one way or another. Rather, it engages with naturalism from a different methodological starting point, namely, the subjective experience of the world. Recent research

---

[6] In this respect, Evan Thompson's latest book *Mind in Life* (2007) is an impressive contribution, because it combines phenomenology, cognitive sciences, and neuroscience in such a way that the explanatory gap between the sub-personal and phenomenological is, if not bridged, then at least diminished substantially. Likewise, the work of prominent phenomenologists such as Dan Zahavi and Shaun Gallagher has made significant contributions to the debate about naturalism and subjectivity (e.g. Gallagher 2005; Gallagher and Zahavi 2008; Zahavi 2004, 2005, 2010). They argue convincingly that phenomenology is not contrary to a naturalistic conception of mind and consciousness. On the contrary, phenomenology makes new perspectives possible on the question of naturalism.

in phenomenology argues that a better understanding of the experiential structure of subjectivity may serve to cast new light on the way we pose the question of naturalism in the first place (Zahavi 2004, pp. 342–5). Our understanding of meaning and values and of how these fundamental features of human life are incorporated into a naturalised conception of the world and human nature depends on how we *experience* such features in the first place. And a clarification of our *experience of nature* should be an integrated element in any philosophical discussion of naturalism. If we start out with a twofold picture of the world, the subjective and the objective, and then try to fit one of them into the other, we risk ending up with either a reductive account of consciousness and mind as merely physical, or else a rationally enchanted conception of nature with no connection to the physical world, or—as a third option—an unsustainable Cartesian picture of two ontologically separate, but equally important, aspects of human nature. As mentioned above, we are not opposed to Thornton's McDowellian idea of a 'relaxed' naturalism, and in many ways we sympathise with his solution although we have doubts about the cognitive emphasis of the account. We believe, though, that an analysis that begins with a phenomenological grounding can provide a much stronger case for this kind of answer to the question of naturalism without the risk of neglecting the a-rational aspect of our emotional life.

An alternative answer to the challenge of naturalism is to contrive a theoretical framework that is conducive to explanations of *how* and *why* subjective and personal values, norms, and judgements are critical for understanding the function and nature of the human animal. In other words, a philosophy of psychopathology that endeavours to accommodate Papineau's critique of 'relaxed' naturalism by providing an argument for how and why the subjective aspect of human nature—how a human person experiences her own nature—can be integrated with a naturalistic explanation of human thought and behaviour.

Subjectivity does indeed seem to be crucial for our understanding of mental illness. As Thomas Fuchs explains, subjectivity becomes an issue on both the theoretical and the therapeutic level of our approach to mental illness:

> The intentional and qualitative aspects of beliefs and emotions cannot be explained in terms of physical processes in the brain; nor can we do without new subjective and intersubjective experiences if we want to change the patient's maladaptive beliefs and dispositions that have lead to his illness and may lead to relapse in the future [. . .] What is decisive, however, is that a reductionist approach to treatment would undermine the patient's capacity for self-understanding, self-efficacy, and autonomy. To deny his freedom of will, self-determination, and responsibility on the basis of a deterministic view of the brain as the 'real' cause of his illness results in another kind of 'learned helplessness', namely a dependency on expert knowledge of brain mechanisms and brain modification.
>
> (Fuchs 2005, p. 117)

What the debate about naturalism evidences, though, is that human nature, and mental illness in particular, cannot be explained by an account of subjective experience alone. There is more to human nature than conscious experience. So although the theoretical framework that we propose starts with subjectivity, it does not remain on a purely phenomenal level. We shall argue for a necessary development from a phenomenological analysis of subjectivity to a hermeneutical model of personhood that is able to incorporate the implicit experiential structures of subjectivity into the broader context of both our biological constitution and our concrete existence in the world. The notions of emotion and personhood are deeply involved with ontological (What am I?) and normative (What shall I do?) questions, and as such they go beyond the phenomenal level of analysis (What do I feel?) as well as the phenomenological investigations of the pre-reflective structures of subjectivity (for instance, how these experiences are shaped by time, space, embodiment, and otherness). Such questions of ontology, existence, and value are, in the continental tradition at least, normally topics dealt with in hermeneutics.

Hermeneutical Phenomenology

As we shall explain in more detail in the following two chapters, hermeneutics is necessarily rooted in phenomenology, since it begins with subjective experience. And hermeneutics is, or so we shall argue, the necessary partner of phenomenology, because our first-person experience is not merely concerned with self-awareness and experiential objects, but also with how the experienced objects and the sense of being a self are experienced as an integral part of a person's life and entrenched in and constantly shaped by history and the sociocultural context. Or, to put it differently, whereas phenomenology mainly investigates the structures of subjective experience and pre-reflective self-awareness, hermeneutics is concerned with how the subject reflectively understands itself as an embodied human person situated in the world. It struggles with the question 'Who am I?', the answer to which involves both the ontological (What am I?) and normative (What shall I do?) dimension of being a person. We could say that hermeneutics deals with how we respond to and interpret the questions that our subjective experience of the world, other people, and ourselves give rise to. As noted above, phenomenological investigations of subjectivity have become more sensitive to the significance of the empirical sciences in relation to our understanding of human experience, as can be gleaned from the words of one leading phenomenologist:

> For phenomenology, science is not simply a collection of systematically interrelated justified propositions. Science is performed by somebody; it is a specific theoretical stance towards the world. This stance did not fall down from the sky; it has its own presuppositions and origins. Scientific objectivity is something to strive for, but it rests on the observations and experiences of individuals; it is knowledge shared by a community of experiencing subjects and presupposes a triangulation of points of view or perspectives. Thus, according to this view, rather than being as such a hindrance or obstacle, consciousness turns out to be a far more important requisite for objectivity and pursuit of scientific knowledge than, say, microscopes and scanner.
>
> (Zahavi 2010, p. 6)

Neither hermeneutics nor phenomenology denies that the empirical sciences provide important contributions to our understanding of human nature, even though they both reject the idea that empirical sciences are somehow endowed with a privileged access to human nature. Both approaches therefore insist on a non-reductive account of human subjectivity, but hermeneutics is more comprehensive in its investigation of subjectivity than phenomenology. It aims, among other things, at an integration of subjective experience with the broader dimension of human embodied personhood in order to understand how the human person feels, thinks, and acts as a self-conscious self, rooted in nature and embedded in the world. Hermeneutics does not begin with a rigid notion of what is real and what is not real in nature; on the contrary, it examines the *meaning for human life* of both phenomenological and scientific explanations of *what there is*. In this sense, it pleads for a hermeneutical sensibility for the multifarious facets of 'reality' that enhances our access to the world and ourselves. The hermeneutics that we are going to propose in this book is suspicious of phenomenology's pre-reflective 'givenness' as well as of scientific claims of 'hard facts'—without letting this suspicion attenuate the solid gains of both kinds of investigation. It merely uses this suspicion to question the rather quaint claims concerning explanatory priority that neither phenomenology nor the natural sciences are shy to advance. With respect to the claims about 'hard facts' coming from the natural sciences, Shaun Gallagher has made a wise observation:

> Some people think that science is restricted to quantitative accounts, and if something cannot be quantified, it doesn't allow for scientific study [. . .] I think that it is better to think of science as using any means possible to explain *what there is*. And if *what there is* includes such things that cannot be reduced to computational processes or the subpersonal activation of neurons, or cannot be quantified, or objectified without loss—such things that nonetheless have meaning for human life, and therefore fall into the province of hermeneutics—then to turn away from them and deny their actuality is in fact being unscientific.
>
> (Gallagher 2004, p. 173)

Understood in this way, as a comprehensive approach to the question of naturalism and human nature, the version of hermeneutics that we are going to propose in this book is clearly an attempt to make a synthesis between two major ramifications of our contemporary body of knowledge, that is, the 'hard' scientific disciplines as well as the more 'soft' reflective disciplines. If intellectual history has taught us anything, though, it is that engaging in broad over-arching syntheses is a risky business. The first half of the twentieth century abounded with complex philosophical anthropologies with the explicit aim to provide a unified description of the human person; among the most important are those of Max Scheler, Karl Jaspers, Helmuth Plessner, Arnold Gehlen, Stephan Strasser, and Paul Ricoeur. One of the principal risks that such endeavours inevitably face is that of becoming blurry and obscure in wanting to encompass everything about human nature. To want to account for the biological, subjective, personal, social, and ethical dimension of human existence is a big mouthful, and most philosophers would say too big a mouthful for any single person or even any research programme. How can we possibly integrate all details of every aspect into one single account? Will we not necessarily downplay some aspects and overemphasise others? Do we know enough about human nature to even begin such a project? These are surely legitimate concerns, and it is proper to be critical at any attempt to make broad explanations of human nature. However, we can think of at least three reasons why such comprehensive theories should nevertheless be attempted.

First, and more generally, although ambitious philosophical anthropologies have lost much of their appeal and respect in academic philosophy, attempts to provide a unified explanation of human nature flourish in other disciplines such as neuroscience, cognitive science, and evolutionary psychology. In fact, the 'plethora of naturalisms' (Kim 2003, p. 84) alive in the academic world today thrusts upon researchers, especially those affiliated with the natural sciences, an unflagging demand for a unified and complete explanation of all aspects of human nature. The naturalistic framework, however vague and obscure the notion of naturalism is in itself, does not accept 'relaxed' versions of naturalism that allow for a qualitative distinction between the realm of hard, objective facts and the realm of soft, personal values. And in order to counter the strong reductionist attitudes prevalent in much scientific research today, those opposed to such attitudes cannot stop at merely pointing out the weaknesses in the naturalistic bulwark. They need to clarify that non-reductive approaches are not inherently anti-scientific and do not necessarily make use of methods contrary and hostile to those of the natural sciences, but that they can provide valuable alternatives to predominantly scientistic methodologies.

Secondly, the attempt to think together the two aspects of human nature is especially important in psychopathology given the current naturalistic tendencies of psychiatry. To convince mental-health professionals to take the phenomenological and existential claims of psychopathology seriously, it is simply not enough to emphasise the importance of non-reductive approaches to subjective experience or judgemental norms with regard to value and meaning. We need a framework that enables a unified account of human nature, neglecting neither the objective nor the subjective aspect of being human; that is, a framework that attempts to explain how subjective values constitute the life of a human person, not neglecting the fact that these subjective values are conditioned and shaped by the objective, anonymous values that arise by the sheer fact of living and breathing as a biophysical organism. Subjective values and objective values are not two separate realms. They stand in a mutual relationship of influence and conditioning without being reducible to one another.

And finally, contrary to some of the philosophical anthropologies of the past and many forms of synthesis done in cognitive science and evolutionary psychology today, our hermeneutical proposal is not intended to be conclusive in any way. It is an attempt to establish a methodological framework that allows us to appreciate the fast growing bulk of scientific insight into human nature and, theoretically, to integrate this insight with our particularly human way of experiencing, being, and acting in the world. The challenges that naturalism poses to subjectivity will not disappear. If we want to promote more 'relaxed' forms of naturalism that countenance the importance of subjectivity, we need a thorough account of how to accommodate subjective experience, and the rational capacities characteristic of human beings, with the anonymous, a-rational laws and functions at work in mammalian life. We are animals, peculiar animals to be sure, but still animals, and as such our lives are shaped and conditioned by the same a-rational biological norms that govern other higher primates. We have to provide a sensible answer to Papineau's question about why and how judgemental norms, subjective feelings and emotions, rationality, and personal values exert a 'peculiar force' on creatures like us when they do not seem to be of any concern whatsoever to other animals in nature. Consciousness would, of course, be the most obvious answer. But consciousness is a highly complex and debated problem in its own right, as anyone merely superficially familiar with the current discussions in philosophy of mind would know. So instead of venturing into theoretical discussions about how to explain the nature of conscious experience, thought, and rationality, or how such colourful phenomena are related to the dull matter of the brain, we have chosen to focus on the more concrete problems involved in the encounter of subjectivity and naturalism: why is subjectivity important for our understanding of, and therapeutic approach to, mental illness? How does the ambivalence of personal values and biological norms affect our thinking? How do we experience and cope with the apparently cognitively impenetrable nature of bodily feelings? What does it mean that our emotions are embodied, and to what extent is that embodiment governed by evolutionary forces? What are moods—a product of rationality, or of biology, or a conglomerate of both—and what role do moods play in our vulnerability to mental illness? What is the relationship of rationality and a-rationality in human thought, feeling, and behaviour?

We believe that one profitable way to approach problems of this sort is to focus on the complex relation between emotions and personhood against the backdrop of a hermeneutical theory of subjectivity.

Why Ricoeur's Theory?

To say that we employ a hermeneutical framework for our investigation of emotions and personhood is not a very precise or informative description of our approach. Hermeneutics has come to mean close to everything or nothing during the twentieth century, so if a hermeneutical approach is to have any philosophical weight at all, it must be qualified further and singled out within the confused cornucopia of hermeneutical theories.

Broadly described, hermeneutics is a theory of interpretation that dates back to ancient philosophy (Bruns 1992; Grondin 1994). But hermeneutics is not confined to philosophy. Throughout the history of western thought it has been, and still is, instrumental in the development of biblical exegesis and legal interpretation. In philosophy, however, hermeneutics gained momentum in the early nineteenth century with Romanticism and Friedrich Schleiermacher, and at the turn of the twentieth century, with the work of Wilhelm Dilthey, it became an integral part of the methodological discussions concerning the relation between the natural sciences and the humanities. It was Heidegger, though, who with his *Being and Time* in 1927 turned hermeneutics into one of the major philosophical currents of the last century. Being a theory of interpretation, hermeneutics had previously been ineradicably linked with texts and language. Heidegger broke with this tradition. He argued with his existential analysis of subjectivity that hermeneutics is not confined to textual or linguistic analysis, but is deeply rooted in the ontological constitution of human selfhood. Human beings are interpretative creatures. It is a fundamental part of our being human that we interpret ourselves as being a particular, embodied self situated in a certain pragmatic, cultural, and social context. We are meaning-seeking animals whose existence is constituted by our capacity to interpret and understand our being in the world. Hermeneutics, on this view, is an existential task with which the self is necessarily engaged by the simple fact of being a thinking being. The self is thrown into the world (*Geworfenheit*) and finds itself in a totality of involvement (*Bewandtnis*) of pre-reflective, pragmatic significance (*Bedeutsamkeit*) that it must interpret and understand in order to exist as a human self with a past and a possible future. The pragmatic facticity of selfhood, its being-in-the-world shaped by a past and endowed with certain capacities, must be interpreted and appropriated to realise the possibilities of existing as a human self. In short, *I interpret therefore I am*; or said with Heidegger's rather cryptic terminology:

> As understanding, Dasein projects its being upon possibilities [*Sein auf Möglichkeiten*]. This *being towards possibilities* that understands is itself a potentiality for being [*Seinkönnen*] because of the way these disclosed possibilities come back to Dasein. The project of understanding [*Entwerfen des Verstehens*] has its own possibility of development. We shall call the development of understanding *interpretation* [*Auslegung*].
>
> (Heidegger 2010, p. 148)

Heidegger's seminal elaboration of an ontological hermeneutics initiated an eruption of philosophical hermeneutics that has lasted to this day, and hermeneutics has left an indelible mark on contemporary philosophy and has spread rapidly throughout the humanities in general.

This immense popularity has come with a cost, though. The word 'hermeneutics' has been diluted and transformed so many times over that it has become difficult for many philosophers to acknowledge hermeneutics as a serious philosophical theory. Often it is considered as a lightweight version of popular philosophy, diffuse and comprehensive enough to be applied in disciplines so diverse as literary studies, cultural anthropology, theology, art theory, economy, sociology, and many others—including psychology and psychopathology. This critique of hermeneutics has some serious truth to it. Taken as a loose theory of interpretation with unsubstantiated slogans such as the hermeneutical circle, fusion of horizons, narrative identity, and textual model, hermeneutics does not amount to much of a coherent or theoretically useful theory. This is a sad development, since influential philosophers after Heidegger such as Hans-Georg Gadamer, Gianni Vattimo, Richard Rorty, and Paul Ricoeur have developed elaborate hermeneutical theories with substantial philosophical validity and scope. Key notions such as the hermeneutical circle, narrative identity, and fusion of horizons still possess significant philosophical value well beyond their status of hackneyed slogans, and the first task of a philosophical hermeneutics today is to dissipate prevailing distortions of its central notions. Another, equally important, task is to make the sometimes obscure and unnecessarily knotty arguments of philosophical hermeneutics accessible to readers who are perhaps more familiar with the analytical tradition. Philosophical hermeneutics is often, like phenomenology, suffocated by text-exegetical dogmatism, a fetishist scrutiny of a particular philosopher's idiomatic arguments, and extensive use of secondary literature, to such an extent that the philosophical insights risk being lost among page-long footnotes of cross-references and circumstantial details. This is not to say that detail and minute analysis are not important, only that much hermeneutical philosophy could learn from the succinct and clear form of mainstream analytical philosophy. Accordingly, a philosophical hermeneutics that aspires to contribute to the philosophy of psychopathology must provide a framework substantial enough to avoid distorting labels and, at the same time, it must present the theory in a way that promotes a dialogue with analytical philosophy and contemporary science. In our attempt to work out such a framework, we have chosen the philosophical hermeneutics developed by the French philosopher Paul Ricoeur.

Ricoeur's philosophy is complex and his production enormous; still, his patient investigations of the conflictual nature of human subjectivity and the fragility of personhood have a solid theoretical core, which we have tried to isolate and reformulate in a way that makes his theory of subjectivity accessible to the non-specialist reader and a cogent basis for clinical practice. Obviously, this reformulation of Ricoeur's theory will not satisfy readers who are familiar with his work and the way in which it is normally presented. For over half a century, Ricoeur worked out his philosophy through an impressively patient dialogue with contemporary and traditional philosophers from the continental as well as the analytical tradition, theologians, neuroscientists, literary theorists, and political scientists. Thus, expositions of his philosophy often use these dialogue partners to articulate his thoughts and arguments. Despite the obvious risk of distorting the picture of his philosophical endeavour, we will not follow his hermeneutical methods in that direction. Apart from the following section, where we briefly present his heritage from Husserl and Kant in relation to the experiential structures of subjectivity, we have tried to provide an analytically strict account of his hermeneutical theory of subjectivity, with very few references to the rest of his philosophy or the traditions he was in dialogue with. We have chosen this approach because of the specific aim of this book, which is not about philosophical hermeneutics, or Ricoeur for that matter. This is a book about philosophy of psychopathology, with the ambition to provide clinicians with appropriate tools to grasp the nature of their patients' emotions, to find the place of emotions in the patients' life stories, to make sense of them, and in general, to provide insights for the practice of mental health care. Our reformulation of Ricoeur's theory of subjectivity reflects these aims.

Ricoeur's hermeneutical phenomenology contains the fundamental ingredients for a philosophy of psychopathology: a descriptive *theory of subjectivity* that shows the vulnerable constitution of the human life rooted in conflict, a *normative theory* of 'the good life' that helps to deal with the vexed distinction between normality and pathology; and a *theory of practice*, that is, a method, devised for philosophical purposes but flexible enough to be used by clinicians, to explore human subjectivity and make sense of it through the construction of personal narratives. We present his ideas and arguments in such a way as to promote a framework for our further investigation of the relationship between emotions and personhood.

Ricoeur implements his hermeneutics as a hermeneutical phenomenology, which for him means that 'phenomenology remains the unsurpassable presupposition of hermeneutics' (Ricoeur 1991, p. 38 [61]). This is an important feature of Ricoeur's version of hermeneutics that distances him from other hermeneutical theories and emphasises his close relation to Husserl and Heidegger. Contrary to more historically (e.g. Vattimo) or textually (e.g. Gadamer) orientated versions of hermeneutics, Ricoeur maintains the focus on subjectivity through the long development of his theory. Although he spends considerable time and energy on symbols, metaphors, and textual models, these efforts remain an integral part of his general investigation of subjectivity and human nature. His theory has both a phenomenological and an ontological ambition in that it is intended to clarify both the experiential structures of subjectivity and the complex constitution of human nature. He adopts various elements from Husserl's phenomenological method and works out his ontology in a close reading of Heidegger's existential analysis in *Being and Time* of being-there (*Dasein*), being-in-the-world (*In-der-Welt-sein*), and care (*Sorge*). In many ways, Heidegger is more influential in his theory than Husserl because of this ontological emphasis. Husserl remains fundamental to Ricoeur, though. The ontology that Ricoeur develops would be incomprehensible without the intrinsically Husserlian background of self-awareness and intentionality. This continuity with the phenomenological tradition makes his theory especially apt for the philosophy of psychopathology, since much psychopathology, both traditional and contemporary, is done against a phenomenological background.

Moreover, Ricoeur's hermeneutics provides an excellent framework for the discussion of naturalism with respect to human feelings and personhood. Despite the heavy influence from Heidegger's ontology, Ricoeur's ontology remains more Kantian than Heideggerian. Ricoeur is in many ways a Kantian thinker. His philosophy is inspired by Kant's lifelong project of explaining how the human self can be both an anonymous part of a larger physical nature and a human person. Working from this Kantian grounding, that is, trying to think together the physical and ethical aspects of being human, Ricoeur confronts this fundamental problem of human existence by investigating the fragility of human identity and the normative nature of human feelings, thoughts, and actions in a physical world that knows nothing of normativity or humanity. Accordingly, his ontology is shaped mainly by two fundamental pillars of Kant's philosophy: the conception of subjective experience as a synthetic product of the two heterogeneous faculties of sensibility and reason, and the idea of personhood as a normative concept. These two themes run like a red thread through Kant's works, and the spirit of his philosophical impetus is beautifully captured by the famous words from the conclusion of the *Critique of Practical Reason*:

> Two things fill the mind [*Gemüth*] with ever new and increasing admiration and reverence, the more often and more steadily one reflects on them: *the starry heavens above me and the moral law within me*. I do not need to search for them and merely conjecture them as though they were veiled in obscurity or in the transcendent region beyond my horizon; I see them before me and connect them immediately with the consciousness of my existence [*dem Bewußtsein meiner Existenz*]. The first begins from the place I occupy in the external world of sense [*Sinnenwelt*] and extends the connection in which I stand into an unbounded magnitude with worlds upon worlds and systems of systems, and moreover into the unbounded times of their periodic motion, their beginning and their duration. The second begins from my invisible self [*meinem unsichtbaren Selbst*], my personality, and presents me in a world which has true infinity but which can be discovered only by the understanding [*dem Verstande*], and I cognize [*erkenne*] that my connection with the world (and thereby with all those visible worlds as well) is not merely contingent, as in the first case, but universal and necessary.

(Kant 1996, pp. 161–2)

Kant's anthropology is rooted in his conception of human nature as a conflictual tension between sensibility and reason. Our existence as human persons is a continuous struggle with the complexity of our own nature.[7] We are both *rational* beings and part of an *a-rational* nature,[8] that is, both part of humanity and of physical nature, and our lives are shaped by our reflective thoughts as well as by our pre-reflective perceptions, sensations, feelings, and instincts. The human self is thus constituted by the complex and extremely fragile workings of autonomy and heteronomy, freedom and necessity, endemic to human existence.

Ricoeur develops this Kantian idea of ontological fragility and conflict in human nature. He patiently works out an ontology of care that is rooted in the conflict inherent in human selfhood between self and otherness, person and body, nature and humanity. This conflictual nature of human selfhood is the central theme of our reformulation of Ricoeur's theory over the next two chapters. In the following section we shall clarify his use of the Kantian idea of synthetic experience, so we will not go further into those issues now. We will, however, end this section with an explanation of why we believe that Ricoeur's ontology of care provides a better framework for a philosophy of psychopathology than the Heideggerian alternative.

Ricoeur's ontology of care is, as mentioned, deeply inspired by Heidegger's fundamental ontology, but it also contains some significant differences. He concurs with Heidegger's turn from a pure phenomenology to a more ontological investigation of selfhood:

> At this point, the retrieval of the 'I am' [*la reprise du 'je suis'*] must be not only of phenomenological concern—that is to say, in the sense of an intuitive description—but concerned with interpretation, precisely because the 'I am' is forgotten [*le 'je suis' est oublié*]. It has to be recovered by an interpretation which brings it from concealment. Dasein is ontically the closest to itself, but ontologically farthest. And it is in this distance that the 'I am' becomes the theme of a hermeneutics and not simply of intuitive description. Therefore, a retrieval of the *cogito* is possible only as a regressive movement beginning with the whole phenomenon of 'being-in-the-world' and turned toward the question of the *who* of that being-in-the-world.
>
> (Ricoeur 2004, p. 226 [229])

---

[7] Allan W. Wood's explanation of the basic interplay between autonomy and heteronomy in Kant's anthropology fits perfectly with Ricoeur's view on their ambivalent interplay in human selfhood: 'If we had reliable access to the natural causes of our behaviour, then it would be quite untenable to claim that the real causes are different from these and transcend all experience. Kant's view that we are psychologically opaque has more to do with a set of ideas more often associated with later thinkers, such as Nietzsche and Freud. Kant holds that most of our mental life consists of "obscure representations," that is, representations that are unaccompanied by consciousness; if we ever learn about them at all, we must do so through inference. This is partly because many representations are purely physiological in origin, and never *need* to reach consciousness. But in some cases, Kant thinks, we have a tendency to *make* our representations obscure by pushing them into unconsciousness' (Wood 2003, p. 50).

[8] There is an important difference between 'a-rational' and 'irrational', which will have significant bearings on our understanding of the notion of rationality, and subsequently on our approach to human emotion. In the final section of this chapter, we are going to explain this difference in more detail. As will become clear, we are indebted to Ronald de Sousa's treatment of rationality.

Ricoeur's theory is in this sense obviously Heideggerian, but two features in particular separate Ricoeur's hermeneutics from that of Heidegger: his emphasis on the biological dimension of human existence and the question of the other person.

As we saw earlier, Heidegger's philosophy is not exactly characterised by a friendly attitude to the empirical sciences. Heidegger concentrates his investigation on the a priori structures of embodied selfhood, and he therefore explicitly disavows any connection to the philosophical anthropologies flourishing in his time and their investigation of the empirical dimension of human nature (Heidegger 1995, pp. 108–214; Heidegger 2010, p. 17). Ricoeur, on the contrary, believes that human nature can only be approached by a 'long way' (*voie longue*) over 'lived' symbols, metaphors, and linguistic interpretations of being-in-the-world. His ontology is nurtured by a constant dialogue with different kinds of philosophical anthropology and empirical sciences. We cannot approach human subjectivity without taking into account the biological and the social nature of the human self. Moreover, as the later Heidegger turns towards language and poetry, his ontology also becomes gradually less interested in human existence (*Dasein*) and almost entirely occupied with being-in-itself (*Sein*). Ricoeur's ontology of care, on the contrary, is constantly focused on subjectivity and remains rooted in the complexity of human selfhood as it is experienced by a self existing in a concrete, social as well as physical, world shared with other people.

Ricoeur's permanent insistence on the other person constitutes perhaps the most significant difference from Heidegger's ontology. Contrary to Heidegger's normative focus on the authenticity of the individual self, Ricoeur's ontology revolves around the normative relationship between the self and the other self:

> It is thus the growth of his own understanding of himself [*la propre compréhension de soi-même*] that he pursues through his understanding of the other [*compréhension de l'autre*]. Every hermeneutics is thus, explicitly or implicitly, self-understanding by means of understanding others.
>
> (Ricoeur 2004, p. 16 [20])

Ricoeur works out his hermeneutics and his ontology of care with an explicit focus on the presence of the other person in my self-awareness and self-understanding. Otherness, responsibility, and recognition are key notions in his understanding of the self in terms of personhood, and as we shall see, they are among the motives behind his move from Husserlian phenomenology to a hermeneutical phenomenology. In fact, the ontological nature of human personhood is to be found in the constitutive dialectic between self and otherness, where the pole of otherness covers the multitude of subjective experiences that reveal the involuntary aspect of human existence (e.g. my body, the world, and other persons). The fragile and vulnerable character of human personhood is, for Ricoeur, primarily due to the problematic relation between the self and other persons inherent in our being a person. Our existence in the world is pervaded by normativity. Our biological constitution promotes certain immediate and pre-reflective values such as eating, drinking, sleeping, reproduction, self-preservation, and many others, but our being human persons coexisting with other persons elicits complex values as well such as courtesy, forbearance, self-esteem, love, friendship, envy, respect, hatred, and recognition. These complex and heterogeneous values condition and shape human existence, and to understand human selfhood we have to understand how the self orientates itself and acts by means of these values. For Ricoeur, the most important values in a human life remain interpersonal values. Our world is first and foremost a human world, and our lives are lived together with other human persons. Thus, Ricoeur's ontology of care is primarily constituted by the presence of the other person in human personhood. This is something that is neglected, or at least is not foregrounded, in Heidegger's ontology of care with its emphasis on the authenticity of the individual self. As Jaspers notices in his reading of *Being and Time*:

> Buried under the straightforwardness of [Heidegger's] Authenticity is the authentic [self] that is really existential: [the self] in communication. The infinite task that cannot be objectified in any way: to be able to be a friend and to love [*Das Freundseinkönnen. Liebe*]. Instead of this, the promotion of an unconcerned 'courage to be oneself' ['*Mut zu sich selbst*'] [. . .] Hence, the solipsism, which obviously is not intended or willed, becomes visible. The existence is always individually conceived [*Die Existenz wird zwar 'je' eine genannt*], but the communication between the individual existences is never articulated as a problem. It is always the singular individual that is under scrutiny, and the prevailing approaches only allow the Other to appear for the individual as Other [*nur als der Andere für den Einen*]. Existence is, in spite of its character of thrownness, conceived as absolutely independent [*schlecthin eigenständig*]. Its authenticity is somewhat isolated. That communication merely occurs as the idle talk of 'They' ['*das Man*'], and that relationship between people only exists as company [*Gesellschaft*], is a symptom of that monistic monotony.

(Jaspers 1978, pp. 31–3; our translation)[9]

Contrary to Heidegger's endeavour to arrive at this lonesome state of 'Authenticity', Ricoeur's insistence on the other person in human self-awareness and self-understanding makes his hermeneutical ontology particularly relevant for a philosophy of psychopathology, since much work done in psychopathology today shares the Heideggerian tendency to neglect this fundamental normative feature of human selfhood. In contrast to a Heideggerian ontology, Ricoeur's hermeneutical ontology helps to understand the human person as an embodied biological self, provided with basic drives and an array of emotions as well as with interpersonal values, embedded and engaged in interpersonal relationships.[10]

Finally, and perhaps most pertinent to the psychopathological ambition of this book, Ricoeur's theory is worked out by means of two distinct but interdependent methodological strategies: on the one hand, a *diagnostic* effort to thoroughly describe the conflictual nature of the human self and, on the other, a *therapeutic* endeavour to reconcile the conflict and thus to restore the well-being of the self (1966, pp. 17–20 [20–3], 468–9 [440–1]; 2007b, pp. 302–4 [375–7], 306 [379]). His phenomenological analysis

---

[9] We thank Professor Claudia Welz for her help translating this difficult passage.

[10] We will return to a concrete example of this Heideggerian propensity to downplay the importance of interpersonal values and the normative challenges involved in our interaction with other people when we discuss Matthew Ratcliffe's Heideggerian account of 'existential feelings' in Chapter 7.

of subjectivity uncovers a self that is fragile and inherently troubled by tension and conflict, and his turn to hermeneutics can be read as the development of a *therapy of the self*:

> Under the pressure of the negative, of negative experiences, we must reachieve a notion of being which is *act* rather than *form*, living affirmation, the power of existing and of making exist [*affirmation vivante, puissance d'exister et de faire exister*]. (2007b, p. 328 [405])

In this sense, Ricoeur's philosophy is characterised by the same normative resiliency that we find of particular concern to the great philosophers of the past, who animate and inspire his work, such as Plato, Aristotle, the Stoics, Spinoza, Kant, and Kierkegaard. The aim of his philosophy is not simply to uncover the truth by diagnosing false beliefs and errant judgements. It is also deeply concerned with the flourishing of human life, that is, with diminishing sorrow and augmenting happiness. As he writes: 'Philosophical reflection is purifying in this: that it discerns the nucleus of affirmation shrouded in anger, the generosity concealed in the implicit will of murder' (2007b, p. 323 [400]). For Ricoeur, the self can only come to terms with itself through the negativity that it experiences in the conflict with itself. The self must become the person that it is through the otherness that is part of its own being, that is, to be a self is a task of becoming oneself. As we shall see in the next chapter, he describes this interrelation between *phenomenological diagnosis* and *hermeneutical therapy* by combining a Freudian and Hegelian terminology, as a dialectic 'between the subject's archeology and its teleology, that is, between two dispossessions of consciousness' (1977, p. 460 [444]; translation slightly modified). The former is worked out by means of a phenomenological description of the conflictual structure of selfhood, and the latter is, in its turn, characterised by a hermeneutical endeavour of reconciling this conflict.

Before we delve into our reformulation of Ricoeur's theory it might a good idea to say a few words about how we are going to proceed.

The following two chapters attempt to reconstruct Ricoeur's development of a phenomenologically grounded hermeneutical theory of subjectivity through a reading of several of his major works on subjectivity, from the earliest work in 1950 to the latest one published the year before his death in 2005.[11] This is not meant as an original interpretation of Ricoeur, nor do we give their due to the enormous variety of topics covered in his numerous other works or his elaborate dialogues with other philosophers.

---

[11] On the cost of being tedious at times, we have, however, tried to be as faithful and scrupulous as possible with regard to Ricoeur's texts and arguments. To that end, we have worked out our reformulation through a close reading of several of his most theoretically dense works, from early to late in his production, and furthermore furnished our interpretation with plenty of references to the individual works, both the English translation and the French original, so that the reader can turn to Ricoeur himself when this is needed for clarification or further scrutiny. We shall concentrate mainly on the following works: *Freedom and Nature* [*Le volontaire et l'involontaire*] (1966/1950), *Fallible Man* [*L'homme faillible*] (1987/1960), *Freud and Philosophy* [*De l'interpretation*] (1970/1965), *Time and Narrative, vol. 3* [*Temps et récit, tome III*] (1988/1985), *Oneself as Another* [*Soi-même comme un autre*] (1992/1990), and *Course of Recognition* [*Parcours de la reconnaissance*] (2005/2004). In addition to the major works, we shall draw on various minor texts and occasional writings from different periods of his philosophical career.

We reformulate his ideas and arguments in such a way as to promote a framework for our further investigation of the relationship between emotions and personhood. It is impossible, though, to avoid terseness and at times even dense and complex sections when treating Ricoeur's theory in the relatively concise form that we have attempted here, and for that we ask for the reader's forbearance and patience. Some sections may at first seem irrelevant and unnecessarily gnarled, but hopefully their relevance to the central theme of the book will become clearer in later chapters.

Our reformulation is structured according to the dialectic of diagnosis and therapy at work in Ricoeur's theory of subjectivity. The last section of this chapter and the first section of the following Chapter 2 are both dedicated to the phenomenological diagnosis of the conflictual nature of selfhood. The remaining four sections of Chapter 2 explain Ricoeur's reasons for leaving the methods of Husserlian phenomenology and developing his own hermeneutical phenomenology. The entire Chapter 3 then unfolds this hermeneutical therapy of selfhood. One could say that in this chapter we trace the hermeneutical journey from selfhood to personhood.

Before that, however, we are going to look at the philosophical heritage from Kant and Husserl. Besides clarifying the two most important sources of Ricoeur's philosophy, the section is also meant as an additional clarification of his approach to the question of naturalism.

Reason and Sensibility

Ricoeur's investigation of subjective experience is heavily inspired by Kant and Husserl. There is a difference, however, in Ricoeur's use of the two philosophers. Whereas the influence from Husserl is mainly found in his methodological approach to subjectivity, Kant echoes in almost every aspect of his theory. As he writes: 'Husserl *did* phenomenology, but Kant *limited* and *founded* it' (2007a, p. 201 [250]). He uses Husserl as a methodological guide to the description of the structures of subjectivity and Kant as the speculative engine in his thinking about what it means to be a human person. Still, his use of the two philosophers is quite unorthodox, and it is not as an interpreter of Kant or Husserl that he has gained recognition. He coins his own notions from their forms and performs both minor and major semantic changes in the use of their concepts. It would take us too far afield to go into the details of his critique and use of Kant and Husserl. The aim of this section is to provide an outline of those of his early thoughts about human subjectivity that have an impact on his development of a hermeneutical phenomenology. This requires that we make some introductory remarks about his peculiar use of the Husserlian analysis of intentionality and the Kantian notion of transcendental synthesis. He introduces both concepts in the early phenomenological analysis of human experience, but they remain the theoretical foundation in his turn to hermeneutics.

The concept of intentionality is very complex and has a long history of interpretation.[12] For Ricoeur, three basic interdependent features of the concept are of particular importance: object-directedness, self-awareness, and immediate meaning.

---

[12] For a clear and concise introduction to the concept of intentionality, see Gallagher and Zahavi (2008, pp. 107–28).

First of all, the intrinsic intentional nature of consciousness means that our mental states are characterised by being object-directed; in other words, to be directed at an object is a constitutive feature of human experience. Consciousness is always consciousness of something. If our experiences were not experiences *of* something, they would not be experiences at all. We would not have experiences, but simply be unconscious like a crystal or a lemon tree. When we perceive, we always perceive something, and when we love, feel or desire, we always love, feel, or desire somebody or something. The structure of subjective consciousness can be understood only if we take into account the objective correlate, that is, the perceived, the beloved, the felt, the desired. The multifarious variety of real and possible objects of consciousness discloses a significant feature of human consciousness. An object can be experienced as physical, such as raindrops on my hand, or as beings of a non-physical nature, for example, the hope for liberty and equality or the sudden desire for a cold beer when I am in a boring meeting. In other words, the world experienced by humans is not limited to the physical world that we can touch, observe, and smell.

Moreover, our experiences are not merely registrations of an external, outer world different from ourselves. Our experience of the world around us is entangled with the experience of ourselves, that is, with the objects of our thoughts, ideas, and feelings. The intentional character of consciousness, its object-directedness, discloses the complex character of the experienced world of humans. The objective correlates of my experiences are not limited to the physical world alone, such as the movie that I watch or the sounds that I hear from the other room; I also experience, more or less explicitly, a multitude of bodily, mental, and atmospheric states. Perhaps I feel an annoying headache, an irritation over a character in the movie, my thoughts about that character, a growing determination to switch off the TV soon and go for a walk instead; I might also spontaneously picture my trip to the country last weekend or the dinner that I am going to tomorrow. To appreciate this complexity, we have to acknowledge this heterogeneous character of the objective correlates of experience. Our conscious life is wrought together by all sorts of objects whose existence cannot always be explained by pointing to something out there in the physical world.

The second feature of intentionality that Ricoeur uses in his analysis is intrinsically related to the previous one. The fact that consciousness is always consciousness *of* something not only discloses the objective correlate but also its subjective correlate, namely, the subjective dimension of the experience to which the object is a correlate. We cannot sever self-awareness from our experience of an object. Human consciousness cannot be adequately described, let alone clarified, by focusing only on either the objective or the subjective correlate of experience. Experience is constituted by the interdependent cooperation of these two basic features. With regard to self-awareness in perception, Ricoeur writes:

> What perception does not in any sense include is an explicit judgment of reflection, such as 'It is I who perceives, I am perceiving.' But apart from such explicit reflection, perception includes by its nature a diffuse presence to the self [*une présence diffuse à soi-même*] which is not yet a conscious grasp. In terms of this it *lends itself to* a more complete reflection which is not an added operation, grafted onto perception from without, but the explanation of an intrinsic moment of perception. It is this conception of unreflected

consciousness which justifies the use of the word consciousness to designate perception itself. As Husserl says, consciousness is consciousness of... Intentionality and consciousness belong together.

(Ricoeur 1966, p. 387 [363–4])[13]

Experience of the world always involves a pre-reflective, and often diffuse, awareness of a self. When I am experiencing something I have an immediate awareness that it is *my* experience, and not the experience of another. Accordingly, this pre-reflective awareness of a self means that our experiences are always *qualified* in some way or another. Subjective experience is not a stable and pre-configured registration of an object. Experiences of the same object may change from time to time due to a variety of environmental and subjective factors. My experience of an object is not merely a question of *what* I experience, but also *how* this object *appears* to me and *how* it *affects* me in my act of experiencing it. There are several aspects to this subjective dimension of experience, but Ricoeur is particularly interested in the perspectival and affective aspects of human experience.

We always experience an object from a specific perspective and in a particular context. Our experience of an object is always bound to a certain perspective and never appears in isolation but always against a certain background and in context with other objects. This means that our experience is embodied (conditioned by our bodily constitution; e.g., we do not have eyes in the back of our head) and situated (objects are experienced as *things,* part of the larger context of the human world). An important feature of this perspectival character of human experience is that it is intimately connected with the question of meaning. We will return to this in a moment. It is, however, the affective feature of the subjective experience that interests Ricoeur (and our investigation in the rest of this book) the most. The next chapter will deal explicitly with the affective dimension of experience, so for now a few preliminary words will suffice. That human experience is qualified by feelings means that the subject does not perceive the objects by mere neutral registration as, for example, a video camera or a computer does. Experiences are always qualified in some way or another. They *matter* to the experiencing subject; we are always, more or less dramatically, *touched* and *motivated* by what we experience. Our experiences are

---

[13] Commenting on this passage, Dan Zahavi further clarifies the relation between self-awareness and intentionality: 'as Ricoeur points out, the very suggestion that intentionality and self-awareness might be exclusive alternatives – that we are either so preoccupied with ourselves that every connection with the world is severed or so completely carried outside ourselves that perception becomes unconscious – is based on a quasi-spatial and completely inadequate conception of consciousness: If I am directed toward the outside, I cannot at the same time be directed toward the inside [...] Thus, self-awareness is not to be understood as a preoccupation with the self that excludes or impedes the contact with transcendent being. On the contrary, subjectivity is essentially oriented and open toward that which it is not, be it worldly entities or the Other, and it is exactly in this openness that it reveals itself to itself [...] It is by being present to the world that we are present to ourselves, and it is by being given to ourselves that we can be conscious of the world [...] Self-manifestation and hetero-manifestation are strictly interdependent, inseparable, and co-original' (Zahavi 1999, p. 124).

therefore permeated by the heterogeneous values at large in human existence (much more about this in the next chapter).

The third feature of intentionality that interests Ricoeur is the fact that our experiences seem to possess an immediate meaning. Our experiences are seldom experiences of raw perceptual *objects*. Most of the time, our experiences are experiences of *things*, that is, we understand an object as a certain kind of *thing* in a particular context. Although our perception of an object is always bound to a particular perspective, our experience of the *object* is (most of the time) immediately meaningful as an experience of a certain *thing*. The intentional nature of our experiences is characterised by a pre-reflective continuity between perception and thinking. In this sense, our experience of the object reveals something about the nature of the experiencing subject. Ricoeur's favourite example to clarify this interdependence of subject and object is precisely the nature of perception (1986, pp. 256–7; 1987, pp. 26–7 [44–5]; 2007b, pp. 307–11 [381–5]). As mentioned above, when we perceive an object we are always bound to a certain perspective. The object is always seen from a limited perspective, from the front, side or the back; we are never capable of seeing the object in its totality. Perspectivity thus accounts for the limits and general narrowness of human perception. The conception of the perceived object points back to the nature of the perceiving subject as confined to a certain perspective. However, our experience of the object is not completed in the passive aspect of perception, but reveals an active component in the way we perceive objects in the world. We are immediately aware of our confined vision of the object as a result of our pre-reflective awareness of other possible perspectives on the object. This awareness somehow transcends our own perspective and reveals an understanding of the totality of perspectives on the object. This totality is the *meaning* of the perceived object. If, for example, I look at a plastic chair at the end of a long table, I only see a small part of it, say, the top of its back. Nevertheless, I pre-reflectively form an idea of that piece of matter as being part of a thing that we name a chair. This capacity to form an idea of totality from a fragmentary perception is what Ricoeur calls our 'intention to signify', that is, the fact that 'I say more than I see when I signify' (1987, p. 28 [46]). The subject is capable of talking about the object in its totality, even in its absence. In this way, the pre-reflective understanding of the object as a thing reveals not only the restricted nature of human perception, but also the human capacity to transcend that restriction in the act of expressing a meaning. The subject is open to the object through its bodily senses, but in the act of understanding the object as a thing the subject is revealed as more than just restricted perception.

The interpretation of these three features of the concept of intentionality leads Ricoeur onto a path different from that trodden by Husserl. Whereas Husserl is mainly interested in clarifying the structures of human experience, such as pre-reflective self-awareness and what has later been called the 'minimal sense of self' intrinsically present in every experience (Zahavi 2005, pp. 106, 146), Ricoeur turns his attention to the complexity of that immediate sense of self. It is important, though, to understand that although Ricoeur concentrates on the troubled sense of selfhood, he still subscribes to the Husserlian insistence on a minimal sense of selfhood. A sense of self is foundational to human experience, and indispensable for any further investigation of selfhood. Dan

Zahavi, who is one of the most assiduous advocates for a minimal sense of self, has recently described how we should understand such a pre-reflective sense of self:

> [T]here is subjectivity of experience and a minimal sense of self, not only when I realize that *I* am perceiving a candle, but whenever there is perspectival ownership, whenever there is first-personal presence or manifestation of experience. It is this pre-reflective sense of self which provides the experiential grounding for any subsequent self-ascription, reflective appropriation, and thematic self-identification. Had our experiences been completely anonymous when originally lived through, any such subsequent appropriation would become inexplicable.
>
> (Zahavi 2011, p. 334)

Ricoeur would be in perfect agreement with this description. He would nevertheless insist that this minimal sense of self is unstable and easily troubled. And although experiential troubles are more obvious on a reflective level of subjective experience such as doubt, hesitation, and confusion, Ricoeur nevertheless finds them to be rooted in the subject's pre-reflective experience. The complexity stems from the ontological constitution of the human subject. The phenomenological analysis of intentionality, on Ricoeur's reading, reveals the twofold character of human experience as constituted by bodily sensibility and rational understanding, and Ricoeur takes this as a warrant for rooting his phenomenological analysis (How do I experience?) in an ontological conception of the human being (What and who am I?). One could say that Ricoeur is more interested in how we as concrete persons live with our experiences of the world and of ourselves than merely clarifying the subjective structures of consciousness per se:

> Consciousness spends itself in founding the unity of meaning and presence 'in' the object. 'Consciousness' is not yet the unity of a person in itself and for itself [*l'unité d'une personne en soi et pour soi*]; it is not one person; it is no one. The 'I' of I think is merely the form of a world for anyone and everyone. It is consciousness in general, that is, a pure and simple project of the object. (1987, pp. 45–6 [63])

Husserl's investigations remain ontologically or metaphysically neutral (Zahavi 2002, pp. 102–4). He is primarily interested in the experiential structures of subjectivity—*how* a subject experiences the world and itself, and not *what* the world is or *what* a human subject is. Ricoeur, on the other hand, wants to follow the twofold picture of human experience onto an ontological level, and to do this he turns to the Kantian idea of human experience as the result of a transcendental synthesis of two heterogeneous aspects of human nature.

The human subject is an intermediate being, constituted by sensibility (*la sensibilité*) and reason (*la raison*): 'He is intermediate because he is a mixture, and a mixture because he brings about mediations' (1987, p. 3 [23]). The subject and the world are understood only by turning the attention away from the experienced world and back to the subjective structures that make this experience possible in the first place. This focus on the dynamic nature of subjectivity is Kant's strategic move known as his Copernican Revolution, and it plays a critical role in Ricoeur's account of subjectivity

(1966, pp. 32 [35], 471 [443]). Similarly, in his use of the concept of transcendental synthesis, Ricoeur continues to follow closely on the heels of Kant.

The transcendental synthesis is conceived as the first step in understanding the subject as well as the world. Transcendental here means the basic structures of the human subject that make experience of reality possible (1987, p. 5 [25]). Our experience of reality is a result of the mediations performed by the subject. This is not to be misinterpreted as a kind of idealistic solipsism that reduces the reality of the world to the subjective representation of the world. On the contrary, the world is there and affects the subject through the body: 'existence of the body is the decisive fact which forces us to elucidate concrete life at the limits of intelligibility' (1966, p. 135 [129]). For Ricoeur, as well as for Kant, it is the undeniable presence of the world that prompts a synthetic conception of experience. Through the physicality of body and the perceptive capacities of the bodily senses, the subject is confronted with the existence of a world different from itself that it constantly has to make sense of:

> What is precisely bewildering in the mediating role of the body [*corps*] is that it opens me to the world [*il m'ouvre sur le monde*]; in other words, it is the organ of an intentional relation in which the world is not the boundary of my existence but its correlate. (2007b, p. 307 [380–1])

My existence becomes a part of the world through my body. My body roots me in the physical world by being physically constituted, and my self-awareness is therefore saturated with the world through my body. The subject does not, however, coincide with its sensibility; it does not become one with the world. It is turned back upon itself in the experience of the sensible objects because of the resistance that it experiences from the world (1987, p. 21 [39]). The world does not obey my will and desire. It is in this being turned back upon itself, in the separation from the world, that the subject discovers itself as an intermediate being. A human subject is not constituted by the external world alone but, besides being passively receptive, it possesses a spontaneity capable of representing things and ideas different from those perceived as present. This spontaneity coincides with the workings of our reason without the input from sensible data. The human subject is neither mere sensibility nor unrestricted reason, but a synthesis of the two.

The transcendental synthesis of reason and sensibility is that which makes consciousness possible in the first place, but it only provides us with the basic structure of consciousness, because '[t]he consciousness philosophy speaks of in its transcendental stage constitutes its own unity only outside itself, on the object' (1987, p. 45 [63]) and, on this level, 'the universe of things is still only the abstract skeleton of our life-world [*l'ossature abstraite de ce monde de notre vie*]' (1987, p. 47 [65]; translation slightly modified). Through the experienced object the subject understands itself as constituted by sensibility and reason, but nothing more. It is an empty consciousness that has no idea of *how* or *why* it exists. However, the transcendental synthesis provides a basic scheme for the analysis of human subjectivity and is therefore the necessary first step in understanding the nature of the subject (1987, pp. 5 [25], 45–6 [63]). As we shall see in the following chapter, contrary to Kant, Ricoeur turns his attention to a dimension of human experience that Kant excluded from the theoretical part of his critical philosophy, namely, our feelings.[14] Feelings, for Ricoeur, are that which enables us to transform the formal notion of consciousness into the concrete and lived consciousness that characterises human experiences.

But before taking up Ricoeur's treatment of feelings in the next chapter, we shall close this chapter with an explanation of how this synthetic conception of subjectivity bears on the question of naturalism by looking more carefully at how it affects our conception of rationality. How to understand rationality is a central problem in contemporary philosophical discussions of naturalism, and the way in which we conceive of our rational capacities is fundamental to our understanding of psychopathology.

Wounded Thinking

We are rational creatures. Thinking enables us to attenuate the fetters of our sensible condition, if not to free ourselves entirely from them. Our rational capacities transform mindless reactions to inputs from the external world into thoughtful actions calibrated in the light of our beliefs, desires, feelings, and our thinking about past and future. We calculate our chances of success, reflect upon what is appropriate and what is not, and deliberate on our decisions before acting. We are not entirely reasonable or purely rational, though. Human experience, thought, and behaviour are characterised by what Peter Strawson, in a famous book on Kant, called the bounds of sense (1966). We are biological creatures. Even though we flourish by means of our rational capacities to control and shape our existence, we are deeply enmeshed in the mindless, or a-rational, workings of the rest of nature. We are able to understand Aristotle when, in the *Metaphysics*, he writes that the law of non-contradiction is the most certain of all logical principles. We also understand Whitman, though, when in *Song of Myself* he writes 'Do I contradict myself?/Very well then I contradict myself/(I am large, I contain multitudes)' (1993, p. 113). We are able to understand, and even sympathise with, both thinkers because we are complex creatures. All of us contain multitudes of inclinations, desires, feelings, instincts, and ideas that are not bridled by our rational capacities. In other words, our rationality is precarious, or as Ricoeur puts it, '[t]he Cogito is internally fractured [*Le Cogito est intérieurement brisé*]':

> Reasons for this intimate rupture become apparent when we consider the natural inclination of reflection dealing with the Cogito. The Cogito tends to posit itself [*tend à l'autoposition*]. Descartes' genius lies in having carried to the limit this intuition of a thought which makes circles with itself in positing itself and which takes into itself only an image of its body and an image of the other [...] Now this tendency on my part to be going in circles with myself cannot be overcome simply by willing to deal with the body as a personal body [*corps propre*]. Extension of the Cogito to include the personal body in reality requires more than a change in method: The 'I' [*le 'moi'*] must more radically renounce the covert pretention of all consciousness, must abandon its wish to posit itself, so that it can receive a nourishing inspiring spontaneity which breaks the sterile circle that the self forms with itself [*le soi forme avec lui-même*]. (1966, p. 14 [17]; translation modified)

---

[14] Contrary to all too common misconceptions of his philosophy, Kant did, in fact, explore quite carefully the affective dimension of thought and action in both his practical philosophy and in his extensive writings on anthropology, pedagogy, and aesthetics.

In a sense, the rest of the book is an exploration of this intimate rupture of the 'I think', of our rationality, in terms of the disruption of the self by that which is not itself (diagnostic) and, subsequently, the reappropriation of the self as a person through the dialectic of otherness and selfhood (therapeutic). We are convinced that in order to understand the disruption of thinking, or what with Ricoeur we could call the 'wounded Cogito [*Cogito blessé*]' (1977, p. 439 [425]), at work in mental illness, we should start by looking at the constitutive precariousness of human rationality. As we shall see, we follow Ricoeur's insistence on locating this precariousness in the ambivalence of biology (vital desires) and rationality (spiritual desires) at work in our emotional life, but in order to understand our digging at the emotional roots of rationality, we first need to make clear how we understand the notion of rationality.

We owe our take on rationality to Ronald de Sousa. He argues that we use the notion of rationality in two basic senses: a categorical and a normative sense (1987, pp. 160–1; 2007, pp. 6–12). In the *categorical* sense, 'rational' contrasts with 'a-rational' or 'non-rational', that is, a kind of behaviour which cannot be judged by degrees of rationality or even in terms of teleology. An a-rational behaviour cannot be explained in terms of choice or free will, but merely refers to caused events. Causality is here used to explain how one event, or a series of events, causes another event without any interpolation of rational deliberation or goal-oriented action. In the *normative* sense, however, 'rational' contrasts with 'irrational'. Here our notion of rationality opens up a normative space of more or less rational thought and behaviour, whereby a belief or an action can indeed be judged by degrees of rationality or by the more fluid standards of what is reasonable, appropriate, becoming, authentic, understandable, and so forth. In other words, this normative sense of rationality covers a tightly woven web of peculiarly human reasons, norms, and values.

The difference between 'a-rational' and 'rational' can be illustrated with two variations over one story. Say that one late afternoon my wife and I decide that we want to make an omelette. Unfortunately we are out of eggs, so my wife offers to cook the omelette, if I go out to buy the eggs. Half an hour later, I return abashed with an empty egg pack. When she asks why the pack is empty, I tell her one of the two following stories. On my way home from the grocery store, a massive branch of the old chestnut tree at the corner of our street broke off and tumbled down over my head. I managed to jump away from under the falling branch, but the egg pack slipped from my hand, and all the eggs broke when the pack hit the ground. This is one story. The other version goes like this. When I turned the corner from the grocery store, I caught sight of my former boss. Ever since the bastard first humiliated me in front of everybody and then fired me eight months ago, I have nursed an intense grudge against him, so when I saw him on the other side of the street I could not control myself. I became so enraged that I started to throw the eggs at him.

Now, it is glaringly obvious that my wife will react very differently to my two stories. In the first case, she will, or so at least I hope, be relieved that I am not hurt and consider the business of the broken eggs a freak incident which could have ended tragically, but fortunately turned out well. In fact, she might even be impressed and commend me on my agile and attentive reactions. The fact that the eggs are broken is due to a series of events which were out of my control and had nothing to do with rationality whatsoever.

On the contrary, it can only be ascribed to an a-rational, causal chain of chance and necessity—to use Jacques Monod's poignant expression (1970). It goes without saying that the reaction of my wife will be quite different when I tell her the second version. I can be pretty sure that she will not be impressed or commend my behaviour. Being the level-headed person she is, she will probably sigh and tell me that it was an irrational or stupid thing to do, since it will not bring about any good. It will certainly not give me my job back, help me regain my self-respect or convince my previous boss of anything save that it was a good decision to get rid of me in the first place. If I try to argue that in spite of this, it made me feel good, my wife can point to the obvious fact that I cannot go around doing things just because they make me feel good. All kinds of behaviour might feel good without therefore being rational. At this point, it seems difficult, if not impossible, for me to reply to her argument. I could try to blame her for her cold-hearted lack of empathy and her obnoxiously bourgeois reasonableness in a circumstance where all I need is to be cuddled and understood. But no matter what I say to justify my behaviour or to express my disappointment at her, in my eyes, insensitive rational thinking, I cannot argue against the irrational nature of my action.

The difference between 'a-rational' and 'rational' that we want to illustrate with these two stories is surely obvious, but not philosophically trivial. In fact, it evidences the obscure line that separates what is human from what is not human. **An a-rational behaviour or event refers to what occurs in nature without the noisy interference of human reasons.** By saying that something is rational, our explanatory enterprise makes a categorical shift from what is 'a-rational' and unaffected by human reasoning to what is rational and thus thoroughly saturated with the noise of human, sometimes all too human, meaning. Once we allow this human noise into the workings of nature by considering the rationality or irrationality of some behaviour or event, our scientific endeavours change drastically. The explanatory focus turns from the a-rational workings of nature to the, more or less, rational dispositions of human nature.

Now, having made clear the difference between the categorical and the normative sense of rationality, it is time to look at what happens when we want to explore the normative sense. When we introduce rationality into our explanations, it is because we want to make sense of the particular human noise in nature. This can also be framed as a question: what does it mean to be a human being situated and deeply entrenched in a nature which is not, to put it mildly, particularly human? We are part of nature, and yet our behaviour seems to be drastically different from any other kind of behaviour found in nature. One principal reason for this difference can be found in the fact that our behaviour is governed by rational dispositions besides mere a-rational causality. Thus, when we say that some kind of behaviour is rational or irrational, we enter the particular human world with its complex web of heterogeneous values, norms, conventions, and meanings—and the different ways they may, or may not, help us to govern and regulate our thoughts, feelings, and actions.

There are at least two kinds of rationality in play in our use of the normative sense of rationality: a *thin* (skeletal) kind and a *thick* (fleshy) kind. The thin kind of rationality pertains to the functioning of the logical structures of our cognitive abilities. It is a rather clear and very stable kind of rationality, but its functioning is also unfettered from the larger normative web governing ordinary human behaviour. It is the kind of rationality to which it is not contrary, as Hume famously said, 'to prefer the destruction of the whole world to the scratching of my finger' (1958, p. 416). However, in our usual employment of the notion of rationality to characterise ordinary human behaviour, this notion thickens and becomes more interestingly fleshy. When we judge behaviour to be rational or irrational in this thick sense, our judgement does not merely refer to the norms governing the logical function of our cognitive capacities, but also includes the broader, and more complex, norms of situated and embodied human behaviour. Where the thin kind of rationality is stable because of its strict formality, this thick kind is unstable because of its normative nature. It is an embodied, personalised, and context-sensitive kind of rationality, where 'rational' behaviour cannot be distinguished from 'irrational' behaviour merely by means of what is logical and what is not. This becomes obvious if we return to our story of the broken eggs. In the second version of this story, I said that my wife was right to deem my throwing the eggs at my boss irrational. If we view my behaviour from the standpoint of the thin notion of rationality, though, my behaviour was perfectly rational. I felt a desire to get back at my mean boss, and I found myself holding a pack of eggs which I believed was perfectly suitable for that purpose, so it was indeed rational to break the eggs for that purpose. Nevertheless, my wife can give several reasons why it was an irrational thing to do: it is an inconsiderate waste of perfectly good eggs, it makes me look like an idiot, it is immature and inappropriate for a man of my age, it is not a normal way of behaving, it is not a reasonable way to deal with problems, and physical aggravation in whatever form is simply wrong. What is important to notice here is that when my wife judges my behaviour irrational she needs to scaffold her use of rationality with several densely normative adjectives such as 'inconsiderate', 'immature', 'inappropriate', 'normal', 'reasonable', and the explicitly ethical one 'wrong'. This scaffolding brings out the normative instability of the thick notion of rationality. Simply to say that a certain kind of behaviour is rational is either close to being empty (the thin kind of rationality) or an expression of certain norms, values, and conventions that calls for further explanation and argument (the thick kind of rationality).

In the rest of the book, we will focus on this thick kind of rationality, arguing that a basic reason for the precariousness of rationality is that it does not respect the distinction between a-rationality and normative rationality. The reason for this conflation is that human rationality is emotional, and as such it is deeply embedded in the bodily, a-rational functions of human nature. In Part II, we shall carry through the argument that our emotions are the most embodied of our mental phenomena, and thus the ambivalence of a-rationality and rationality is fundamental to how we understand ourselves as persons. We find the conceptual framework for this view of emotions, and the importance of emotions for human personhood, in Ricoeur's hermeneutical theory of subjectivity, and the remaining chapters of this part of the book will unfold this theory. In Part III, we shall then argue that human vulnerability to mental illness can, for a large part, be explained by the instability of rational dispositions as it is manifested in our emotional life.

As a preliminary illustration of how the precarious character of rationality bears on psychopathology, we can imagine a third version of the story with the broken eggs. Suppose I tell my wife that I arrived safely back at our front door, but when I was about to open the door, I was suddenly overtaken by a feeling of despair immediately followed by an agonising feeling of emptiness and spleen. It felt as if my heart splintered in pieces, and the meaning of my life was shattered in an instant. I cannot explain why, I say to my wife, but I took the eggs out of the pack and dropped them, one by one, down the three steps leading up to our door. It was as if something inside me, like a piece of my brain, caused me to do so. It simply happened. I try to explain myself, but find no words to express the strangeness of this anonymous event which had taken place inside myself. It was simultaneously *my* body and *a* body, something external and internal at the same time that made me behave like this. It felt as a kind of otherness in myself, impersonal and personal at the same time, with no clear-cut distinction between my self and that otherness. I also felt that it was me who was the owner of this piece of my brain, but not its possessor; something that belonged to me but that it was not under my control. It was as if it acted *through* me.[15]

How is my wife supposed to react on hearing this story? Surely, she will be shocked and become deeply concerned for me, but how is she supposed to understand what has happened? Are we talking about a-rational events, like those in the first story? Or can my behaviour be explained in terms of a radical degree of irrationality, akin to the second story? How we choose to explain my behaviour, despair and spleen in general or even clinical disorders, depends (in part at least) on how we understand the interplay of rational and a-rational factors constitutive of our emotional life. We shall argue that our emotions are permeated by rationality, but that the rationality we find in our emotional life is an unstable rationality entrenched in, and to a certain degree constituted by, the a-rational changes of our bodily landscape. This instability, though, is not something that can be done away with by recoiling into either a rationalistic or a biological conception of human emotions. We are fragile beings because of this ambivalence of a-rational and rational factors of our emotional life, and we believe that our investigation into Ricoeur's wounded Cogito will help us understand this fragility, and hopefully shed some light on why human persons are vulnerable beings.

As mentioned in the beginning of this chapter, systematic investigations of naturalism have not played the same prominent role in continental philosophy as in the analytical tradition. Moreover, classic Husserlian phenomenology has, as noted above, made an effort to remain ontologically neutral and to avoid the encounter with the empirical sciences. In fact, 'Husserl himself is known as a staunch anti-naturalist' (Zahavi 2004, p. 333). Ricoeur's position on the question of naturalism is more complex. One thing is certain, though: he is not a naturalist in the strict sense, since one of the basic presumptions of his philosophy is that '[t]he body of a subject and the body as an anonymous empirical object do not coincide' (1966, p. 12 [15]). Understanding the embodied nature of subjectivity cannot take the form of an empirical investigation of the body as a biophysical object on par with other, non-human objects in the world, because '[t]he dependence of my body on my self which wills in it and through it has nothing corresponding to it in the universe of discourse of empirical science' (1966,

---

[15] This narrative is fictional, of course, but it draws on several self-reports made by our patients.

p. 12 [15]). In an extended discussion with the prominent neuroscientist Jean-Pierre Changeux, he explains further that 'a person is not housed in his body as a captain in his ship: a wounded person will say "my leg" whereas the captain will go on seeing the hole in the hull of his ship as something external to himself [. . .] The body of a human being [*Le corps d'un homme*] ceases to be just another body [*un corps quelconque*]' (Changeux and Ricoeur 2000, pp. 38–9 [47]). Despite this sharp methodological distinction between empirical and phenomenological investigations of human nature, Ricoeur is nevertheless compelled, due to the ontological nature of his investigations, to deal more explicitly with the naturalistic challenges than is common in traditional phenomenology. In fact, his insistence on the biophysical character of the embodied self is among the reasons for his turn from phenomenology to hermeneutics. The ambivalence of biology and subjectivity is at the heart of his understanding of the troubled feelings of selfhood.

Ricoeur insists on the fractured nature of our Cogito, that is, our rationality or our reflective capacity to make sense of the world and ourselves. The subject is constituted by both biophysical mechanisms and mental states and must therefore be analysed with a methodology different from the one used in natural sciences without, however, recoiling into an introspective mysticism: 'Inversely, knowledge of subjectivity cannot be reduced to introspection [. . .] Its essence is to respect the originality of the Cogito as a cluster of the subject's intentional acts' (1966, p. 10 [14]). The concept of intentionality reveals the conscious subject as an ambivalent being. It belongs to nature and yet it is able to go beyond the immediate reaction to its surroundings. To approach such an ambivalent being, we must contrive a method that embraces as many aspects as possible of this particular being. Ricoeur finds such a methodology in his interpretation of the two inherited concepts, intentionality (Husserl) and synthesis (Kant). In the concept of intentionality, he discovers an argument for the twofold nature of subjective experience that he labels with a quotation of Maine de Biran's famous dictum 'Homo simplex in vitalitate duplex in humanitate'[16] (1966, p. 228 [213]; 1987, p. 91 [107]).

Ricoeur breaks off from Husserlian phenomenology by insisting on this twofold picture of consciousness. Whereas Husserlian phenomenology focuses on a pre-reflective self-awareness and a minimal sense of self as an integral and constitutive feature of human experience, Ricoeur insists on the troubling ambivalence of this awareness of being a self. Ricoeur does not deny that I always have pre-reflective sense of self whenever I experience something, so in this sense his account presupposes the Husserlian minimal sense of self. But he maintains that this sense of self is fragile and often conflictual in nature. He finds support for the idea of selfhood as fragile and conflictual by turning to the nature of human feelings—which has seldom been central to traditional phenomenological investigations of subjectivity. Our pre-reflective awareness of a self is pervaded by a multitude of confused and unsettling feelings that prompts the subject to a reflective understanding of itself as a self. It is in this sense that Ricoeur would agree to a notion of a minimal self inherent in our experiential relation to the world. He

---

[16] The dictum can be roughly translated as 'A human being is simple by the fact that it is alive, ambiguous by virtue of being human'.

would, however, add that this notion of a self is not yet a *human* self, but only a fragile conceptual presupposition for any talk about a self.

The human self is not a self simply in experiencing the world. Pre-reflective self-awareness is an important presupposition for any notion of self, but even the most minimal notion of a self must take into account the affective and motivational nature of such self-awareness. The fragile and conflictual nature of our minimal sense of self makes it clear that 'the self is in its acts' (1966, p. 58 [56]). A human subject experiences the world in order to act in this world: '[t]o exist is to act' (1966, p. 334 [316]), or as he explains more explicitly:

> In any case the world is not just a spectacle, but also a problem and a task, a matter to be worked over. It is the world for the project and for action. Even in the most immobile project the feeling of power, of being able, presents the world to me as horizon, as theatre, and as matter for my actions. (1966, p. 212 [198])

This motivational nature of pre-reflective self-awareness becomes visible in the affective dimension of human subjectivity. And Ricoeur's hermeneutics is basically an attempt to explain how the human self is a being that must *become* itself as a person through a lifelong interpretation of what it experiences and cares for in the world. In other words, the subject has to *reappropriate* itself in the world in which it finds itself at a loss:

> Appropriation signifies that the initial situation from which reflection proceeds is 'forgetfulness.' I am lost, 'led astray' among objects [*je suis perdu, 'égaré' parmi les objets*] and separated from the center of my existence, just as I am separated from others and as an enemy is separated from all men. Whatever the secret of this 'diaspora', of this separation, it signifies that I do not at first possess what I am [*je ne possède pas d'abord ce que je suis*]. (1977, p. 45 [53])

This reappropriation of selfhood through interpretation will be the central theme of the next two chapters.

Chapter 2

A Hermeneutics of 'I Am'

We have seen in the last chapter that Ricoeur approaches the complexity of subjective experience by combining the Husserlian concept of intentionality with the Kantian idea of the twofold nature of the human subject. He turns from phenomenology to a hermeneutical conception of ontology. The affective nature of subjective experience reveals a fragile and problematic self-awareness, which cannot be clarified only by a phenomenological investigation of the experiential structures of subjectivity. Our troubled self-awareness goes beyond our experience of the world. It is rooted in our peculiar ontological constitution. We are fragile beings because of the ambivalence of reason and sensibility at play in our experience, thoughts, and behaviour. We are rational creatures, but our rational capacities are bound to our senses and enmeshed in the a-rational, causal functioning of our body. This means that 'our Cogito is internally fractured', as Ricoeur says, and our rational capacities are deeply precarious and easily wounded. We possess an immediate sense of being a self, but this minimal sense of self is characterised by ambivalence and confusion which can only be dealt with through an ongoing interpretation of the self's existence in the world. The self finds itself situated in a world in which it has not placed itself, and it is in this world, by interacting with otherness (that which is not itself), that it must reaffirm itself as an individual person: 'the self [*le moi*] must be lost in order to find the "I" [*le "je"*]' (2004, p. 19 [24]). The self continuously struggles with the question '*Who am I?*', and in order to reappropriate itself, it is compelled to measure itself with the insecurity stirred up by the otherness that constitutes its being:

> The hermeneutics of the *I am* can alone include both the apodictic certainty of the Cartesian *I think* and the uncertainties, even the lies and the illusions, of the self, of immediate consciousness. It alone can yoke, side by side, the serene affirmation [*l'affirmation sereine*] *I am* and the poignant doubt [*le doute poignant*] *Who am I?* (2004, p. 259 [262]; translation slightly modified)

In this chapter, we attempt to clarify this 'hermeneutics of the *I am*'. We start out by explaining how Ricoeur's investigation of selfhood is rooted in the affective dimension of human nature. The values that inform and orient our existence are generated by the multitude of heterogeneous feelings that characterise human experience. Ricoeur proposes that we approach these feelings in terms of the two basic roots of selfhood, namely, reason and sensibility. He argues that the core of human selfhood, which he calls the heart, is in a permanent restless tension between vital desires (sensibility) and spiritual desires (reason). This affective fragility of selfhood calls for an interpretive approach to our troubled selfhood. We then deal with Ricoeur's turn from a 'pure' phenomenology to a hermeneutical phenomenology, and end the chapter with a brief introduction to the notion of narrative identity that will play a central role in the following chapter.

Some of Ricoeur's concepts and ideas, especially his early account of affectivity to be treated in the first two sections, might strike the reader as obscure and belonging to another age. We have nevertheless chosen to include these early investigations, since they are essential for understanding how feelings and emotions call for a hermeneutical approach to selfhood.

The Affective Generation of Values

Human subjectivity is constituted by sensibility and reason. This implies, as we have seen, that the self is always bound to a certain point of view that limits its openness to the world. The self is able, however, to transcend this perspective and try to make sense of its limited perception of the world. This basic transcendental structure reveals a intimate fracture at the core of subjectivity, and subjective experience and action is a continuous mediation between the two heterogeneous aspects of human nature. The relation between the two aspects is marked by a disproportion, though. The self is an embodied mind and not a reasonable body. Although Ricoeur never underestimates the importance of the body in the constitution of subjectivity, he has no doubt about the primacy of reason. The subject is intelligible only from the perspective of its capacity to understand (1966, pp. 56–7 [54–5], 341–2 [319–20]; 1987, pp. 44–5 [62], 64 [81]). He therefore argues that the human subject is characterised by a disproportion. The mind dominates the body, but is nevertheless bound to it and limited by it. The idea of disproportion is important to Ricoeur, because it leads him to another idea central to his argument for a hermeneutical development of phenomenology, namely, that fallibility is an intrinsic feature of being human. The subject's understanding of the world and itself is characterised by its being liable to fail, to be inaccurate, inappropriate, problematic, and simply wrong.

Disproportion and fallibility are uncovered in the experiential structures outlined above. Our experiences reveal an unstable sense of selfhood rooted in the complex nature of our pre-reflective experience. Our understanding of ourselves (and the world) is always at risk of being problematic, because '[t]he bond with the body [*le lien avec le corps*], even though indivisible, is polemic and dramatic' (1966, p. 227 [212]). This tense and difficult situation is a result of the disproportion of sensibility and reason. On the one hand, reason is the capacity by which the subject dissociates itself from the workings of the world and, thereby, makes room for freedom. On the other, the body is that which, inescapably, binds the subject to the workings of the world. Hence, we are our body whether we like it or not: 'It is to the extent to which the entire world is a vast extension of our body as pure fact [*fait pur*] that it is itself the terminus of our consent' (1966, p. 343 [321]). The body affects and restricts the subject's access to the world. And the subject cannot ignore or in any way escape this 'pure fact'. In other words, the body is both access (we are open to the world through our senses) and limit (this openness is always determined by a specific perspective) to the world.

Ricoeur finds the origin of our unstable experience of the world and ourselves in the affective dimension of our experience. Human existence is generally 'pathetic', because our problematic relation to the world, other people, and ourselves is *felt* before it is *understood* (1987, p. 81 [97]).

My feelings reveal the importance of being the self that *I* am. It is through our feelings that we become aware of the normative feature of selfhood in the sense that feelings are what makes my thoughts and experiences *matter* to me:

> [F]eeling [*sentiment*] interiorizes reason [*raison*] and shows me that reason is my reason, for through it I appropriate reason for myself [...] In short, feeling reveals the identity of existence and reason: it personalizes reason. (1987, p. 102 [118])

Subjective experience is permeated and qualified by feelings, and, for Ricoeur, the term 'feeling' covers a number of various functions: 'affective regulations, disturbing emotions, affective states, vague intuitions, passions, etc.' (1987, p. 83 [99]).

The function of feelings is best explained in relation to understanding. As we saw in the previous chapter, the intentional nature of consciousness has both an objective and a subjective aspect, that is, we understand in terms of the opposition between subject and object. When I try to understand what I experience, I relate myself to the experienced object as a thing different from myself which I then try to make sense of. For example, I understand the apple on the table before me as something different from myself. Now, feelings inverse this objective form of understanding because 'feeling is the felt manifestation of a relation to the world more profound than that of a representation which instantiates the polarity of subject and object' (1986, p. 253; our translation); or said more explicitly:

> The universal function of feeling is to bind together. It connects what knowledge [*connaissance*] divides; it binds me to things, to beings, to being. Whereas the whole movement of objectification tends to set a world over against me, feeling unites the intentionality, which throws me out of myself, to the affection through which I feel myself existing. Consequently, it is always shy of or beyond the duality of subject and object. (1987, p. 131 [147])

I am not a free-floating mind that represents reality from a third-person perspective. Rather, I am a situated and embodied self that strives to interpret a reality to which it is a priori bound, 'because by means of feeling, objects touch me' (1987, p. 89 [105]). Feelings disclose the fact that I exist as a self already situated in the world that I attempt to understand. I am involved with the world before I understand the world or myself. The apple on the table is not just an indifferent object. It affects me and kindles certain feelings through which it matters to me, that is, it is invested with significance and possible actions (I may ignore it, eat it, be disgusted by it, paint it, squash it, or give it to my child).

Obviously, feelings and reason are not two separate functions at work in subjectivity, but work together simultaneously as an experiential unity (1986, p. 252). Feeling discloses the felt motives and values of our rationality (*why* something matters to us), and our rational capacities clarify the intentional structure of feeling (*what* it is that we are feeling). This intrinsic connection of feeling and values discloses the *normative* nature of human selfhood. Being the self that I am is always normatively qualified. When I consider a particular action, experience a situation or meet another person, my feelings reveal the value of these phenomena to me, that is, how they matter to me. I may feel that the person is lovable, the action repugnant or the situation embarrassing. Feeling exposes my interiority by manifesting 'pre- and hyper-objective connections with the beings of the world' (1987, p. 86 [102]).

We can call this relation the personal relation to the world. It is personal because feeling is what qualifies experiences as *my* experiences. It is *my* love, *my* repugnance, and *my* embarrassment. On the other hand, feeling is always a feeling of something. The qualitative dimension of feeling is always bound to an object, physical or mental. Feelings are characterised by an intentional structure that points to something other than just the quality of *my* feeling: 'Our "affections" ["*affections*"] are read on the world they develop, which reflects their kinds and nuances' (1987, p. 84 [100]). The intrinsic interplay of feeling (interiority) and reason (intentionality) in our emotional life discloses a critical feature of human selfhood: the coexistence of *self* and *the other than self* in my sense of selfhood. The subject is affected both by itself and by that which is different from it. Feelings are central to understanding self-awareness because of this dual aspect: *they are simultaneously generated by the world and the subject itself*. They manifest an intrinsic dialectic between selfhood and otherness, the voluntary and the involuntary, activity and passivity, in the subject's pre-reflective sense of being a self. My feelings bind me to the world and other people, and it is exactly through that emotional binding that the world and other people influence and shape my existence as a self. This affective qualification is what reveals that my existence in the world matters to me. I find myself in a world pervaded by values generated and shaped by myself, other people, and the world. My feelings make me aware that I 'am-already-in' a world pervaded by heterogeneous values. It is not something that I can choose to be part of or abstain from. It is not I alone who make up the values by which I live my life. It is simply part of my being a self to be situated among and constituted by values that are not of my choosing. Thus, the values that my feelings reveal are heterogeneous and often discordant.

The complex character of values that inform and shape my existence is expressed by feelings, since the affective dimension of subjectivity reveals the complex interrelation of self and otherness in our experience:

> That is to say that consciousness is not consciousness of an object but self-consciousness [*conscience de soi*]. This affectivity is the elementary form of the apperception of the 'I' ['*moi*']. As all self-consciousness, it accompanies in an original way all consciousness of something, sometimes muted, sometimes as an exalting or painful orchestration of the presence of the world. (1966, p. 412 [387]; translation modified)

In other words, affectivity reveals an active, living consciousness in which the world and the subject are interwoven 'by all the secret threads that we call "inclinations", which are "strung out" ["*tendus*"] between us and the [other] beings' (1986, p. 253). Inclinations are constitutive of our values and motivations. They disclose the original *why* of the predicates 'good' and 'bad'. An inclination holds this power to qualify since, through feelings, it elicits a self in direction of a certain action. Moreover, my inclinations stress the involuntary aspect of my values by linking them to basic needs such as eating, drinking, sleeping, and reproduction. It is the pre-reflective values pertaining to our instincts, bodily sensations, and vital needs which bind a human self to its bodily constitution, and thus make the body the inarticulate bedrock of our values. Our body is the flesh of our existence, the organ for our actions, and the recipient for (some of) our sufferings:

> Need [*besoin*] is the primordial spontaneity of the body; as such it originally and initially reveals values which set it apart from all other sources of motives. Through need, values *emerge* without my having posited them in my act-generating role: bread is good, wine is good. Before I will it, a value already appeals to me solely because I exist in flesh [*j'existe en chair*]; it is already a reality in the world, a reality which reveals itself to me through the lack [*le manque*] [. . .] The mystery of incarnate Cogito ties willing to this first stratum of values with which motivation begins. (1966, p. 94 [90])

It is through the body that we first feel a motivation to do something, to act, because '[t]he first non-deducible is the body as existing, life as value [*la vie comme valeur*]' (p. 94 [90]). Despite this intimate relation of human values to our biological constitution, there is a difference between affective values in humans and in other animals. Whereas feelings in animals seem to coincide more readily with their instinctual behaviour, the feelings that motivate human behaviour are drastically different. This becomes clear when we look at the feelings involved in human inclinations and desires. The human self is affected by an obscure confusion of feelings due to the intimate fracture of reason and sensibility in its being.

Fragility of the Heart

Our feelings, inclinations, and desires—and the values revealed by them—often put us in a state of conflict or tension. In fact, an important function of feelings can be understood in relation to this tension:

> Feeling points out how far along we are toward the resolution of tensions. Its modalities and its felt nuances mark the phases of action launched by a certain disequilibrium seeking a new equilibrium. Feeling is thus a function of the recovery of the living creature's equilibrium [*la rééquilibration du vivant*]. To understand its role in this process is to understand feeling. (1987, p. 99 [115]; translation modified)

Feelings express a basic conflict between sensibility and reason in subjective experience. They express 'the intimate conflict of human desire [*le conflit intime à la désirabilité humaine*]' (1987, p. 92 [108]; translation slightly modified).

According to Ricoeur, all human conflicts originate in the 'affective node' of subjectivity, which is the radical and dramatic manifestation of the primary dual aspect of human selfhood; the disproportion felt as conflict (1987, p. 106 [123]). To clarify the intimate affective core of subjectivity, Ricoeur makes use of Plato's treatment, in book IV of the *Republic*, of the relationship between the heart (*thymos*), the vital desires (*epithymia*), and the spiritual desires (*erōs*). Vital and spiritual desires keep the self in a continuing tension between the feelings of 'pleasure' and 'happiness' because of our existence in the world as both a biological and a spiritual being. Our desires drive us towards a complex satisfaction of values generated by both of these aspects of human selfhood. However, the self is not divided into two separate parts, a pure reason and an obscure sensibility, but acts as a unity by means of a mediation of vitality and spirituality, and as Ricoeur writes, '[h]ere we encounter Plato's valuable idea of the heart [*thymos*], the median function par excellence in the human soul. The heart is the living transition from bios to logos. At one and the same time it separates and unites vital affectivity or desire and the spiritual affectivity' (1987, pp. 81–2 [98]). The heart is here meant as a unifying symbol for the heterogeneous multitude of feelings involved in existing as a human self, and as such 'the "heart", the restless heart [*le cœur inquiet*], would be the fragile moment par excellence' (1987, p. 82 [98]) because it is intended to ensure an ontological unity of (vital) pleasure and (spiritual) happiness. By acknowledging vital pleasure as a constitutive part of being human, Ricoeur rejects the basic idea of Kantian and other philosophical anthropologies (the Thomist and the Cartesian), which argue that the subject has to obey only the rational part of its nature in order to become a person (1987, pp. 77–8 [92–3]). For Ricoeur, the humanity of the subject, personhood, is not constituted only by its rational capacities; on the contrary, it makes no sense to speak of a pure reason, since human reason is always rooted in sensibility, just as sensibility is always shaped by reason.

Ricoeur separates the manifold of feelings into two basic categories, the schematised and the atmospheric feelings. The schematised feelings are those involved in our relation to things and other people in our existence in the world. By the term 'schematised', Ricoeur refers to the intentional structure of our feelings as involved in our practical engagement with the world, that is, the feelings involved in the decisions, norms, and actions that constitute our coexistence with other people: 'we must specify and articulate the relationship of the self to another self by means of the objectivity that is built on the themes of having, power, and worth' (1987, p. 113 [129]). Human feelings can only be understood in the intentional relation to the other person through the dimensions of politics, economics, and culture. These different relations to otherness awake a multitude of feelings at the heart of the subject. They disclose the feelings involved in our concrete existence with other people.

Not all feelings, though, are expressed by an intentional relation. We experience feelings that do not seem to refer to any distinct object at all. They are more like an atmosphere or a tonality accompanying our being situated in the world without relating to anything in particular. Ricoeur calls these feelings atmospheric. They are the formless background against which we conduct our lives. Their origin is the 'being-already-there' of our existence, and they are the felt expression of the involuntary or passive aspect of human subjectivity. They are experienced as *moods* (being in a good mood, a bad mood, lightness, heaviness, sadness, well-being, uneasiness, happiness, joy, and so on), gathered as the totality of our sentiments in 'the fundamental feeling [*le sentiment fondamental*]' (1987, p. 105 [121]).[1] It is in this fundamental feeling that the schematised feelings originate, from which they develop into distinct feelings with an intentional content, and into which they dissolve themselves again. This fundamental

---

[1] The definition of 'mood' vs 'affect' will be developed in Chapter 6.

atmosphere of the heart is the internalisation of the subject's relation to the world as a totality that constitutes our sense of being a self. This sense of being a self is, however, characterised by a troubling unrest:

> [B]y interiorizing all the connections of the self to the world, feeling gives rise to a new cleavage, of the self from the self [*de soi à soi*]. It makes perceptible the duality of reason and sensibility that found a resting place in the object. It stretches the self between two fundamental affective projects, that of the organic life that reaches its term in the instantaneous perfection of pleasure, and that of the spiritual life that aspires to totality, to the perfection of happiness. (1987, pp. 131–2 [148])

This cleavage or fracture in the self discloses the ontological status of being a human self. Our being a human self is characterised by a basic conflict inherent in the constitution of our nature. In this way, it is in the affective dimension of subjective experience that Ricoeur finds the core argument for his turn away from a phenomenological analysis of human experience to an ontological investigation into the nature of being a human self, which in turn requires a hermeneutical approach:

> We may now embrace the whole range of the dialectic of feeling and knowing. While we oppose ourselves to objects by means of the representation, feeling attests our coaptation, our elective harmonies and disharmonies with realities whose affective image [*l'effigie affective*] we carry in ourselves in the form of 'good' and 'bad.' The Scholastics had an excellent word to express this mutual coaptation of man to goods that suit him and to bads that do not. They spoke of a bond of connaturality [*un lien de connaturalité*] between my being and other beings. This bond of connaturality is silently effected in our tendential life; we feel it in a conscious and sensory way in all our affections, but we do not understand it in reflection except by contrast with the movement of objectification proper to knowing [*connaître*]. Consequently feeling can be defined only by this very contrast between the movement by means of which we 'detach' over against us and 'objectify' things and beings, and the movement by means of which we somehow 'appropriate' and interiorize them. (1987, p. 88 [104])

We are inescapably bound to the world, other people, and ourselves through our feelings. In this sense, our shared ontology, our 'connaturality', with the world and other people is what makes our existence matter to us. Feelings, however, are inarticulate and often obscure. Thus, in order to understand how or why something matters to us, to clarify the values that shape and inform our existence, we must distinguish between selfhood and otherness (that which is not me) by means of our rational capacities in order to interpret these affective values and eventually to reappropriate our selfhood through that interpretation of otherness.

Being an embodied self situated in the world is, as should be clear now, always characterised by feelings. Feelings basically function as affective regulations that aim at 'the re-equilibration of the living', and to understand their function in this process is to understand the feelings themselves. How, then, do feelings regulate the being of the self? To answer this question, we have to look more carefully at the notion of disproportion.

The disproportion of reason and sensibility is intrinsic to the basic structure of subjectivity, that is, in our experience of the world as well as in our intimate feeling of being a self. The intimate feeling of being a self is experienced as an atmosphere, a fundamental feeling, rooted in two heterogeneous aspects of the subject, the vital (sensibility) and the spiritual (reason), each of which awakes certain inclinations and desires: vital desires thrust us towards satisfaction of immediate pleasure, whereas spiritual desires aim at the existence as a totality of meaning, that is, a self desiring a meaningful existence in the world shared with other people. These two kinds of desire are in tension in the heart of the self and are experienced in the fundamental background feelings, our moods, through which we engage with the world and other people. These can be feelings of anxiety, sadness, joy, satisfaction, boredom, happiness, and so on (1987, p. 106 [122]). Our felt relation to the world, the schematised feelings, is qualified through this diffuse background tonality, which motivates our actions by clothing human values with their embodied and personal meaning.

It is the 'heart' that mediates between the two heterogeneous desires. In the heart we find the basic conflict that characterises human selfhood: the fragile relation between self as body and self as reason. This non-coincidence is felt as a conflict in the subject:

> If one does not take into consideration the primordial disproportion of vital desires and intellectual love (or of spiritual joy), one entirely misses the specific nature of human affectivity. The humanity of human beings [*l'humanité de l'homme*] is not reached by adding one more stratum to the basic substratum of tendencies (and affective states) that are assumed to be common to animals and human beings. The humanity of human beings is that discrepancy in levels, that initial polarity, that divergence of affective tension between the extremities of which is placed the 'heart'. (1987, p. 92 [108–9]; translation modified)

Our feelings regulate this conflict in the sense that they personalise experience and transform the objective structures of our experience of the world into a personal world, in which we find ourselves embedded and in which we engage with things and other people through a multitude of heterogeneous values.

The core of the self, the heart, is 'restless and fragile' because of the conflict between the two heterogeneous aspects of its being, vital desires and spiritual desires, and feelings are what reveal 'this non-coincidence of self to self' (1987, p. 141 [157]). The objective disproportion between limited perspective and unlimited meaning that we noticed earlier in the structure of subjective experience now finds its 'ontological "locus"' (1987, p. 134 [150]) in the complex or synthetic constitution of the self. It is through our feelings that we become aware of the ontological status of the human being as an intermediary being (1987, p. 108) constituted by sensibility and reason.

But even though conflict is constitutional of human subjectivity, Ricoeur, as noted earlier, has no doubt as to the relation between the two aspects of our nature. We have to understand the self from its capacity to rationally cope with the conflictual nature of its being. Our rational capacities to make meaning of confusion, sense of nonsense, and to mitigate the conflictual nature of our being, are what makes the subject a *human self*. The power of the self to affirm itself through and despite the negative features of its existence is virtually infinite. Despite the narrowness of our experiential perspective and vital desires, despite our ossified habits and sometimes wilful character, human meaning is endlessly abundant: 'Feeling alone, through its pole of infinitude, assures me that I can "*continue my existence in*" the openness of thinking and of acting' (1987, p. 137

[153]). Our effort to think and act springs from what Ricoeur calls the 'originating affirmation [*l'affirmation originaire*]' or, with Spinoza, 'the effort to exist [*l'effort pour exister*]' (1987, p. 137 [154]) that characterises our being.[2] However, 'the originating affirmation *becomes* human only by going through the existential *negation* that we called perspective, character, and vital feeling' (1987, p. 137 [153]; translation modified). This 'existential negation' is the fact that my being is contingent and, in some respects, out of my hands:

> Existence is discovered to be *only* existence, *default of being-through-self* [*défaut d'être-par-soi*] [. . .] I did not choose to exist, existence is a given situation: that is what language brings out in the rational sign of non-necessity or contingency. I am here, and it was not necessary; a contingent being who reflects on his existence in the categories of modality must think of it as non-necessary; and this non-necessity exhibits the negativity shrouded in all the feelings of precariousness, of dependence, of default of subsistence, of existential dizziness, which come of the meditation on birth and death. In this way there arises a kind of coalescence between this lived dizziness and the language of modality: I am the living non-necessity of existing [*je suis la vivante non-nécessité d'exister*]. (1987, p. 139 [155])

With Ricoeur we can thus characterise the human self as a being in conflict between an originating affirmation (a will to exist) and an 'existential negation' (perspective, character, vital desires). The human self is not a being immediately given to itself, but *becomes* who and what it is by working through the conflict constitutive of selfhood (1987, p. 141 [157]).

The self is the fragile synthesis between these two aspects of its selfhood: 'Fragility is the human duality of feeling [*La fragilité est la dualité humaine du sentiment*]' (1987,

---

[2] The term *originating affirmation* is one of the more obscure points in Ricoeur's early works. It seems to be more of a conviction about human nature than part of an actual argument. It is somewhat similar to Spinoza's concept of *conatus* in the sense that it hints at a primitive and original will to live constitutive of being a self. In all its actions, the human self is characterised by a primitive will to exist: 'This will is no longer the object of statistical inquires, of inductive generalization; rather, it is recaptured as the primitive act of consciousness' (2007a, p. 218 [66]; translation slightly modified). The affirmation is primitive in the sense that it is part of the nature of the subject, not a product of its activity. It is that which enables the subject to act in the first place, and thus it has to be considered as an intrinsic feature of subjectivity. It is a dynamic force that drives the self to engage itself with the world and other people. In other words, the interaction with otherness, the encounter with, reflection upon, and dialoguing with the world and the other people, is elicited by this basic feature of human subjectivity. Despite the often problematic, *negative*, character of the interaction with the world and other people, the originating affirmation makes us want to continue our existence with and through that which is not ourselves, i.e. otherness. As Ricoeur writes: 'Under the pressure of the negative, of negative experiences, we must re-achieve a notion of being which is *act* rather than *form*, living affirmation, the power of existing and of making exist' (2007b, p. 328 [405]). We return to the notion of originating affirmation in Chapter 7, where we will argue that the concept can be substantiated in the light of Spinoza's notion of *conatus* and recent developments in affective neuroscience. In Chapter 8, we shall use the notion to make sense of the lack of vitality involved in the particular mood that characterises schizophrenic persons.

p. 125 [142]). On the one hand, the self is rooted in the vital will-to-live, which determines its desires and actions in the direction of self-preservation. I am only a self as long as I breathe. On the other, the self is a person intertwined with other persons due to its humanity, and can only become a self by realising the desire to become a person through and in this humanity. Through our emotional attachment to other people, we understand that we *are* this humanity; that our being is an existence in the light of the idea of humanity because 'then reason is no longer an other: I am it, you are it, because we are what it is' (1987, p. 137 [153]). Our feelings reveal this complexity as a conflict between my vital desire to be what I am, the continuing existence of this particular self, and my spiritual desire to be a person among persons, that is, a self understood as more than just itself, as a part of humanity:

> [T]he demand for justice is like hunger and like thirst. This means that the faculty of desiring is broader than organic concern. I am a lacuna and a lack of something other than bread and water [. . .] In the last analysis, it is the other who counts. We must always return to this. It is thus the good of the other which I lack. The "I" [*le "moi"*] is empty with respect to the other "I" [*l'autre "moi"*]. He completes me, just as food does. The being of the subject is not solipsistic; it is being-in-common [*il est être-en-commun*]. In this way the sphere of intersubjective relations can be the *analog* of the organic sphere, and the world of needs [*le monde des besoins*] can provide the fundamental *metaphor* of appetite: the other "I", like the "not-I" ["*non-moi*"]—as for example nourishment—comes to fill up my lack [. . .] The community is my good because it leads towards making me whole within the "we" [*dans le "nous"*] where the lacuna of my being would be filled. In some moments of precious communion I sense tentatively that the isolated self is perhaps only a segment torn from such others who could have become a you for me [*devenir pour moi un toi*]. (1966, pp. 127–8 [122]; translation slightly modified)

The self cannot successfully disregard either of these aspects. It is both this particular self *and* a part of humanity. A major part of human fragility stems from this ontological status of the self as a complex or 'mixed' being (1987, p. 140 [156]). And this peculiar nature determines the self's actions because '[h]uman freedom is a dependent independence, a receptive initiative' (2007a, p. 228 [79]).

It is important, however, not to misread the notion of existential negation. It is not a flaw in or a degeneration of the subject. It is an inescapable ontological trait of human subjectivity, perhaps better understood as an 'existential difference' (1987, p. 135 [152]) that qualifies the self as this particular self. It is the contingency and the otherness that characterise the existence of the human self. It is that by which we differ from each other, but also that which, together with the originating affirmation, 'makes possible the understanding of language, the communication of culture, and the communion of persons' (1987, p. 138 [154]).

The notion of existential negation or difference is critical for the further development of Ricoeur's hermeneutical phenomenology, because the self only finds itself through this difference. Since the being of the subject is marked by a non-coincidence endemic to selfhood, the subject must turn towards that which can restore its being in existence, namely, the existence together with other subjects in time, language, and society. We saw how the fundamental feeling of being, the atmosphere of existence, transforms into schematised feelings through the intentional relation to the world and other people, i.e. that which is not the self. These schematised feelings are characterised by their object-directedness in the sense that their meaning is produced in the encounter between the self and otherness. The self is driven towards the world and the other in order 'to fill the lacuna' in its own being. In other words, the self discovers that its being is constituted both by *what it is* and by *what it is not*.

So Ricoeur makes a change in methodology in order to approach this detour over the meaning of the encounter with otherness. He turns away from the structural analyses of Husserlian phenomenology and Kantian transcendental philosophy to a hermeneutical investigation of the reappropriation of the self as a person through the dialectic of selfhood and otherness. This journey from selfhood to personhood is the theme of the rest of this chapter and the following.

Interpretative Recovery of Selfhood

The uncovering of the affective fragility at the heart of selfhood leads to the acknowledgement that the self has no immediate *knowledge* of itself, despite the fact that subjective experience is characterised by an intrinsic *awareness* of self. This has a strange, almost paradoxical, ring to it. If the self were supposed to know anything at all, this something should be itself, or at least its capacity to affirm itself through thinking. This was the assertion of *self-transparency* constitutive of the Cartesian Cogito that subsequently became the metaphysical anvil on which the modern self was coined and developed. But something happened with 'the school of suspicion' in the decades leading up to and around the turn of the twentieth century (1977, pp. 32–3 [40–1]). The ideas of Marx, Nietzsche, and Freud changed self-knowledge from an assertion to a question. Immediate consciousness could no longer be conceived of as the unvarnished bedrock of truth. Consciousness must be teased out from the encroaching human texture of treacherous ideologies, lies, and repressive desires. Consciousness, in other words, became a 'task' (1977, p. 44 [51]). We are no longer persuaded by the idea of an invincible first truth about the self as an adamant intellectual intuition, a piece of psychological evidence or a mythical vision. Such impervious certainties are doomed to remain abstract and empty, or even worse, they may be used to lead us astray and into illusions about ourselves. The methodological lesson to be drawn from 'the school of suspicion' is that the self may posit itself as a Cogito, but that Cogito is deeply problematic:

> [I]t is a wounded Cogito [*Cogito blessé*] that results from this adventure—a Cogito that posits itself but does not possess itself; a Cogito that sees its original truth only in and through the avowal of the inadequacy, illusion, and lying of actual consciousness. (1977, p. 439 [425])

Immediate self-knowledge can no longer be used as a firm philosophical fundament. The self has to be included as part of the philosophical question and not as its presupposition. To accomplish the 'task' of coming to know itself, the self must refrain from the pretension of immediacy and understand itself as 'the watchful "I" [*le "moi" vigile*], attentive to its own presence, anxious about the self and attached to the self' (1977, p. 54 [62]; translation slightly modified).

We saw how the pretension of immediacy was already weakened in the previous section, where the self was shown to be a fragile mediation between the two heterogeneous aspects of subjectivity, namely, sensibility and reason. The self first becomes an integral self in the mediation of these two aspects of its nature. Also, the self must find itself through its bodily existence, that is, it has to understand itself as being situated in a world of persons, things, and events that affect it through the body. It is through my body that I enter the world as a space of meaning: 'A meaning that exists is a meaning caught up within a body, a meaningful behavior' (1977, p. 382 [372]). The self is thus a restless self lost in the world that it has to make sense of in order to reappropriate itself. This process of becoming who and what we are is not a result of a pure choice, though, but an interaction in and through time with the things and persons in the world. They affect my actions, just as my actions affect them. The answer to the question 'Who am I?' is to be sought in an interpretation of the self's interaction with the world. It is not only the self who gives meaning to the world; on the contrary, it already finds itself situated in a world impregnate with meaning: it is 'this inversion of thought which now addresses itself to me and makes me a subject that is spoken to' (1977, p. 31 [39]). Time, events, and other persons reveal my existence as an embodied self, embedded in a world already saturated with meaning, which challenges my understanding of myself. My existence as the self that I am is not immediate or transparent, but 'remains an interpreted existence' (2004, p. 23 [27]).

The rejection of immediacy entails that the subject has to approach itself by an interpretive detour over the things and persons that constitute its being in existence, and since these mainly reveal themselves through language, a reflective recovery of selfhood is necessarily hermeneutical in nature.

We have seen that the self, in its inmost core, is characterised by an originating affirmation, a basic desire-to-live, and that this affirmation is conditioned by an 'existential difference' (body, world, and other people). The 'existential difference' is what makes the self a human self. I am a self situated in a world whose meaning is derived not only from me, but also from the world and other persons. I find myself embedded in a world of heterogeneous values that matter to me and I can therefore only come to know myself through an interpretation of those values. How and why do the world and other people matter to me? What do I care about and how am I supposed to make sense of and cope with my concerns? I have to understand myself by making sense of the values that are revealed by my feelings and emotions. The question of meaning is therefore inescapably connected to the affective origin of values. Now, we saw that the values that inform and orient my existence are not produced by me alone, but that they are a result of emotional engagement with the world. My body, the world, and other people affect me, elicit an array of heterogeneous feelings which make things and people matter to me, make me value them. My values and concerns are equivocal, though, and often conflictual. I am often confused and insecure about what my values mean to me, what I care about or how to understand my concerns. Language thus becomes the medium through which the meaning of my values is articulated and that which allows me to reflect upon the values that shape my existence. I interpret my existence through the meaning generated in the coexistence with other people in the world. The meaning of my existence is not immediately given, but has to be recovered in an interpretation of my being-in-the-world:

> [B]y passing through a hermeneutics, reflective philosophy emerges from abstraction; the affirmation of being, the desire and effort of existing which constitute me, find in the interpretation of signs the long road of awareness [...] The appropriation of my desire to exist is impossible by the short way of consciousness; only the long path of interpretation [*la voie longue de l'interprétation*] of signs is open. Such is my working hypothesis in philosophy. I call it *concrete reflection*, that is, *the cogito mediated by the entire universe of signs*. (2004, pp. 257–8 [260])

The aim of hermeneutics is therefore to situate the self in the world and approach the conflictual nature of selfhood by means of interpretation. Because of the fractured character of the Cogito, that is, the non-coincidence of the self, identity is possible only through an interpretation of the self's normative interaction with the world and the other persons. The self must reaffirm itself in an interpretation of its coexistence with otherness; or '[e]ven better, it could be said that what is one's own and what is foreign are polarly constituted in the *same interpretation*' (1991, p. 51 [80]).

The job of a hermeneutical phenomenology is, then, to articulate and reappropriate the fragile sense of self. Ricoeur proposes a hermeneutical method that combines two seemingly antithetical approaches, the Hegelian and the Freudian, establishing a dialectic between archaeology and teleology in order to deal with two fundamental dispossessions of consciousness (1977, p. 460 [444–5]). Freud and Hegel represent two complementary models of approaching the non-coincidence of the self. Both these thinkers conceive of subjectivity as different from the immediate self-assertion of the conscious subject. Whereas Freud undertakes an archaeology of the unconscious to understand the behaviour of the conscious self, Hegel embarks on the struggle for recognition, that is, the inscription of one consciousness into the consciousness of another with the aim of becoming a human person (1977, p. 474 [458]). This combination of Freudian archaeology and Hegelian teleology allows Ricoeur to develop a dialectic through which the self may be able to reappropriate itself as a self. The two basic aspects of the reappropriation of selfhood are therefore, on the one hand, the unconscious, libidinal action of the self rooted in its vital nature and limited by its bodily perspective, its character, and habits; on the other, the conscious action that aims at coexistence with other persons in a human world:

> In order to have an *arché* a subject must have a *telos*. If I understood this articulation between archaeology and teleology, I would understand a number of things. First of all I would understand that my idea of reflection is itself abstract as long as this new dialectic has not been integrated into it. The subject, we said above, is never the subject one supposes. But if the subject is to attain its true being, it is not enough to discover the inadequacy of its own self-consciousness [*l'inadéquation de la conscience qu'il prend de lui-même*], or even to discover the power of desire that posits it in existence. The subject must also discover that the process of 'becoming conscious,' through which it *appropriates* the meaning of its existence as desire and effort, does not belong to it, but belongs to the *meaning* that is formed in it. The subject must mediate self-consciousness through the mind [*médiatiser la conscience de soi par l'esprit*], that is, through the figures that give a telos to this 'becoming conscious.' (1977, p. 459 [444]; translation slightly modified)

This interpretative reappropriation of selfhood means that human values are not only bound to immediacy, the present, but extend back into the past and forward into the future. Furthermore, values cannot be reduced to the unconscious, libidinal workings of one individual self (archaeology), but must include the conscious inscription of the actions of oneself into the actions of another (teleology).

To assist the 'wounded' and dispossessed Cogito's endeavour to reappropriate an integral sense of selfhood, Ricoeur introduces another idea in his analysis, namely, that of narrative identity. Explaining the hermeneutical turn, Ricoeur claims that:

> The man who speaks in symbols is first of all a narrator [*un récitant*]; he transmits an abundance of meaning over which he has little command and thus makes him think [*donne à penser*]. This thickness of manifold meaning is what solicits his understanding; interpretation consists less in suppressing ambiguity than in understanding it and in explicating its richness. (1977, p. 49 [56]; translation modified)

Here we will merely introduce this idea of the narrating self by briefly explicating the relation between narratives and temporality, which should prepare us for the more extensive development of narrative identity in relation to the other person in the following chapter.

Narratives of Time

Narratives are first introduced by Ricoeur as a way to articulate the problematic character of human temporality, more specifically in the 'mediations between the discordant concordance of phenomenological time and the simple succession of physical time' (1988, p. 22 [42]). Human existence is marked by time, and therefore to fully understand human selfhood we must clarify how the self is characterised by time.[3] Ricoeur challenges what he calls the aporetics of temporality. Human temporality cannot be reduced to personal, phenomenological time nor to impersonal, cosmic time. Once again he confronts himself with (among others) Kant and Husserl. Whereas Kant emphasises the anonymous or objective time of nature as the transcendental condition for conscious experience, Husserl investigates the phenomenological time of intentionality, i.e. subjective time experience. Ricoeur, however, thinks that neither Kant nor Husserl is able to fully explain the temporal character of human experience because their respective analysis focuses on only one aspect of temporality. On the contrary, the particular nature of human time depends on both the subjective and objective conception of time and finds its explanation in what Ricoeur calls 'third-time [*tiers temps*]' (1988, p. 245 [441]). This third-time is time configured both by the way time affects the self involuntarily (cosmic time) and by how the self voluntarily understands and shapes time (phenomenological time), and these two aspects come together in the practical category of narrative identity. The two aspects

---

[3] 'In this regard my basic hypothesis is the following: The common character of human experience, which is marked, articulated, and clarified by the act of storytelling in all its forms, is its temporal character' (1989, p. 63; our translation).

of narrative identity are interlaced in a dialectical relation between historical and fictional narratives:

> From these intimate exchanges between the historicization of the fictional narrative and the fictionalization of the historical narrative is born what we call human time [le temps humain], which is nothing other than narrated time. (1988, p. 102 [185])

History is bound to what has really happened, a concrete event that occurred in a specific physical place and time. History is something that cannot be undone, reversed or reflected away. And yet history, since it is based on an interpretation of archives, documents, and traces, always contains an imaginary element, a 'fiction-effect [effet de fiction]' (1988, p. 186 [337]) or 'quasi-fictive' element (1988, p. 190 [346]). This fictive element in our historical narratives aligns history with the task of memory in order not to forget past actions and sufferings (1988, p. 189 [342]). We unfold this narrative by engaging in imaginative mediations between cosmological time (exemplified by the calendar and the sundial) and phenomenological time: 'History, I said, inscribes the time of narrative time within the time of the universe' (1988, p. 181 [331]). We tell history to understand human time, and, not less important, we must understand time in order to understand the nature of humanity: 'To think of history as one is to posit the equivalence between three ideas: one time, one humanity, and one history' (1988, p. 258 [461]).

Fiction, on the contrary, is the re-enactment of what might have been, of 'the probability of the universal' (1988, p. 191 [345]). When we engage in fictive narratives, we explore 'certain possibilities that were not actualized in the historical past', and therefore fiction is 'able, after the fact, to perform its liberating function' (1988, p. 191 [347]). Fictional narratives engage in a creative imitation, a mimesis, that liberates the logical structure or meaning of the possible events in a human life. In other words, 'I offer myself to the possible mode of being-in-the-world which the text opens up and discloses to me' (1981a, p. 177 [107]). Fiction possesses a 'heuristic force' to re-describe reality as we know it (1991, p. 175 [248]).

History and fiction are intertwined in a circular relationship in the act of narration, which reconfigures the experience of time in such a way that we come to terms with the aporetics of temporality. By narrating time, lived time (phenomenological time) is reinscribed in the time of nature (cosmic time) so that a bridge is built over the polarity of the two conceptions of time. Human time is neither lived time nor the time of nature, but a complex of the two. We are bound to the time of nature through our body, which is inescapably rooted in the physical workings of the world, and yet lived time is not restricted to the physical aspect of time. Our past is not only measured by the anonymous quantity of days gone by or by the traces of time visible on our faces, it also reveals itself as the intrinsic time of consciousness that we experience in memory. We are not situated in time as helpless spectators; on the contrary, we are involved with time as agents in the constitution of time. Human time springs from the ambivalence of acting and suffering. On the one hand, we are affected by time through the evolving of anonymous cosmic time, the succession of generations, cultural tradition, and the involuntary events of a life story. On the other hand, we ourselves constitute time, because we seek to understand and put into order the experience of temporality. Time becomes intelligible through our attempt to speak about our experience of temporality. We understand our relation to time and how we, as human beings, are situated in time, by speaking about time in terms of narratives and metaphors.[4] Thus the third-time, human time, is time as it is narrated with reference to the identity of the self who suffers time and is able to speak about time. In *The Dry Salvages*, the third poem of his eminent *Four Quartets*, T.S. Eliot captures the disturbing obscurity of time against which we try to make sense of our own temporality:

> And under the oppression of the silent fog
> The tolling bell
> Measures time not our time, rung by the unhurried
> Ground swell, a time
> Older than the time of the chronometers, older
> Than time counted by anxious worried women
> Lying awake, calculating the future,
> Trying to unweave, unwind, unravel
> And piece together the past and the future,
> Between midnight and dawn, when the past is all deception,
> The future futureless, before the morning watch
> When time stops and time is never ending;
> And the ground swell, that is and was from the beginning,
> Clangs
> The Bell.
>
> (Eliot 1944, p. 26)

Temporality is critical to the question about personal identity, or more precisely, we cannot ask about the identity of the self without dealing with the temporal dimension of human existence (1992, pp. 113–14 [137–8]). Nowhere does the non-coincidence of the human self become so critical as in the temporal character of a human life. A person changes over time, gains new character traits, transforms and loses old ones, and yet she remains the same person. Still, it is problematic simply to assert that the person remains the same person over time. Personhood, as we shall describe it more carefully in the next chapter, is not something static or certain, but a permanent task approached in terms of an intrinsic process of appropriation and affirmation (or restoration) of the self.[5]

Narrative identity enables us to cope with the problematic temporal character of human identity, because it integrates the apparent polarity in the identity of the self, that is, persistence and diversity over time. How can I affirm my self-constancy, or deny it for that matter, if I do not make my 'life itself a cloth woven of stories told' (1988,

---

[4] 'Humanity becomes its own subject in talking about itself' (1988, p. 212 [383]).

[5] In Chapter 9, we shall see the importance of this intrinsic process of appropriation in the borderline type of existence, where it disintegrates into the mere presence of disarticulated 'nows'. We shall also see how this disintegration is intimately related to the borderline person's emotional life.

p. 246 [443])? I relate myself to the identity of my existence in time by examining my life as a complex of stories told about my life. Thus, Ricoeur establishes a connection between self-constancy and narrative identity that, as he claims, confirms one of his most persistent ideas:

> The self of self-knowledge [*connaissance de soi*] is the fruit of an examined life [*le fruit d'une vie examinée*], to recall Socrates' phrase in the *Apology* [. . .] And an examined life is, in large part, one purged, one clarified by the cathartic effect of the narratives, be they historical or fictional, conveyed by our culture. So selfhood [*l'ipséité*] refers to a self instructed by the works of a culture that it has applied to itself. (1988, p. 247 [443–4]; translation modified)

The identity of the self cannot be reduced to what happens to the self over time, to the way time works on the self (the cosmological time), but must necessarily include how the self *reflects and acts upon* its being affected by time (lived time). The problem of persistence and diversity, of whether the self remains identical to itself through the diversity of different temporal states or simply disintegrates into a mere flow of different 'nows', is mitigated when we approach the identity of self as 'refigured by the reflective application of narrative configurations' (1988, p. 246 [443]; translation slightly modified).

Narrative identity is a practical category, which means that it deals with the aporetics of time and identity in relation to the concrete existence of the self, that is, with how the self acts and suffers in the actual coexistence with other persons in a human world. Ricoeur acknowledges that narrative identity has its limits with regard to the explanation of both time and identity. Also, he would in no way subscribe to the radical constructivist idea that the identity of a person is nothing but the stories he tells about himself or the actions that he performs. In fact, he explicitly points to the limits of narrativity in relation to the unrepresentability or inscrutability of time, and further emphasises that '[n]arrative identity thus becomes the name of a problem at least as much as it is that of a solution [. . .] and has to link up with the nonnarrative components in the formation of an acting subject' (1988, p. 249 [446–8]). Hence, narrative identity has to be understood in relation to the other aspects of Ricoeur's theory of subjectivity. First, it is part of his hermeneutical turn in the sense that narrative identity places the notion of subjectivity in a concrete, historical context since, it is argued, we cannot understand human subjectivity in isolation from its existence in time, and human time can be reduced neither to anonymous cosmic time nor to lived phenomenological time. Second, it is a way to deal with the problem of identity as it is felt and lived by the self, namely, the problem of the self's persistence and change over time. Third, it is a theoretical instrument coined in order to develop the basic conflict between self (the vital desires of the body) and self (the spiritual desires of reason) on the level of concrete subjectivity. Fourth, it helps to set the whole problem of human identity as an encounter between self, world, and other people, or to put it differently, as the never completed task of integrating selfhood and otherness.

We cannot understand the human self without taking into account the historicity of the world in which the self is situated and embedded. On the one hand, this historicity 'is itself the record of human action' (1991, p. 154 [218]) as we experience it through traces such as archives, documents, generations, and traditions. We create a past by narrating the times past, which, however, does not mean that we are free to create an arbitrary past based on our likes or dislikes, since '[w]e belong to history before telling stories or writing history' (1981b, p. 294 [200]). On the other hand, the historicity of our being-in-the-world is not restricted to an understanding of the past, but is expanded and thickened by fictional narratives that do not limit themselves to re-describing what has been. On the contrary, they liberate our imaginative capacities in that they imitate the actual possibilities hidden in the ontological structure of human action and thereby point towards the future: 'what mimesis imitates is not the effectivity of events but their logical structure, their meaning [. . .] Mimesis, in this sense, is a kind of metaphor of reality' (1981b, p. 292 [197]).

Emotions have a strong influence on the way these narratives about ourselves are constructed. In human existence, the meaning of an experience is set within a temporal dynamic that is highly *non-linear*: indeed, past experiences have influence on the future, but expectations also affect the meaning of past experiences. An example of the way emotions shape narrated time is the phenomenon of hope. Hope, as a future-orientated emotion, is integral to the sense of possibility, and as such a prerequisite for attributing new meanings to one's own past and for overcoming one's past. Hope is a primarily future-orientated expectation of attaining personally valued goals that will give or restore meaning to one's own experiences. The orientation towards the future, essential to the phenomenon of hope, bestows new meaning(s) on the past. The very marrow of the phenomenon of hope is that it restores the unification between past, present, and future that is jeopardised by other emotions, for instance, by despair which is a common feature in mental pathology in general. Hope restores the flux of lived time and of becoming, and therefore re-activates the dialectic of narrative identity.

Interpreted in this way, we see how the idea of narrative identity is a way to articulate and systematise the insights developed in the hermeneutical analysis of subjectivity, which, on their part, draw heavily on the structures uncovered by the reflective-phenomenological analysis of feelings at the beginning of this chapter. The hermeneutical approach to subjectivity elaborates and thickens the notion of a self. It unfolds the symbolic transfiguration and historicity of values and insists on the inescapable presence of the other subjects. In the following chapter, we shall explain how Ricoeur makes use of this hermeneutics to examine the nature of human personhood and to develop an ontology of care.

Chapter 3

Body and Personhood

One of the most persistent ideas in Ricoeur's theory of subjectivity is the body as the primary existential link between self and world. Without the lived body the self could not inscribe itself in the world nor be affected by the world, and world and self would remain two separate entities. Despite this pivotal function, though, the body is more a problem than a simple fact:

> The same doubled allegiance of the lived body founds the mixed structure of 'I – such a one' ['*je-un tel*']; as one body among others, it constitutes a fragment of the experience of the world; as mine, it shares the status of the 'I' understood as the limiting reference point of the world. In other words, the body is at once a fact belonging to the world and the organ of a subject that does not belong to the objects of which it speaks'. (1992, pp. 54–5 [71–2]; translation modified)

Ricoeur uses the analysis of the body from the phenomenological tradition (Heidegger in particular) and confronts the problem that one's own body is at once 'the flesh's intimacy to the self [*l'intimité à soi de la chair*] and its opening onto the world [*son ouverture sur le monde*]' (1992, p. 326 [377]). In other words, it is in the subjective experience of our own body that we find the origin of all experience of otherness: we are exposed to that which is not ourselves through our body. It is through our bodily experience that we first become aware of the passivity inherent in being human. Otherness is that which transcends, conditions, forces, obstructs, or even eliminates our capacity to act, to set our mark on the events of the world, and thereby it reveals a suffering passivity in the existence of the self. The notions of non-immediacy and passivity are disclosed by the otherness involved in the embodied nature of subjectivity; that is, they find their first (personal) expression in the ambivalent experience of one's own body.

In this chapter, we look at Ricoeur's development of an ontology of care. He once again confronts the problem of otherness in subjectivity, the conflict between the self as reason and the self as body, but this time at a *practical* or *therapeutic* level. This move from structural and diagnostic analysis to practical account is characterised by the development of his analysis of subjectivity into a therapeutically oriented hermeneutics of human personhood. We start with his account of bodily ambivalence, the body conceived of as personal as well as physical, and go on to explain his distinction between event and action. This distinction is then used to further develop the notion of narrative identity. Here the concept of responsibility becomes important and is employed in the approach to the complex notion of personal identity and the development of an account of human personhood. We then examine how human practices constitute and shape the nature of human experience of the world. This examination, in turn, enables us to explain how the notion of 'the good life' reveals the other person as fundamental to our understanding of subjective values and personal self-esteem. Finally, we sum up the implications of our reformulation of Ricoeur's theory of subjectivity in an ontology of care that will serve as the theoretical background for the development of our account of emotions and personhood in the following chapters.

Bodily Ambivalence

The human body is an enigma. Of course, all living bodies are enigmatic, but the human body more so than any other body found throughout nature. Echoing Thomas Nagel's famous essay about what it is like to be a bat (1974), the neuroscientist Todd M. Preuss invites us to consider *What It is Like to Be a Human*, and in particular, how strange the human body actually is from an evolutionary point of view:

> Our physical form and life history provide ample testimony to the strangeness of humans. Humans have a kind of locomotion—striding bipedalism—that is unique among known animals, and our pelvis and lower limb has been radically remodeled in relation to this, to the point that we have lost one of the hallmarks of the primate order, a grasping big toe [...] Alone among anthropoid primates, which subsist mainly on fruit and leaves, humans have included in their diets a substantial component of meat. Human females can survive for decades after menopause; in other primate species, the cessation of ovulary cycling essentially coincides with senescence and death. Humans, too, have the capacity to live much longer than other primates: under the best circumstances, few chimpanzees or gorillas make it to age 50, whereas in hunter-gatherer societies, a woman has a decent chance to live to age 65. In addition, the human disease profile differs in important respects from that of other primates. Even ignoring our intellectual abilities and cultural accretions, people are most peculiar beasts.

> (Preuss 2004, p. 5)

Ricoeur's development of a phenomenological investigation of subjectivity into an ontology of selfhood obliges him to deal with this strangeness of the human body. The enigma of the body is a crucial aspect of the question of naturalism. How are we to accommodate the strangeness of the human body with the rest of nature? How do we explain the peculiar nature of what seems to be the ambivalence of the human body, that is, both part of and different from the rest of nature? Consciousness is of course the root of this problematic difference. We experience our body as well as being our body. We are a body and we have a body. We move our body and we are moved by our body. The human body is both a subject and an object, that is, the centre of a fragile entwinement of activity and passivity. Whereas much contemporary debate about naturalism approaches the problem of the body from the third-person, empirical perspective of how the functioning of the brain can give rise to consciousness, or how to place consciousness in the physical world, Ricoeur remains true to his phenomenological origin and approaches this aspect of naturalism from the perspective of embodied subjectivity: what does the biophysical nature of our body mean for our experience of being a self?

An ontology of selfhood is rooted in the ambivalence of the body: 'How am I to understand that my flesh [*ma chair*] is also a body [*un corps*]?' (1992, p. 326 [377]). My body is mine, i.e. the affective bedrock of my most intimate experiences and the organ by means of which I am able to engage with the world. On the other hand, my body is a part of that which is not mine, i.e. the otherness experienced in being subjected to biophysical causality and the impersonal events operating in the world:

> To the extent that the body as my own body constitutes one of the components of mineness [*mienneté*], the most radical confrontation must place face-to-face two perspectives on the body—the body as mine, and the body as one body among others. (1992, p. 132 [159])

The non-coincidence that we uncovered at the core of subjectivity finds its primary experience in the ambivalence of the body. Our decisions must be carried out by means of the body to become actions and, furthermore, the world reveals itself only through our bodily senses. I cannot escape my body, neither by abstracting from it nor by ignoring it. My decisions might be made without paying attention to my bodily constitution, but in the attempt to realise such decisions my own body reveals the limits of my possibilities by transforming some of them into *actual* possibilities and others into impossibilities. My practical knowledge of the world is shaped by the bounds of my senses and the abilities of my body. And consequently, my self-understanding must be balanced with my practical knowledge of the world. That is to say, I understand myself as an individual self with these specific capacities and situated in this particular world through the appropriation of my own body. In bodily experiences, the subject experiences an otherness that is part of itself. The self cannot dispose of this otherness, but is, by plain fact, compelled to integrate this experience in the understanding of itself.

The body that I find my self bound to, my flesh, is *my* body in the most intimate way. My body assumes an instrumental character by means of which I liberate myself from the pure passivity of not-acting. I set my mark on the events in the world by using my body. The body also escapes my initiative, though, by the fact that it situates me in a given context, disobeys me, confines me within certain limits, and determines the scope of my actions. In this sense, the world works on me, affects my being this individual self through my own body. I am bound to a certain perspective and given this particular physical constitution (e.g. these ears, this hair, this colour of skin, and this tone of voice) without my own consent; I am subject to pain, sickness, ageing, and eventually death because of my body. Or said more plainly, my body does not always behave the way I want it to behave. For instance, I reach out for a cup of coffee and end up with a pen in my hand or turn red in the face when I am nervous or embarrassed. Therefore, I live 'with the otherness of the flesh that I am [*avec l'altérité de la chair que je suis*]'. (1992, p. 326 [377])

However, the ambivalence of the body is not limited to the neat distinction between praxis and pathos, acting and suffering, but includes the dialectic of selfhood and otherness in action in the way I use my body to affirm my selfhood. The moment I transform my decision into action, i.e. inscribe my intimacy into the world, I am no longer in complete command of my decision. I cannot control how my actions inscribe themselves in the events of the world and in the understanding of the others. My body opens up to the world, but does not have power over the world. It is an integral part of the workings of the world, and as such it blends in with the world in such a way that the scope and effect of my action necessarily escapes my initial intention.

In my bodily existence, the person that I am is not something immediately given. I must gain control over my body. I learn to walk, speak, eat with knife and fork, ride a bicycle, drive a car, and so on. Moreover, I have to pay attention to how my body manifests itself in the world: I must control my voice in conversation, sit still at dinner, not laugh when inappropriate, etc. I might also eat excessively, perhaps smoke and drink too many beers, which are all ways to impair my body. And then I may feel that I have to go on a diet and begin to exercise as a means to get a better and healthier body. But more generally, I have to accept that my body is not only an object of my will, but also a part of that over which I have no control. My actions are realised through *my* body, but are already part of an otherness in the action itself (because of the otherness in my body). To become the person that I am I must accept and consent to the being of my body. My body is also what opens up to the world, my particular access to the world, and in this way it transforms the world from something totally foreign to the primary otherness of human finitude 'insofar as it is sealed by embodiment [*l'incarnation*]' (1992, p. 327 [378]). Or put differently: 'one's own body is revealed to be the mediator between the intimacy of the self and the externality of the world' (1992, p. 322 [372]). The embodied nature of human subjectivity shapes the experience of the world and the self-awareness of the self in such a way that the world in which the self is situated is transformed from something completely foreign, something without relation to the being of the self, to an otherness that is part of the self's existence in the world. The world becomes something that the self cares about:

> Only a being that is a self is *in* the world; correlatively, the world in which this being is, is not the sum of beings composing the universe of subsisting things or things already-to-hand. The being of the self presupposes the totality of a world that is the horizon of its thinking, acting, feeling—in short, of its *care* [*souci*]. (1992, p. 310 [360])

Therefore, to clarify how the world and the self together configure the human world of the self, we have to consider the passivity inherent in the bodily experience of the world and, more importantly, how this passivity influences the subjective experience of being-in-the-world.

In Chapter 1, we saw how the affective dimension of subjectivity revealed, through the ambivalent nature of human feelings, the non-coincidence in the heart of the self. Through the complexity of our feelings (vital and spiritual desires) we continuously experience, at an intimate and pre-reflective level, a conflict between the originating affirmation and the existential difference or negation (perspective, character, vital desire) constitutive of being a human self. We need to develop the implications of this basic conflict for a hermeneutical understanding of the self in a concrete human world of heterogeneous values. That is, when we are affected *through* and *by* the body, how does the body determine our practical experience?

The fact that we are affected *through* the body, i.e. that the body is our openness to the world, reveals that we are not ourselves the origin of our existence. We do not experience our coming into the world. Our existence is marked by an experience 'of already having been born and of finding oneself already there' (1992, p. 327 [378]). We find ourselves involuntarily present in and exposed to the world through our embodiment. To deal with this thoroughly passive aspect of selfhood, Ricoeur elaborates on the Heideggerian concepts of *thrownness* (*Geworfenheit*), *attunement* (*Befindlichkeit*), and mood (*Stimmung*). He explores what it means to the self to interact with a world in which it has not chosen to live. The affective dimension of this being-already-there is experienced by the subject as certain moods, that is, a feeling of being this individual self in this specific situation. Heidegger's analysis of thrownness, attunement, and mood paves the way for an ontology of the flesh, which, Ricoeur argues, Heidegger himself never developed:

> [A]n ontology of the flesh [*une ontologie de la chair*], in which the latter gives itself to be thought not only as the embodiment of 'I am' but as the practical mediation of that being-in-the-world that we are in each case. This conjunction between flesh and world is held to allow us to think of the properly passive modalities of our desires and our moods [*humeurs*] as the sign, the symptom, the indication of the contingent character of our insertion in the world. (1992, p. 327 [378]; translation slightly modified)

Moreover, in an extreme sense, the contingency of our existence in the world is a burden that the self has to endure in 'the task of having-to-be' (p. 327 [378]), since it has not itself chosen to exist. Our body, which is itself rooted in passivity, places us in the world in a certain way. Our bodily existence precedes every distinction between voluntary and involuntary because 'I will' is firmly rooted in 'I can'. I only have the possibility to choose, to affirm myself in the world, because I am *given* certain bodily capacities in the first place.[1]

---

[1] How does Ricoeur develop this ontology of the flesh that he finds so important for the notion of subjectivity? His analysis leaves the reader rather perplexed. He repeatedly returns to the ontology of the flesh and emphasises the importance of what he calls authentic spatiality as a crucial element of such an ontology. And still, he never arrives at an explicit definition of what he means by an ontology of the flesh. He only leaves the reader with sporadically suggestive hints at the notion of authentic spatiality. For example, authentic spatiality is essentially different from 'the geometric space as a system of indifferent places' in that it is 'the spatial dimension of being-in-the-world [. . .] the backdrop of the spatiality of available and manipulable things' (1992, p. 328 [379]). Or he writes that the self is in relation to the world as to a totality of concerns in the sense that everything concerns the subject (1992, p. 314 [363]). And further, that we need to coordinate the human initiative with 'the movement of the world and all the physical aspects of action' (p. 314 [363]), because only by doing so can we explain the extension of the totality of our concerns from being-alive to the praxis of living well. Still, he does not gather these observations into a structured notion, and therefore the importance of the reflections on authentic spatiality and an ontology of the flesh remains somewhat inarticulate. His shift from phenomenology to hermeneutical phenomenology might be the reason why he does not develop the ontology of the flesh that he nevertheless believes to be so important for an ontology of selfhood. Perhaps it is because of his emphasis on a more hermeneutic (i.e. concrete, historical, and practical) notion of subjectivity that the immediate bodily experience remains inarticulate. We believe, however, that an ontology of the flesh is crucial for Ricoeur's theory of subjectivity, and for our subsequent investigation, and that it can be articulated and made clearer if one puts the somewhat dense analysis of bodily experience in relation to the analysis of affective experience in the last chapter. The rest of this section is an attempt at such an articulation.

The ambivalence of the body, marked by activity and passivity, selfhood and otherness, is the basic (i.e. immediate) experience of the interaction of self and world. The world is the correlate to our actions and our sufferings. We pre-reflectively experience the world as a space saturated with heterogeneous values that express our concerns. It is a spatiality internal to and shaped by the flesh, because our senses place us in a pre-linguistic world that becomes a practicable world through our capacities to interact with the otherness of that world. The self is part of that otherness, because its body is merely a body among others, and yet it is capable of appropriating the otherness of the world in which it finds itself, and of transforming it into a familiar world by means of the capacities to affirm itself that are at work in its own body, in its flesh. The ontology of the flesh is a necessary step towards an ontology of selfhood, since it gives an account of how the being of the self is related to the being of the world. Spatiality is the central concept in an ontology that brings to the forefront the ambivalence of embodiment, i.e. the fact that the self is both part of the physical world (spatially and temporally) and, at the same time, somehow different from the workings of that world. In our immediate interaction with the external world, we feel and experience the dialectic of selfhood and otherness that is endemic to our being an embodied human self.

The phenomenological analysis of the self ends with this ontology of the flesh, since the experience of my own body points to the limit of my self-awareness, to the passivity in my-being-this-body, 'namely, not what it means that a body is my body, that is, flesh, but that the flesh is also a body among bodies. It is here that phenomenology finds its limit' (1992, pp. 325–6 [376]). This otherness transcends our conscious experience, and as such it cannot be investigated by phenomenology. The hermeneutical approach to subjectivity therefore begins where phenomenology ends, namely, with the conflict between otherness and selfhood in the heart of the subject that brings out the mediated or fractured character of subjective self-awareness.

The question of the identity of the self is rooted in ontology. Accordingly, the phenomenological description of the experiential structures of subjectivity must be combined with ontological analysis in order to clarify 'the unity of man with himself and his world' (1966, p. 467 [439]). Although the affective dimension of subjectivity is what 'truly represents man's humanity' (1987, p. 136 [152]), the conflict brought about by vital and spiritual desires can only be dealt with by bringing in the social and cultural context in which the self finds itself situated and strives to affirm itself. Thus, Ricoeur is concerned with the life of the self as a person, but he insists that the term 'life' should not be understood here 'in a strictly biological sense but in the ethicocultural sense [. . .] The word "life" designates the person as a whole in opposition to fragmented practices' (1992, p. 177 [208–9]).

In order to understand the life of the self as a human person, we need an ontology that accounts for the difference between *action* and *event*. If we adopt a strict naturalistic ontology that reduces personal actions to a subclass of impersonal events, we cannot distinguish between action and event and are therefore unable to articulate the relation between agent and action. By assigning personal action to an ontology of anonymous events, we neglect the personal aspect that is the fundamental aspect of human action, namely, the question of 'who' did the action. Thus, we should look for 'another sort of ontology, one more consonant with the search for the self, the genuine place of linkage between the action and its agent' (1992, p. 74 [93]); or to put it differently, an ontology that does not sacrifice the specific difference between human and non-human events in order to reach a seamlessly unified explanation of everything that happens in the world. To uncover human personhood, we have to respect the fact that the action of a person bringing about a change in the world differs substantially from an impersonal event such as an earthquake or a dog causing an accident: 'This different ontology would be that of a being in the making, possessing de jure the problematic of selfhood, just as the problematic of sameness belongs de jure to the ontology of events' (1992, p. 86 [107]).

The difference between personal actions and anonymous events stems from the fact that an action, in principle at least, could have been done otherwise or even prevented by the agent, whereas an event is not a matter of doing or not doing—it simply happens. Contrary to mere events, personal action is characterised by intentions: 'Describing an action as having been done intentionally is explaining it by the reason the agent had to do what she did' (1992, p. 75 [95]).

Now, a personal reason for an action cannot be explained by means of the causal model at work in a strictly naturalistic ontology of anonymous events, and the key-notion for an alternative explanation is the concept of motivation. A *motive* is what connects the action and the agent. The action is ascribed to the agent because the agent must appropriate his or her action. The agent cannot dispose of an action made, but remains the possessor of what he or she makes. The action causes a change in the world, which cannot but find its origin in the self that initiated that change. The 'how' and the 'why' find their common root in the complex question 'who?'. An action differs from an event, because its cause can never derive from an object, but always originates in a self that possesses the capacity to realise or to refrain from a possible action. The self may be an object of external forces, and yet it always remains a self because of its capacity to deliberate on what to do when it is affected by the world in which it is situated: 'Ascription consists precisely in this reappropriation by the agent of his or her own deliberation: making up one's mind is cutting short the debate by making one of the options contemplated one's own' (1992, p. 95 [117]). Hence, we are directed to the self and its motives and not to the forces of an anonymous causality, when we want to know the 'how' and 'why' of a certain action.

We saw a moment ago that the distinction between selfhood and otherness in subjectivity is not as clear-cut as the distinction between motive and cause might make it appear. The self is part of the world, so it is always difficult to discern exactly to which extent one may say that an action depends on the self. Nevertheless, in order to talk about subjectivity, we must not let the nature of action be confused with the causality of an anonymous event, because '[t]he action must be able to be said to depend on the agent in order to be blamable or praiseworthy' (1992, p. 101 [123]).

The nature of personal action is therefore to be sought in the self that initiates the action. Once again, we have to take a closer look at the self that is capable to cause an event in a world governed by laws different from those of the self. We have to identify the dimension of personal action within the anonymous events in the world by restricting our investigation to where we can talk about responsibility. This is not, of course, an easy task, but we may begin by delineating 'a new and properly practical dimension' of subjectivity (1992, p. 101 [121]). The ontology of the flesh is a presupposition for this practical dimension, because it outlines the pragmatic dimension of action. The self is able to act through its body. The self and the world come together in the body, since the 'I can' depends on the body that is simultaneously *my* body and *a* body among the other bodies in the world. Among the actual options that are made possible by its capacities, the self decides on a certain option by realising it through action. These actions may be 'blamable or praiseworthy' according to certain norms or standards (the question of norms will be dealt with later in this chapter), in short, they are characterised by their *imputability*. The agent and the action are related to one another by means of the concept of imputability. The action refers to a self that has chosen to act in one way and not in another, and thereby the self puts itself at stake in the actions that it performs. The subjectivity of action is therefore ultimately a question of the self that initiates the action: 'with imputability the notion of a capable subject reaches its highest meaning, and the form of self-designation [*la forme d'autodésignation*] it implies includes and in a way recapitulates the preceding forms of self-reference [*sui-référence*]' (2005, p. 106 [158]). Or put differently, the difference between action and event is that an action is personal whereas an event is impersonal. And this difference, in turn, reveals the difference between motive and cause. A motive *initiates* an action when chosen and realised by a self whereas a cause *continues* a larger chain of reactions that lacks a definite initiation and therefore cannot be qualified as an action but only as an event. And since the self somehow initiates the action, that is, he or she is the possessor of the action, attention must necessarily shift from the action to the agent. While we cannot place a responsibility with regard to events, actions are always subject to such a judgement because they originate in a self that could have done otherwise:

> Imputability, we shall say, is the ascription of action to its agent, *under the condition of ethical and moral predicates*, which characterize the action as good, just, conforming to duty, done out of duty, and, finally, being the wisest in the case of conflictual situations. (1992, p. 292 [338])

However, before dealing explicitly with this practical dimension of subjectivity, we will look once again at the notion of narrative identity that functions as a bridge between the descriptive and normative aspect of subjectivity by investigating the 'triad – describing, narrating, prescribing' (1992, p. 140 [167]). The notion of subjectivity is neither purely descriptive nor purely normative. It is rooted in both a factual and normative dimension. The self is a part of physical nature, and we must pay attention to the embodied, a-rational character of subjectivity (ontology of the flesh). On the other hand, the self is a member of humanity, which means that it lives a life together with other persons who demand that the self considers its own existence as a coexistence. Moreover, it is situated in a certain sociocultural context, inscribed in a tradition, and governed by specific rules and norms that are irreducible to the laws of physical nature. These two heterogeneous dimensions pertain to different ontologies, namely, one that is grounded in the causality of anonymous, a-rational events, and another that considers the normative nature of subjectivity: 'Are these two ontologies mutually exclusive? I do not think so; they are, in my opinion, simply different by reason of their starting points, which themselves cannot be compared' (1992, p. 86 [107]). Although Ricoeur focuses on a normative ontology, he is well aware of the necessary integration of a normative ontology with a causal one.²

Now, however, we shall take a closer look at the notion of narrative identity in order to clarify how narrating may bridge the apparent gap between description and prescription.

Personhood and the Narrating Self

The difference between cause and motive turns the analysis of action away from the action to the agent who performs the action. The agent is not just a cause among other causes in the anonymous chain of causal events. On the contrary, the agent is an autonomous self (and not merely a part of the world). This leaves us with two different explanations, a factual and a normative. A factual approach to human action must concentrate on *how* the action inscribes itself into the workings of the world, i.e. *how* the self causes a change in the world. The normative approach, on the other hand, turns to the agent and emphasises the *who* of the action: 'An agent is not *in* the far distant consequences as he or she is in a sense *in* his or her immediate act. The problem is then to delimit the sphere of events for which the agent can be held responsible' (1992, p. 106 [130]). We are then left with two distinct approaches to human action that are, as mentioned, seemingly incongruent. We can attempt, though, to connect them by returning to the notion of narrative identity.

This time Ricoeur uses narrative identity to bridge the factual and the normative dimensions of subjectivity, and once again he employs the temporal dimension of existence, namely, the fact that the self has its own history (1992, p. 113 [137]). So, although the fact that the self has its own history might seem intuitive and trivial, Ricoeur develops his conception of personal action from the problems concerning personal identity by investigating the historicity of human existence. How does the self remain identical to itself throughout its existence in time?

In the previous chapter, narratives were used to cope with the aporetics of human temporality. Narrated time duly takes into account how time affects the self, as well as how the self copes with time. Differently from a plant or a dog, a human self does not remain passively receptive to the workings of time. For example, we go to the hairdresser's when our hair becomes too long, stop eating cholesterol-rich food when we become older, or plan our future in the light of our past. We adapt to time, reflect, and work on time. Our being this particular person is therefore thoroughly determined by time. Time poses a challenge to our identity in the sense that it is 'a factor of dissemblance, of divergence, of difference' that we, as persons, have to deal with (1992, p. 117 [142]).

---

² We shall end this chapter with an attempt to show how Ricoeur's idea, unfortunately undeveloped in his own works, may point in the direction of an integration of a causal ontology with a normative one. In fact, a significant part of our effort throughout Parts II and III is dedicated to the exploration of how these two kinds of ontology play a significant role in the fragility of human personhood, and consequently in our peculiar vulnerability to mental illness.

Ricoeur identifies three components in personal identity: *numerical identity*, *qualitative identity*, and *uninterrupted continuity*, which on their part express the main principle of *permanence* in time. A person must fulfil all three criteria over an unspecified period of time in order to be identified as the same person and not two different ones. Numerical identity refers to the fact that a person must remain the same biophysical entity through all kinds of imaginable changes in time. A person might lose all her physical characteristics over the years or completely lose her memory of all deeds done or events that occurred to her and still be the same person in a numerical sense, because she remains the same organic structure evolving through time (which can be verified, for example, by looking at her DNA). Nevertheless, we might find it difficult to accept that her *personal* identity has remained the same if all the characteristics that defined her as a certain person at some point have changed into something completely different. So to understand personal identity, we must also pay attention to both the qualitative and the uninterruptedly continuous aspect of personal identity. We identify a person according to certain character traits. She walks in a certain way, her voice has a characteristic modulation, her temper is bad late in the afternoon. She loves fishing and is faithful to her longstanding principles about monthly charity to the less fortunate, the discipline of hard work and early rising, and the abiding necessity of capital punishment. Now, time plays an even more critical role with respect to this qualitative kind of identity. As we age we remain the same biophysical organism, but normally our dispositions and character traits change, and sometimes drastically at that. Could we say that a person is still the same person if his or her principles, ideas, and overall life-plan have changed beyond recognition? The question is, of course, complicated. For instance, we allow that a cold-blooded murderer can change, serve her sentence and become a better person who has atoned for the crimes done in the past. She is quite literally a different person. And most of the time, we judge a person on how she acts now, and not on past mischief, or beneficence for that matter. On the other hand, we are well aware that she is, in fact, not another person. She is still the murderer, but she has changed into something better. She has, hopefully, learned from her terrible deeds, transformed her principles and worked out a significantly different life-plan for herself. Faced with such difficulties, is it at all possible to speak about the permanence of personal identity through the sometimes dramatic changes over time?

Ricoeur is convinced that '[t]he idea of structure, opposed to that of event, replies to this criterion [permanence] of identity, the strongest one that can be applied' (1992, p. 117 [142]). We must concentrate on the structural permanence of the person and not on the events that seem to dissolve personhood into fragmented pieces of a self. In other words, we must find what remains invariable in the different relations in which the person is through the course of time:

> The entire problematic of personal identity [*l'identité personnelle*] will revolve around this search for a relational invariant [*un invariant relationnel*], giving it the strong signification of permanence in time [. . .] There is a form of permanence in time which can be connected to the question 'who?' ['*qui?*'] inasmuch as it is irreducible to any question of 'what?' ['*quoi?*'] There is a form of permanence in time that is a reply to the question 'Who am I?' ['*Qui suis-je?*']. (1992, p. 118 [142–3]; translation modified)

Ricoeur proposes to explain this 'relational invariant' of personhood in terms of two opposite models of permanence in time: *character* (*le caractère*) and *keeping one's word* (*le maintien de la parole donnée*). These two models of permanence form a dialectic that, articulated by means of a narrative structure, might capture and explain the subtle difficulties involved in the notion of personal identity:

> My hypothesis is that the polarity of these two models of permanence with respect to persons results from the fact that permanence of character expresses the almost complete mutual overlapping of the problematic of *idem* and of *ipse*, while faithfulness to oneself [*fidélité à soi*] in keeping one's word marks the extreme gap between the permanence of the self and that of the same and so attests fully to the irreducibility of the two problematics one to the other. I hasten to complete my hypothesis: the polarity I am going to examine suggests an intervention of narrative identity in the conceptual constitution of personal identity in the manner of a specific mediator between the pole of character, where *idem* and *ipse* tend to coincide, and the pole of self-maintenance, where selfhood [*ipséité*] frees itself from sameness [*mêmeté*]. (1992, pp. 118–19 [143])

To be able to follow his proposal, though, we first have to briefly clarify the terms that he is introducing. The notion of *character* stands in close relation to a person's immutable perspective and opening to the world (what he earlier called the 'existential difference or negation') that the person is not able to change (our birth place, physical constitution, and, to a certain degree, our habits). Ricoeur concentrates on the temporal dimension of character, which brings into question the immutable status of character. Some aspects of our character lose their feature of immutability when considered in relation to time, because our habits and dispositions often change through the span of our life. So, character, he argues, 'designates the set of lasting dispositions by which a person is recognized' (1992, p. 121 [146]). The notion of character functions as a criterion by which we are able to identify a person in terms of the general things or traits that we can describe, without asking about the self behind the different descriptions. We can therefore say that '[c]haracter is truly the "what" of the "who" [*le "quoi" du "qui"*]' (1992, p. 122 [147]).[3]

Contrary to character, the notion of *keeping one's word* 'expresses a *self-constancy* [*un maintien de soi*] which cannot be inscribed, as character was, within the dimension of something in general but solely within the dimension of "who?"' (1992, p. 123 [148]). This kind of permanence in time captures the self that we cannot identify by means of mere character traits, that is, the self that is more than the sum of its descriptively recognisable traits. To keep one's word is to defy the changes of our body, our character, our habits that time brings about. Ricoeur exemplifies this dynamics with the nature of a promise. Say that I have promised a friend to visit him in Berlin within a few months. However, work piles up, money runs low, and my desire to visit him seems to subside in view of other and more interesting agendas. Nonetheless, I have given him my word that I will be coming, and not to do so would therefore be inconsistent with what

---

[3] We shall see in the following chapters, and especially in Chapter 6, that emotions (in the form of temperament) play a key role as rather permanent features of character, that is, as dispositions to act and react in a given way.

friendship stands for, namely, trust, endurance, and sincerity. It is obvious that this kind of permanence in time is an aspect of identity that cannot be accounted for in neutral, descriptive terms but always involves a normative stance, or an obligation:

> [T]o respond to the trust [*confiance*] that the other places in my faithfulness. This ethical justification, considered as such, develops its own temporal implications, namely a modality of permanence in time capable of standing as the polar opposite to the permanence of character. (1992, p. 124 [149])

Ricoeur thus identifies two distinct poles of personal identity: a descriptive form which he names identity of the same (*idem*) and a normative form which is named identity of the self (*ipse*). The first expresses the passive aspect of personhood that remains the same. It fulfils the three criteria for identity through time (numeric, qualitative, and uninterrupted continuity) without any significant activity on behalf of the person itself. The second, however, demands that the person is constantly aware of how to remain faithful to his or her promises and engagements in the light of certain values, norms, and social standards. On the one side (*idem*, identity of the same or character), we have what is seemingly the most stable aspect of personhood, which involves the physical characteristics and longstanding dispositions shaped by genetics, upbringing, education, and convictions, which we can call character or personality. On the other (*ipse*, identity of the self or keeping one's word), we find the more dynamic and impalpable normative aspect, which has to do with how a person acts according to the norms and procedures that govern the social interface between him and other persons.

We should now begin to see how narrative identity may be of help in approaching the difficulties concerning personal identity.

Although character is the most stable form of identity, i.e. that by which we are re-identified and thereby recognised, many of our character traits are still a result of ongoing conscious choices made during our life. Choices become habits and long-term dispositions, which turn into something that we no longer choose; or, said more eloquently, habits are 'the return from freedom to nature' (1992, p. 121 [146]). The formation of habits and seemingly unconscious or automatic dispositions to act is our most obvious and docile tool to cope with otherness, since they internalise otherness (the body, the world, and the other) and make it a part of our person. Our dispositions to act are shaped by how we are brought up and by our social, geographical, and cultural context. If I have grown up in a violent environment, my first reaction to fear and provocation is more likely to be an act of violence than if I have always been taught to avoid the use of violence at any cost. Thus, a major part of our personhood is influenced and conditioned by how our habits and dispositions are developed. A person, however, is more than the sum of his or her habits and dispositions. *A person is a self that can relate itself to his or her character*, and can choose to follow inclinations and dispositions or choose not to. In this sense, the identity of a person depends on the dialectic of self and character:

> The dialectic of innovation and sedimentation, underlying the process of identification, are there to remind us that character has a history which is contracted, one might say, in the twofold sense of the word 'contraction': abbreviation and affection. (1992, p. 122 [147–8]; translation modified)

Narrative identity can contribute to the unfolding of this dialectic. Its task is:

> [T]o balance, on one side, the immutable traits which this identity owes to the anchoring of the history of a life in a character [*l'ancrage de l'histoire d'une vie dans un caractère*] and, on the other, those traits which tend to separate the identity of the self from the sameness of character. (1992, p. 123 [148])

The key-notion here is 'the history of a life'. Narratives help unfold the dynamics of our identity in that they are able to articulate the reasons for our character and dispositions. The narrative defies, so to speak, the immutability of the character, because it makes the otherwise inalterable part of our personhood (the same or *idem*) a dynamic part of our personal history. Through narratives, we may become aware of how we came to have such a nervous character or such violent dispositions, instead of just accepting that, in the end, this is just how we are. The dialectic of selfhood and sameness has a history that is unfolded through otherness—that is, through my body, the world, and in particular other people. We are who we are because the history of actions and sufferings—our own and those of other people—is sedimented into the obscure texture of our identity. Or, as T.S. Eliot writes, still in *The Dry Salvages*:

> Now, we come to discover that the moments of agony
> (Whether, or not, due to misunderstanding,
> Having hoped for the wrong things or dreaded the wrong
>   things
> Is not in question) are likewise permanent
> With such permanence as time has. We appreciate this
>   better
> In the agony of others, nearly experienced,
> Involving ourselves, than in our own.
> For our own past is covered by the currents of action,
> But the torments of others remains an experience
> Unqualified, unworn by subsequent attrition.
> People change, and smile: but the agony abides.
> Time the destroyer is time the preserver
>
> (Eliot 1944, p. 29)

To approach our identity as a narrative structure enables us to distinguish between what we have done ourselves and what is not of our doing but has been produced by other factors such as genetic predisposition, upbringing, friends, birthplace, partner(s), and education. We are always the same person, but our personhood is characterised by a tension between what we do and what we are. I might be a considerate and loving person, but in order to remain so I must continue to act according to that which makes me that kind of person. Or I might be a cruel and violent person, but that does not mean that I am destined to remain such a person. Narratives articulate this dynamics because '[w]hat sedimentation has contracted, the narrative [*le récit*] can redeploy' (1992, p. 122 [148]; translation modified).[4]

---

[4] This is, of course, one of the principal factors that make psychotherapy work.

The self is marked by a fundamental non-coincidence, often a troubling conflict, in the core of its being between vital and spiritual desires. The former tend towards pleasure according to the immediate well-being of the self, whereas the latter seek a more total form of happiness that must include the presence of and coexistence with other people. As we saw in the previous section, responsibility is what renders human action distinct from the realm of mere anonymous events. And yet, as with most human qualities, responsibility is a problem, not a fact. The issue is how to narrow down where responsibility begins. We have seen that narratives may help identify the 'who' in the 'what', that is, they may show to what extent we can be said to be responsible for what we have done and for what we are. For example, how am I to be blamed for my violence, if that is all that I have ever experienced? Can I be praised for my hard work, when I love what I do? Could we blame somebody for his indecision and insecurity, when he has never learned to trust himself? Or am I responsible for my weak will? Of course, narrative identity cannot simply solve these arduous difficulties involved in personal responsibility, but it can bring out nuances and perspectives that are otherwise easily overlooked.

Personal identity is not just a question of what we are or how we remain the same, but also how we relate ourselves to the person that we are. Understanding personal identity becomes a very difficult task when we want to account for identity in other terms than numerical identity. Qualitative identity, or the 'relational invariant', seems to be impossible to grasp, since the person keeps changing throughout the entire duration of his or her life. Ricoeur, however, chooses to confront this problem in terms of responsibility. And according to his reflections on motive and cause, responsibility is originally a question of imputability: 'It is for the other who is in my charge that I am responsible. This expansion makes what is vulnerable or fragile, as an entity assigned to the agent's care, the ultimate object of his responsibility' (2005, pp. 108–9 [162]). My identity as a person is ultimately a question of my actions in regard to the other person. This is where the fragility of my personhood becomes most clearly manifest. If my identity only depended on me, then I could change my opinions, motives, and principles to my heart's desire without ending up in difficulties. I would not have to account for my actions to anyone. Now, we all know by experience that this is not the case. I always act as a person in the eyes of the other. I would be unrecognisable as a person, if I supported capital punishment one day and the next day marched for the abolition of this legal action, or said on Monday that I love cats and hate dogs, and then on Wednesday vigorously claimed that I hate cats but love dogs. In order to maintain personal integrity, I have to remain identical at least in some matters. In other words, I am responsible for what I do and say. Now, problems arise when we have to determine how much and in what matters a person can change and still remain the same 'relational invariant', the same person. This is where narratives come in. There seems to be a gap between describing a person and prescribing what a person must do to remain a person, that is, between the ascription of an action to an agent and the imputation to the agent of an obligation to act in a certain way in order to remain the same person. The key concept that is supposed to bridge this gap is '**narrative configuration**' (1992, p. 142 [169]).

If we consider the structure of action in terms of narratives, we shall be able to extend 'the field of practice' so that the agent's various actions become configured according to a hierarchy of practical units. The practical field is extended and qualified, because narratives view actions from a top-down perspective that differentiates human events from mere physical events and furthermore consider actions over the course of time: 'Telling a story is saying who did what, why and how, by spreading out in time the connection between these various viewpoints' (1992, p. 146 [174]; translation modified). Contrary to a causal explanation of action, narrative configuration concerns the qualitative aspects of personhood that become articulated in the story. While a causal model tends to dissociate the agent from the normative aspect of its action, the narrative model insists on this aspect because a story, 'which is never ethically neutral, proves to be the *first laboratory of moral judgment*' (1992, p. 140 [167]). In using the structure of literary fiction as a model for personal identity, Ricoeur asserts that a story always involves agents and sufferers and opens up a field of evaluations where we judge the value of an action (and thereby its agent) with respect to how it affects another person, who thus becomes a sufferer of the action done. In this way, narrative configurations make explicit what is actually the case with all human action, namely, that 'every action has its agents and its patients' (1992, p. 157 [186]). Of course, this is not to be taken literally, as if, for example, I were to determine the suffering of another human being when I poured myself a cup of coffee. However, our actions (even the most insignificant ones) are, somehow, always inscribed in a larger complex of human relations. This fact becomes clear in narrative configurations, even though it tends to go unnoticed in our everyday experience. In fact, '[i]t is precisely because of the elusive character of real life [*caractère évasif de la vie réelle*] that we need the help of fiction to organize life retrospectively' (1992, p. 162 [191]).

Narratives are an attractive model for explaining personal identity because they do not exclude causal explanations (bottom-up perspective), but seek to integrate them into a wider explanation. It is true that narrative configuration approaches the question of personal identity from a normative, top-down perspective, but it operates with a dialectic that emphasises the complexity of human nature, namely, that a person is part of both nature and humanity. We cannot understand personal identity from one of these aspects in isolation. The person is determined both by its biological constitution and by its being part of personal interrelations:

> The practical field then appears to be subjected to a twofold principle of determination by which it resembles the hermeneutical comprehension of a text through the exchange between the whole and the part. Nothing is more propitious for narrative configuration than this play of double determination. (1992, p. 158 [187])

This play of double determination is fleshed out in narrative configurations of our practical field of experience because, although narratives are structured around what Ricoeur calls '*imaginative variations*' of our personal identity (1992, p. 148 [176]), and these always involve 'an unstable mixture of fabulation and actual experience' (1992, p. 162 [191]), our personal identity remains grounded on 'the existential invariant of corporeality and worldliness [*l'invariant existential de la corporéité et de la mondanéité*]' (1992, p. 151 [179]). Imaginative variations are unstable because they are concerned with the more impalpable features of personal identity: ideas, wishes, dreams, norms, social heritage, upbringing, etc., and are therefore liable to fabulation, self-deception, and denial. This risk is balanced, though, by the invariable nature of corporeality and worldliness in the sense that the stories we (and others) make about ourselves find their verification or appropriateness in relation to our body and to the other persons around us. Our experience of ourselves and others is configured by narratives, but the narratives themselves are always grounded on the non-narrative, pre-reflective dimensions of bodily feelings and the presence of other people. The previous section dealt with the ambivalence of the body as being, at the same time, mine and just another object in nature. The narrative configurations of our self-experience are always determined by this ambivalence, since we may ascribe to ourselves, for example, physical qualities that we do not possess in reality. However, this self-deception will, normally, shatter when confronted with the mirror of otherness (my actual body, the world, and other people). Even though Ricoeur focuses on the normative aspect of personal identity, his model is, as we have seen, compatible with a more descriptive, causal approach.[5]

However, it is the normative aspect that Ricoeur finds most critical to personal identity. Narrative configuration is supposed to bridge the gap between the descriptive and prescriptive levels of personal identity. On the one side, it is conditioned by the descriptive explanation of the body, and on the other, it is determined by the concept of responsibility. Now, the concept of responsibility is unfolded by the narrative configuration, but somehow it also transcends the explanatory power of narratives. Narratives clarify the dynamics of personhood, but do not solve the problem of responsibility: 'The story of a life includes interactions with others [. . .] In the test of confronting others, whether an individual or a collectivity, narrative identity reveals its fragility [*l'identité narrative révèle sa fragilité*]' (2005, pp. 103–4 [155–6]).

Rules and Practices

A self acquires a singular identity as a person through the temporal unity of a life. A person cannot be separated from the actions and sufferings that constitute his or her identity through the changes in and of time. This is exactly what is captured in the narrative configuration of experience. Narratives ascribe actions to an agent and explore the implications and effects of those actions, especially with respect to interpersonal relationships: 'stories are about agents and sufferers' (1992, p. 144 [172]). Personal identity can be articulated in terms of narratives, because our identity as a person depends (partially) on stories that explain the *why*, the *what*, and the *how* of our being this particular person with certain character traits, dispositions, idea(l)s, plans, and more or less stable patterns of behaviour. By providing answers to these questions, narratives help sort out our confusion concerning personal identity. Narrative configurations not only clarify questions regarding personal identity, but may also assist us in our explanation of human action and behaviour. Narrative structures extend the practical field of human action by configuring the otherwise incomprehensible multitude of actions into 'a hierarchy of units of praxis that, each on its own level, contain a specific principle of organization, integrating a variety of logical connections' (1992, p. 153 [181];

---

[5] In Chapter 5, we return in more detail to the question of ambivalence with respect to body, personhood, and identity.

translation modified). We are able to make sense of an action because of these units of practice in the sense that values, motives, and decisions find an explanation in the light of the logic governing a certain practice. For example, I move my arm and finger *because* I have to switch on the light *because* I need to see in an otherwise dark room *because* I have to find the refrigerator *because* I must find the sandwich *because* I am hungry. Each of these *because* refers to a practical unit that explains why I do a certain action. They run from the most basic action, such as moving my finger, to a more global level that involves actions concerning such serious issues as life projects or general ideas of happiness, goodness, and justice. However, the internal dynamics of this hierarchy of practices is highly complex:

> [T]he practical field is not constituted from the ground up, starting from the simplest and moving to more elaborate constructions; rather it is formed in accordance with the twofold movement of ascending complexification [*complexification ascendante*] starting from basic actions and from practices, and of descending specification [*spécification descendante*] starting from the vague and mobile horizon of ideals and projects in light of which a human life apprehends itself in its oneness [*unicité*]. (1992, p. 158 [187])

An action can thus be explained on different levels in accordance with the unity of practice we take into consideration, and different levels may possess different kinds of rules and potential meanings. I move my finger to grab, I grab to pull out a chair, I pull out a chair to sit, I sit to rest, and so on. The rules governing different levels, and the potential meanings involved, are somehow interrelated, although I naturally perform innumerable basic actions without paying attention to my horizon of ideals and projects. Often even simple actions involve the presence of other persons. My action becomes an interaction with other persons, and we are returned to the fact that 'every action has its agents and patients'. When I perform an action, that action is always saturated with normativity due to the rules that govern the practice, and as such every action contains a value both to myself and to other persons. That is, our attempts to make sense of human action are always orientated according to a multitude of heterogeneous values, and since a person's action always involves other people, these values are always constituted by rules that point in the direction of moral rules. It is important, however, to note that these rules are first of all rules of meaning, as, for example, the rules of chess:

> The rule, all by itself, gives the gesture its meaning: moving a pawn; the meaning stems from the rule as soon as the rule is constitutive, and it is so because it constitutes meaning, 'counting as'. The notion of constitutive rule can be extended from the example of games to other practices, for the simple reason that games are excellent practical models. (1992, p. 154 [183])

The rules that constitute the meaning of action are governed by the configuration of experience as a human world, where we experience the external world as an organised whole, a world that means something to us as persons. Actions and events present themselves in terms of values according to the practices in which they are inscribed. Values are defined by the rules that constitute the practice. To put it simply, something is good if it attains the goal of the practice and bad if it hinders or prevents the fulfilment of the practice. For example, if I successfully grab a chair, that action is good in the light of the practice of getting a chair; or opening the refrigerator to get food;

or working to get money. Thus, our experience of the world is characterised by the multifarious values pertaining to things, actions, and persons. When we experience objects, they present themselves as meaningful things or persons according to various practices, and their value is influenced by the fulfilment or failure of the practice. Subjective experience is primarily configured according to these practices. Human subjects do not experience a fragmented succession of indifferent objects, but things and persons inscribed in the, for the most part, coherent unity that we experience as our existence in the world.[6]

This human existence can therefore be approached as a narrative unity experienced as a totality, as a life:

> The term 'life' [*vie*] that figures three times in the expressions 'life plan,' 'narrative unity of life,' and 'good life' denotes both the biological rootedness of life and the unity of the human being as a whole [*l'homme tout entier*], as that human being casts upon itself the gaze of appraisal. From the same perspective Socrates said that an unexamined life is not worth living. As for the term 'narrative unity,' the aspect that we are emphasizing here is less the function of assembling-together, performed by the narrative at the summit of the scale of praxis, than the connection the narrative makes between estimations applied to actions and the evaluations of the characters [*personnages*] themselves. (1992, p. 178 [209]; translation modified)

Now, Ricoeur is naturally more interested in how to get a reflective hold on the narrative unity concerning 'the good life' than the less troublesome actions that govern our practices of getting a chair, using our finger to switch on the light or our hand to open the fridge. This is not to say that these more basic actions are not interesting, which they surely are, but only that our idea(s) about 'the good life' do tend to involve more obviously significant values and concerns. I do indeed care about sitting in a chair or getting the sandwich in the fridge, but I am normally more emotionally involved in questions about how to understand, and realise of course, a good life. So in the remaining part of this chapter, we shall try to clarify the problematic relation between values, care, and conceptions of 'the good life'.

The Good Life

We saw at the beginning of the previous chapter that human values are generated by two broad categories of desire, vital and spiritual ones, which inform and orient our engagement with the world, other people, and ourselves. These desires shape the affective dimension of the subjective experience in the form of feelings. Feelings are heterogeneous and generate a non-coincidence in the heart of the self that is felt as a conflict between a desire for self-preservation (my own well-being) at every cost, and a desire for humanity as a kind of totality that procures global meaning to the manifold actions

---

[6] In Chapter 8, we will describe the disintegration of habitual practices of perception and meaning-bestowing in the schizophrenic mood. Especially in the early stages of schizophrenia there is a fragmentation of *Gestalt perception*, that is, a dissolution of one's habitual way to experience space together with the disruption of one's familiar mode to feel engaged in one's surrounding world and make sense of it.

done by the self. We noticed that this conflict could not be examined at a theoretical level, but had to be understood through the various crystallisations of these basic desires in the concrete existence of the self, that is, a self embedded and situated in, among other things, language, society, culture, history, and economics. Hence, on Ricoeur's model, human values are generated from these two fundamental desires, but we need to approach them in terms of the rules that govern the practices of a self embedded in a certain sociocultural context. Our values are shaped and influenced by our engagement, through practices, with a particular society governed by certain rules and norms of behaviour. Values are partially contingent because of this dependency on context, but at least some values seem to aspire to a kind of universality. Such quasi-universal values are mostly those involved in interpersonal relations. Most of our actions involve and influence the presence of other people; or as Ricoeur puts it: '[p]ractices are based on actions in which an agent takes into account, as a matter of principle, the actions of others' (1992, p. 155 [184]). The presence of other people has critical impact on our personal values, since the values involving the presence of the other seem to claim a greater degree of universality than other values.

To understand why this is so, we have to articulate what the presence of other persons means to the self, and in this connection we need to take a closer look at the notion 'the good life' ('*la bonne vie*').

As explained above, the world that we experience by virtue of being persons is configured according to certain values derived from constitutive rules of practices. I understand actions and events (they having meaning and value for me) in the framework of such practices, that is, 'the self is essentially an opening onto the world' and the self's relation to the world is 'a relation of total concern: *everything* concerns me [*tout me concerne*]. And this concern indeed extends from being-alive to militant thinking, passing the way of praxis and living well [*bien-vivre*]' (1992, p. 314 [363]).

Now, although everything concerns me, some things concern me more than others. My concerns express my values, and as such they can be traced back to the basic desires for (vital) self-preservation and (spiritual) well-being. Because I care about my existence in the world, the world becomes the horizon for the realisation of my selfhood; and self and world are intertwined to the extent that '[t]here is no world without a self who finds itself in it and acts in it; there is no self without a world that is practicable in some fashion' (1992, p. 311 [360]). My experience of the world is primarily configured as possibilities to satisfy these concerns, and among the multitude of my concerns the basic value of living is always counterbalanced by the more complex value of living *well*. I care about living, but just as much about living well. To put it differently, the values that configure my experience of the world as a human world are affected by my concerns, in particular my concern for living well.

The notion of 'the good life' is a qualification of the existence of the self conceived as a singular totality; that is, the self considered as a unique self that seeks to assert itself through and, sometimes, in spite of time. All our actions, practices, and sufferings come together in the qualification of our existence as a totality. The basic desire for living well imposes upon us the need to qualify our existence according to an idea of the good life. Obviously, this is not a simple need to fulfil. How can we grasp our entire existence in a single notion such as 'the good life'? And what is actually meant by 'good'? The values by which we live our life are partially contingent and contextual, which means that such a general notion as 'the good life' seems impossible to clarify, let alone explain. Ricoeur is well aware of the impossible character of such an explanatory endeavour. He is convinced, though, that there is an 'idea of a higher finality [*une finalité supérieure*] which would never cease to be internal to human action' (1992, p. 179 [210]). Human action is always interpreted according to a hermeneutical dialectic between the particular and totality, as was pointed out by the narrative approach to personal identity. With a notion borrowed from the philosopher Charles Taylor, Ricoeur defines the human self as a 'self-interpreting animal' (1992, p. 179 [211]).[7] Our different practices have their own local value according to the logic determining their specific fulfilment. At the same time, though, our practices are influenced by the global idea of the good life, our existence qualified as a totality. The obscure and yet intuitive nature of such an idea needs interpretation in order to become articulate. So, although the specific idea of the good life may change in the course of our lives because of our feelings and ideas (mutable and context-dependent) and our character and dispositions (more stable, to be sure), the general idea somehow remains, and as such it influences the configuration of our experience of the world. Our concerns are experienced as values of more or less importance. Some of these values are more contextual and vague than others; some arise and fade in the moment and depend heavily on haphazard circumstances whereas others seem to have a more universal claim on our concerns. To arrive at an idea of the heterogeneous values that configure our experience, we must consider more closely the relation between the self and other persons.

As we have seen, the subject is a self that continuously seeks to affirm or assert itself as a person in a world shared with other persons. Its being is fundamentally characterised by what Spinoza called *conatus*: 'the effort to persevere in being, which forms the unity of man as of every individual' (Ricoeur 1992, p. 316 [366]). This effort to persevere in being, to assert or affirm oneself in the world, is nevertheless conditioned by otherness and, in particular, by other persons. But why, we could ask, does the presence of other persons necessarily condition the assertion of our own self as a person? Can we not just persevere our own being without regarding the presence of other persons? Ricoeur answers these questions by returning to the presence of otherness in the constitution of the selfhood. The identity of the person is vulnerable and fragile. Besides the effort to persevere its own being, that is, our originating affirmation, the life of the self is characterised by a 'need, hence a lack [*le besoin, donc le manque*], that drives the self toward the other' (1992, p. 185 [216]). As we saw at the beginning of Chapter 2, this need or lack originates in the spiritual desire for happiness (well-being) that counterbalances the vital desire for self-preservation in the heart of the self and expresses itself in our idea of 'the good life'. My identity as a person is qualified by this idea, and therefore my selfhood cannot be sustained in solitude, but requires the presence of other persons.

---

[7] Ricoeur describes this dialectic in the following manner: 'between our aim of a "good life" and our particular choices a sort of hermeneutical circle is traced by virtue of the back-to-forth motion between the idea of the "good life" and the most important decisions of our existence (career, loves, leisure, etc.). This can be linked to a text in which the whole and the part are to be understood, each in terms of the other' (1992, p. 179 [210]).

I am who I am in the context of other persons, and my idea of 'the good life' is necessarily influenced by the other persons with whom I am involved in my existence. Ricoeur then uses two interrelated concepts to unfold this intimate relation between the being of the self and the being of the other: *self-esteem* [*l'estime de soi*] and *solicitude* [*sollicitude*].

Self-esteem is 'the primordial reflective moment of the aim of the good life' (1992, p. 188 [220]; translation slightly modified), since our life considered as a totality is valued in accordance with our own conduct. Our idea of 'the good life' finds its reflective correlate in the concept of self-esteem, because 'it is in appraising our actions that we appraise ourselves as being their author' (1992, p. 177 [208]). My self-esteem is heavily influenced by the actions that I perform. The values that I ascribe to the unfolding of my life (actions as well as sufferings) are part of a more global evaluation of my existence. Accordingly, the concept of self-esteem is inescapably connected with the concept of solicitude:

> To self-esteem, understood as a reflective moment of the wish for the 'good life,' solicitude adds essentially the dimension of *lack*, the fact that we *need* friends; as a reaction to the effect of solicitude on self-esteem, the self perceives itself as another among others [*un autre parmi les autres*]. (1992, p. 192 [225]; translation slightly modified)

The other considered as a person like me and yet autonomous with respect to me is constitutive for the idea of 'the good life'. My concern for the other does not, or not only, originate in a desire to dominate the other, but in a lack in my own existence that generates a need for the other. We need the other person not as a means to satisfy our own desires but as an autonomous person that constitutes our global idea of 'the good life'. This need for others drastically affects the values by which I act in the world. When the other person addresses me 'in the second person, I feel I am implicated in the first person' (1992, p. 193 [225]). Hence, my self-esteem, which is a dominant part of the global idea of 'the good life', depends on the presence of other people that fulfil and satisfy the basic need of others. This need is felt as solicitude for the existence of the other. Selfhood is not constituted solely of mineness: '*To say self is not to say myself* [*Dire soi n'est pas dire moi*]' (1992, p. 180 [212]). The other person is fundamental to my identity in the world, since the world is a common world whose meaning is derived from the coexistence of different persons. My identity as a person depends on the other's *recognition* of my being so. The others recognise my actions as actions of a person with an individual history and unique ideas and plans for the future. Therefore, the unity and coherence of my various actions with respect to the idea of myself as an individual person is deeply influenced by the reception of these actions by other persons. I feel a need to be recognised and vice versa: 'Becoming in this way fundamentally equivalent are the esteem of the *other as a oneself* [*l'autre comme un soi-même*] and the esteem of *oneself as an other* [*soi-même comme un autre*]'. (1992, pp. 193–4 [226])

The presence of other persons is therefore critical to my values. My values must reflect this recognition of the other as myself and myself as an other. My actions and practices in the world are rooted in this basic condition of selfhood, namely, that the self is constituted by otherness in all its efforts to assert and affirm its own existence. The global idea of 'the good life' involves this otherness and requires careful attention on the part of the self to be realised. It is in this sense that the values that involve our relation to other persons have a somewhat more universal claim on us than other values in our existence. The solicitude for the well-being of the other person defies the mutable and contextual nature of my other values. I cannot disregard the other in my actions and practices. My identity as a person depends on the presence of him or her.

An Ontology of Care

Now we shall try to gather together the previous analyses in order to form the notion of an ontology of care showing how care for otherness is constitutive for becoming a person. That is, the therapy of the troubled self becomes a hermeneutical reappropriation of the self by means of the notion of personhood.

In the previous chapter we reformulated Ricoeur's phenomenological diagnosis of the troubled sense of selfhood. We uncovered a tension in the self between an originating affirmation and an existential difference or negation that brings about a conflict between vital and spiritual desires. This led to an outline for an ontology rooted in a continuous encounter between selfhood and otherness. The human self is fragile and vulnerable to conflict due to this complex ontological nature. The subject does not repose in its own self-awareness, but is in constant search of restoring the identity of its own self. This restoration of selfhood, of who I am, is experienced as a conflict between selfhood and otherness in becoming a person. My identity as a person is constituted not only by my self-affirmation but also by the otherness that continuously challenges (and threatens) my effort to preserve my selfhood in the course of my existence. The feelings that qualify my existence and motivate my interaction with otherness—my body, the world, and other people—are shaped and informed by vital and spiritual desires. I relentlessly seek to affirm or assert my own (well-)being at every cost, but I also need otherness, especially the other person, because my existence as a person is an existence in and through that which is different from myself. We must turn to a hermeneutical method because the conflict in the heart of selfhood cannot be adequately dealt with at a phenomenological level.

In this chapter, we have sought to articulate Ricoeur's therapeutic solution to the problem of the troubled sense of selfhood. The feelings of otherness are crystallised through the subject's practical interaction in the world through time. The self is lost in the embedded and situated character of its existence in time. Otherness manifests itself through history, society, culture, institutions, etc., and these various manifestations need ongoing interpretation to be understood and appropriated by the self as the human world. This interpretation is always rooted in care[8] or concern for oneself *and* for otherness. That is, the subject cares for the other, because it can only become a person through the reappropriation of itself in and through that otherness. Care is what binds together selfhood and otherness in the notion of personhood.

---

[8] Ricoeur's terminology is slightly unstable with regard to the notion of care. He uses the terms 'solicitude' (*'sollicitude'*), 'care' (*'souci'*), and the Heideggerian notion '*Sorge*' (the German word for care) interchangeably. We do not see any substantial difference in his use of the different terms, so we stick with the term 'care', unless one of the other terms occurs in a direct quote.

This ontological status of care is particularly clear with respect to the other person. The subject cares for its place among other persons (its idea of 'the good life') and feels a strong desire to be part of a human society. This desire for humanity is fundamental for its identity as a person among other persons. The self needs the other person to affirm its own identity as an integral and irreplaceable person. Self-esteem is part of our identity, and the other's recognition is critical to how we esteem ourselves as a person. We are responsible to the other person, because the other person responds to our actions, and we, on our part, act and suffer in accordance with that response. We care about what the other has to say about who and what we are. Accordingly, our identity as persons depends on the recognition of the other person, and not merely on biological continuation of our being. Ricoeur was well aware of this intricate and primary relationship between the self and the other in his earliest work on subjectivity:

> I form the consciousness of being the author of my acts in the world and, more generally, the author of my acts of thought, principally on the occasion of my contacts with an other, in a social context. Someone asks, who did that? I rise and reply, I did. Response—responsibility. To be responsible means to be ready to respond to such a question [...] And yet we sense that the other introduces nothing external but only evokes, like a special revelatory power [*comme un révélateur privilégié*], that aptitude for imputing my acts to myself which is embedded even in my least reflective acts. (1966, pp. 56–7 [55]; translation slightly modified)

Once again, it is here important to remember that Ricoeur's emphasis on the other person as the centre of our care should not in any way overshadow the vital importance of the kinds of otherness that we find expressed in our body or our situated existence in the world. In fact, much of the effort in the following chapters will be spent on trying to explain how our body and our situated existence influence and complicate our sense of identity. For now, we can conclude our reformulation of Ricoeur's theory of subjectivity by saying that an ontology of care attempts to make sense of our troubled sense of selfhood by articulating the relation between selfhood and otherness in the constitution of human personhood.

We shall end this part of the book with a brief outline of how we are going to use this reformulation of Ricoeur's theory in developing our own account of emotions and personhood over the next four chapters. We shall also hint at the use we will make of the idea of an ontology of care in the concluding Chapter 10.

Becoming a Person through Otherness

In the previous chapters we have traced the journey from troubled selfhood to fragile personhood. The self can only become who she or he is by becoming a person through the dialectic of selfhood and otherness. Or to put it differently, the self has to reappropriate itself as a person through otherness in order to come to terms with who and what she or he is. It is a normative journey through negativity, that is, through the conflict of selfhood and otherness at the heart of selfhood. The principal virtue of Ricoeur's theory, we believe, is that it investigates human subjectivity through the interconnection of three distinct levels: the phenomenological (how do I feel?), the ontological (what and who am I?), and the normative (what shall I do?). The conviction that all three levels are indispensable for understanding the journey from selfhood to personhood remains the methodological impetus in the following chapters. The single most important insight that we take with us when we embark on the investigations in the next part of the book is Ricoeur's argument for personhood as rooted in the affective conflict of selfhood and otherness. Only through reappropriation of the otherness involved in what and who we are can we hope to overcome the conflict constitutive of selfhood. Once again T.S. Eliot, in the *Four Quartets*, has eminently resounded this dialectical movement of selfhood and otherness (and our repetitive insistence on this constitutive feature of personhood). Towards the end of the second poem, *East Coker*, he writes:

> You say I am repeating
> Something I have said before. I shall say it again.
> Shall I say it again? In order to arrive there,
> To arrive where you are, to get from where you are not,
>   You must go by a way wherein there is no ecstasy.
> In order to arrive at what you do not know
>   You must go by a way which is the way of ignorance.
> In order to possess what you do not possess
>   You must go by the way of dispossession.
> In order to arrive at what you are not
>   You must go through the way in which you are not.
> And what you do not know is the only thing you know
> And what you own is what you do not own
> And where you are is where you are not.
>
> (Eliot 1944, p. 20)

Besides the dialectic of selfhood and otherness, there are four principal, interrelated features of Ricoeur's theory of subjectivity that we are going to use as the theoretical background for the four chapters in Part II: emotional experience, ambivalence, narrative identity, and values. His theory of becoming a person through the dialectic of selfhood and otherness will serve as the general background, but these four features will have a notable bearing on the explorations that follow. The exploration of prominent philosophical and neuroscientific theories of emotion in Chapter 4 and the investigation of ambivalent personhood in Chapter 5 eventually result in a theory of emotions and personhood in Chapter 6. We close this part of the book with a chapter dedicated to an exploration of values, in which we shall use Ricoeur's analysis of the affective generation of values to steer a middle course between, on the one side, a strictly biological account of values, and, on the other, a purely phenomenological account.

As we have seen, Ricoeur's main concern, from beginning to end, is the otherness of the other person as experienced in one self as another. This pivotal significance of the other person is carried over into our own theory. Our own emphasis, however, shall be on the otherness involved in the embodied nature of emotional experience. We spend considerable time in the following chapters investigating the ambivalence of the biology and phenomenology of the human body, and the significance of this ambivalence for our understanding of human personhood. Ricoeur provides the framework for investigating emotions and the biological dimension of bodily experience, but his actual investigation of these issues remains rather scanty. So we shall develop these issues in constant exchange with contemporary philosophical and neuroscientific theories of emotion, and try to incorporate them into a full-fledged account of emotions and personhood. In fact, we shall argue that nowhere is the conflictual dialectic of selfhood and otherness more manifest than in emotional experience. The fragility of human personhood is rooted in the ambivalence of phenomenology and biology that characterises our emotions and feelings. We shall trace the inescapable resonance of this ambivalence through our endeavour to come to terms with our identity as individual persons. Once again, narratives play an important role in this process. We elaborate on Ricoeur's theory of narrative identity with insights from present day narrative theories of emotion. This enables us to develop what we call a hermeneutics of care that provides us with a language capable of making sense of the heterogeneous character of our emotional experience, which, in turn, will help us live with the challenges of our emotional life.

Part III makes use of the combination of diagnosis and therapy at work in Ricoeur's theory to develop the traditional idea of a dialectical model of psychopathology. Equipped with our investigations of emotions and personhood in Part II, we explore the emotional life-worlds of schizophrenia and borderline personality disorder with the explicit aim at arriving at a hermeneutical strengthening of the dialectical model of mental illness. Ricoeur's theory of the conflictual dialectic of selfhood and otherness provides the theoretical background for our descriptive diagnosis of these disorders in Chapters 8 and 9, and then emerges into the foreground in the final section of Chapter 10 where we, by way of conclusion, attempt to outline the therapeutic implications of our theory. We shall argue that a hermeneutics of care can prove a strong therapeutic tool for the clinician's work with mental illness, schizophrenia and borderline personality disorder in particular, but also with disorders more generally speaking.

Part II

Fragile Personhood

Chapter 4

Conceptual Clarity Amidst an Abundance of Feelings

Human feelings are multifarious and, at times, notoriously difficult to understand and cope with. We are easy victims of our feelings, so even when we are convinced that we act appropriately upon a certain emotion or are able to make sense of a diffuse feeling, we might just be delving deeper into a misunderstanding or be consolidating an unfortunate self-conceit. Understanding our feelings is influenced by how we understand ourselves as a person and what it means to be a person. On the other hand, to obtain a satisfactorily comprehensive notion of personhood, we need a thorough account of human emotions; how feelings and emotions continuously influence and shape human thought and behaviour, and how to cope with this emotional dimension of being human. In Part I, we spent considerable time establishing a hermeneutical framework to approach and understand this relationship between emotions and personhood. In the next four chapters, we will develop the claim about this intricate relationship between emotions and personhood and argue that a hermeneutical approach to human emotions provides a philosophically valid alternative to other accounts of human emotions.

In the present chapter, we will look at the evident problems about getting a conceptual grasp of the diffuse jostle of human feelings. We present three currents in contemporary philosophical theories of emotions and two neuroscientific theories of the emotional brain. The chapter ends with an introduction to our own account against the backdrop of these theories.

People have always been trying to understand their own emotions and those of others. Emotions have left distinct traces in every kind of relic of human history. From solitary cave drawings to the grandiose epics of Gilgamesh or Homer, from Plato's *Philebus* to the memorable movie lines such as 'Frankly, my dear, I don't give a damn', we find an astonishing continuity in expressing and interpreting the emotional lives of human beings. In many ways, some of our prevalent emotions and feelings are universal and ahistorical. They express basic human reactions to the environment and, in particular, to other people. Many of these emotional reactions are deeply ingrained in our biological makeup and, to some extent, the result of the sub-personal mechanisms of the mammalian brain. Despite this undercurrent of continuity, emotions and interpretations of emotions do nevertheless seem to vary from period to period, from community to community, and sometimes even from person to person. Thus, in order to get a preliminary idea of the complexities that face philosophical and neuroscientific theories of emotion, we begin this chapter with a discussion of the difficult task of naming, categorising, and making intelligible our elusive understanding of emotions and bodily feeling, that is, the daunting task of interpreting how feelings and emotions influence human behaviour.

To Name or Not to Name a Feeling

We feel more than we can understand or express in words. This is something that every person knows and lives with, more or less happily. A major part of our lives is constituted by the inexpressible and cognitively impenetrable nature of feelings. Poets and artists through the ages have worked hard at articulating human feelings, and the simple fact that there are still poems to write, paintings and sculptures to make, and new love songs to compose, reminds us of the cornucopia of feelings that constitute human life. As Cordelia laments in the opening of *King Lear*, 'Unhappy that I am, I cannot heave my heart into my mouth' (Act I, sc. 1). But we do not need to read Shakespeare in order to be convinced that feelings are difficult to understand. The humdrum of everyday life abounds with feelings that are difficult to handle, such as when I get out of bed on the wrong side and remain in a bad mood all day with the effect that my thoughts are clouded, my words come out wrong, and I am easily annoyed or irritated; or if my friend hurts me with an inconsiderate remark that leaves me dumbstruck, but with an indistinct feeling of anger and sadness. I can also sincerely want to comfort my mother who is lonely and devastated after my father passed away, but I nevertheless lack the energy to return her phone calls, and I just watch a movie instead.

A major difficulty and, as we shall see, a major problem about human feelings is that our understanding of them reveals that we are often wrong about what we think we feel, and when we form an appropriate opinion we often feel that we have only grasped a paltry part of what is actually going on in our emotional life. Naturally, we have a good grip on many of our feelings, and our lives would dissolve into an indistinct jumble of bodily sensations and feelings, if it was not for our ability to rationally understand, name, and categorise a considerable part of our feelings. However, our attempt to conceptually encompass and understand our feelings and how they influence our behaviour is a risky endeavour. We have to navigate carefully between clear-cut reductionist explanations and inarticulate confusion. The procrustean bed of conceptual analysis and rational structures seems to provide only a pale rendering of the multifarious facets of our emotional life. Music and poetry do a better job of catching the tonality, colour, and atmosphere of our lived emotions, and novels yield more cogent descriptions of why we feel sad, in love or helpless than a book like this one. Music, paintings, and literature moves us exactly because in these art forms our emotional life is conveyed and made resonant, and not encumbered with detailed analysis or overt interpretations. Art can express and describe our feelings without ever naming them as this or that emotion.

The value of a philosophical approach, on the other hand, lies not in providing better descriptions of love, joy or despair, but in the systematic interpretation of such emotions in relation to a more comprehensive understanding of human nature. This comprehensive task of philosophy of emotion is one of the reasons why philosophical theories have such a hard time agreeing on the nature and function of our emotional life. The interpretative grip on our emotions and feelings relies heavily on our more general understanding of human nature. In this sense, John Cutting's characterisation of the state of emotion research more than a decade ago still holds true today:

> The current concept of emotion is a loose agglomerate of aspects of a number of realms of human affairs, and, according to most commentators, is not necessarily bound to every one of these. Body, mind (thinking and remembering), world, and will are all linked, to a greater or lesser extent, in the extant formulations. The tendency is to explain away emotion in terms of some other realm of human affairs.
>
> (Cutting 1997, p. 391)

Emotions are endemic to every aspect of human nature, and as such they are interlaced with our interpretation of these aspects. On a pre-reflective level, emotions permeate, in the form of more or less articulate feelings and drives, most aspects of human life and influence the way we perceive, move our body, and interact with the world. And, when we ponder our situation, or our life for that matter, some of us might recognise the sentiment of Mrs. Ramsey in *To the Lighthouse* who 'often felt she was nothing but a sponge sopped full of human emotions' (Woolf 1941, p. 54). Surely, all of us sometimes have the feeling that our thoughts and ideas are mere bouncing balls for our emotions and feelings. It is difficult to deny the significant role that emotions and feelings play in our endeavours to understand ourselves, other people, and the situations that we find ourselves in. Accordingly, the way we rationally understand and interpret our personal nature and behaviour is already affected by the emotions that we want to understand. The traditional watershed between reason and emotion began to leak decades ago, and today many philosophers agree that rationality is never completely without feelings and emotions are never completely thoughtless (de Sousa 2007, pp. 149–53; Solomon 2007, pp. 205–6; Stocker 1996, pp. 99–104). Finally, and perhaps most importantly, emotions are saturated with a pervasive normativity. We are touched and moved by our feelings. Our experience and understanding of the world, other people, and ourselves is marked by an emotional quality that pervades our perception and rational capacities. The emotional quality makes what we experience matter to us in the sense that we are *touched* and *moved* by our experiences. Our experience of the world is never merely a neutral registration of what goes on around us. Emotions and feelings engage us and make us an active part of what we experience, and they influence how we understand and value the world and our being a part of this world. We think about and act on our understanding because we care about what we understand about the world and ourselves. Thus, as we argued with Ricoeur in Chapter 1, emotions play a fundamental role in the generation of the values that make up and orient our lives as human persons.

If our emphasis on the ubiquitous nature of emotions is correct, it obviously makes it difficult to disentangle what is specifically emotional about an emotional experience from what is not. Traditionally, or at least since the end of the nineteenth century, it has been common practice to distinguish between the categories of emotion and feeling (Deigh 2010). On this picture of our emotional life, the churn of our affective nature can be approached by means of two conceptual categories: (intentional) emotions and (bodily) feelings. Emotions refer to the structured and propositional affective states which include a more or less explicit intentional attitude that we find in complex emotions such as love, pride, shame, and jealousy. Feelings, on the other hand, cover the pre-reflective, bodily felt aspect of an affective state, where we perceive something going in our 'bodily landscape', often without our being in control or exercising an influence over these feelings. Central to this category of affective states are clearly embodied feelings that are physically manifested such as fear, anger, surprise, joy, and aggression. Whereas the category of emotions is primarily concerned with explicitly human affectivity, bodily feelings are considered to be found across various species, or at least in other mammals. We will go into a more detailed presentation of three influential theories of emotions in a moment, but first we will look at some more general problems with this picture of human emotions.

In recent years, this traditional view on our emotional life has been heavily disputed. Here we shall mention only two of these criticisms, which are of particular relevance to our own account. It has been argued that the conceptual distinction between structured emotions and bodily feelings is not tenable. Peter Goldie has insisted that feelings are not merely the registration of bodily changes, but are also characterised by being a 'feeling towards' the world, that is, feelings can be intentional as well as physiological. Our engagement with the world is partly revealed through our feelings, because '[w]hen we have an emotion, we are disposed to have feelings toward a variety of things in a variety of ways' (Goldie 2000, p. 81). More recently, Matthew Ratcliffe has argued along the same lines, albeit somewhat more radically. Whereas Goldie distinguishes between 'bodily feelings' and 'feelings toward' and thus seems to acknowledge some independent, merely physiological, function of bodily feelings, Ratcliffe claims that all feelings are intentional. On his phenomenological account, 'distinctions between world-directed and bodily feelings involve double-counting; bodily feelings just are feelings toward' (Ratcliffe 2008, p. 35). We shall return to both Goldie and Ratcliffe in more detail later, but for now, suffice it to say that the distinction between emotions and bodily feelings is no longer accepted as being so clear-cut as was the case only a few decades ago. This blurring of the categories brings us to the second type of criticism. Thomas Dixon has recently investigated the development of the strict category of emotion out of the realm of variegated notions such as passions, appetites, affections, and sensations in English-language psychological thought. He claims that the scientific spring cleaning of our psychological vocabulary, resulting in the creation of a secular category of emotion during the nineteenth century, is an important factor in sharpening the distinction between affectless reason and thoughtless emotions:

> In the absence of categories such as 'affections' and 'sentiments' that bridged the gap between thinking and feeling, secular psychologies of emotion were left with a simple and sharp dichotomy between cognition and emotion.
>
> (Dixon 2003, p. 17)

He argues that this is not simply a harmless transformation of an outdated psychological vocabulary into a new, more scientifically accurate one. Rather, the slimming of the psychological vocabulary about our affective nature from various categories to the categories of emotion and feeling is the expression of a categorical shift in worldview on the part of the expanding scientific community. The anti-theological attitude that dominated the scientific endeavours in the second half of the nineteenth century dispensed, in the name of scientific progress, with the rich material of the long tradition of philosophical theories of emotions. This resulted, among other things, in an ontological and epistemological transformation:

> The ontology of the new psychology of emotions, as developed by Spencer, Bain, Darwin and, ultimately, James in the 1850s–80s, was one in which there were only two real psychological agencies—the evolutionary past and the body (especially the nerves and viscera). Introspection into one's soul was replaced by observations of others' bodies and behaviours as the favoured epistemology.
>
> (Dixon 2003, p. 241)

Dixon admonishes us to take the history of emotions seriously in order to avoid that our scientific standards are built on (anti-theological and other) prejudices that may end up hampering our understanding of human affectivity. This admonition need not entail a recoil into anti-scientific attitudes or social constructivist theories. An appreciation of the historical aspect of emotions may simply advance a critical awareness of the implicit ontological and epistemological presuppositions of the vocabulary with which we understand and explain our emotions today.

We are not going to plunge into the fascinating intellectual history of emotion in this book, but we will use this historical awareness, together with the hermeneutical theory of subjectivity developed in Part I, to question the validity of the exclusive categories of emotion and feelings. The categories of emotion and feeling have in many ways helped us to think more clearly about our emotional life, and the resulting focus on the physiological and cognitive aspect of emotions has indisputably furthered our understanding of why and how emotions play such an important part in our thoughts and behaviour. Yet, as a consequence of the focus on physiology and cognition, philosophical interest in other aspects of human emotional life that occupied philosophers in the past has also diminished. Concepts such as sentiment, appetite, passion, affection, melancholy, happiness, and mood that were central to such prominent philosophers as Aristotle, Aquinas, Hobbes, Spinoza, and Hume only rarely find their way into contemporary theories of emotion. The disappearance of these concepts from much contemporary philosophy of emotion does not mean that people have stopped using them when thinking and talking about their everyday experience of emotions. On the contrary, we still explain the multifarious nuances of our emotional life by means of a vast array of concepts and names that are left out of the scientific investigation of our affective life. We are well aware that a systematic analysis of emotional experience cannot, for obvious reasons, encompass every word or concept that is employed in our affective vocabulary, but we believe that Dixon is right to argue that more than two broad categories are needed in order to appreciate, and hopefully make sense of, some of the complexity of our emotional life.

Accordingly, in Chapters 6 and 7, we propose an alternative account that attempts to make room for feelings that are not adequately explained by either physiology or cognition. This is not meant as a wholesale critique of existing theories in the philosophy of emotions. It relies heavily on insights from both philosophical and neuroscientific theories of emotion and feeling, and should be read as an attempt to use those insights to understand feelings that are not at the forefront of the contemporary debate. In our approach to human feelings, we focus on the concept of personhood with the hope to articulate the implicit ontological presuppositions of our account of human affectivity. If John Cutting and Thomas Dixon are right, as we believe they are, that explanations of emotions are carried out in terms of other realms of human affairs or on the background of a particular worldview, it may prove valuable to make such presuppositions explicit in our theorising about emotions. The choice of personhood as the Archimedean point for our account of emotion is motivated by what we learned from Ricoeur's theory of subjectivity in Part I. Following these lines, we believe that the notion of personhood has the advantage of articulating an ontology of human nature that pays equal attention to both the phenomenological and biological aspects of being human. To be a person is, among other things, to live with the fact that we are conscious selves who care about our body, the world, and other people. This care, as we argued with Ricoeur in Chapter 3, reveals otherness in the heart of human selfhood. In other words, the notion of personhood articulates the voluntary and involuntary aspects of being a human self. Furthermore, it foregrounds the pervasive normative feature of emotions which, as we will argue, is a fundamental aspect of human emotional experience. But before we develop our own account, we begin with a short presentation of some current philosophical and neuroscientific theories of emotions that provide both insights and material for critique for our own approach.

Feeling Theories

The cluster of theories that normally go under this name insist on the predominance of the (neuro)physiological dimension of human emotions. On this account, emotions are a special kind of experiences like perception (hearing, tasting, smelling, seeing, and touching) and proprioception (registration of changes in the body such as dizziness, nausea, exhaustion, energy, tiredness, and hunger). Emotions differ, though, from other kinds of experience by means of the explicit qualitative feature of their manifestation, that is, they are vested with a specifically felt quality.

The theory found its classical, and most radical, expression in the James–Lange theory of emotion. William James and Carl G. Lange, independently of one another, proposed a theory that reduced emotions to perceptions of bioregulatory changes in the body. Emotions are not manifestations of our cognitive relation to the world. Naturally, we are able to cognitively relate ourselves to what we feel, but only *after* the feeling has manifested itself. Feelings are the result of the workings of our autonomous nervous system, and are not mixed with or caused by our cognitive capacities. James illustrated the central claim of the theory with his famous example of how we become afraid of a bear. Common sense tells us that we see the bear, become afraid, and then run. James, however, turns this picture upside down saying that this way of understanding our emotions is all wrong. We fear the bear because we try to run from it. Emotion is not a result of our cognitive relation to the perception of the bear as if I see a bear, recognise that it is dangerous, become afraid, and then run. On the contrary, our emotions are the experience of feelings caused by the perception of a set of bodily responses. I see the bear, my body reacts to the danger that I perceive, and I have the feeling of what we have come to understand as fear because I perceive the visceral reactions of my body. James argues beautifully for this seemingly counterintuitive claim:

> What kind of an emotion of fear would be left, if the feelings neither of quickened heartbeats nor of shallow breathing, neither of trembling lips nor of weakened limbs, neither of goose-flesh nor of visceral stirrings, were present, it is quite impossible to think. Can one fancy the state of rage and picture no ebullition of it in the chest, no flushing of the face, no dilatation of the nostrils, no clenching of the teeth, no impulse to vigorous action, but in their stead limp muscles, calm breathing, and a placid face? The present writer, for one, certainly cannot.
>
> (James 1884, pp. 193–4)

Although hardly anybody would claim that emotions are ever experienced without some kind of bodily manifestation, only few were initially convinced of this radical reduction of our emotional life to mere perception of bodily changes. During most of the twentieth century the theory was criticised for not being able to distinguish between different kinds of emotions caused by the same visceral reactions. The first important criticism, carried out on a purely physiological basis, was expressed by the physiologist Walter B. Cannon, who in 1927 argued that:

> [T]he responses in the viscera seem too uniform to offer a satisfactory means of distinguishing emotions which are very different in subjective quality. Furthermore, if the emotions were due to afferent impulses from the viscera, we would expect not only that fear and rage would feel alike but that chilliness, hypoglycemia, asphyxia, and fever should feel like them.
>
> (Cannon 1927, p. 110)

The same bodily state may be involved in two (or more) different emotional experiences such as, for instance, fear and rage. The experience of fear differs from that of rage in obvious ways, and we are hardly able to account for that difference by visceral changes alone. There is obviously something more to the emotions than the perception of bodily changes (Kenny 1963, pp. 39–42). After this frontal attack, the feeling theory was discredited in philosophical and psychological research on emotions throughout most of the twentieth century.

A couple of decades ago, though, the theory gained new popularity with the compelling studies of the neuroscientist Antonio Damasio (1994, 1999, 2003, 2010). Whereas James and Lange came to their idea of emotions as feelings mainly from the visible physiognomic expression of emotions, Damasio scrutinises emotions inside the brain, that is, in the neurobiological properties and dynamics of emotions. He broadly concords with the James–Lange theory and develops their thesis by reflecting on new evidence provided by a combination of clinical practice and cognitive neuroscience, and he convincingly defends the feeling theory from the criticism launched by Cannon and others. He shows, among other things, how the body is not always distinctly present in the feeling of an emotion. The brain is able to somehow 'by-pass' the body through what he calls 'as-if'-feelings by means of which '[w]e conjure up some semblance of a feeling within the brain alone'; immediately afterwards he qualifies this idea, though, by noting 'I doubt, however, that those feelings feel the same as the feelings freshly minted in a real body state' (Damasio 1994, p. 156). The cogency of his argument for a reappraisal of the feeling theory comes from the fact that he is able to show that there is not always a direct link between a specific body state and a certain feeling of emotion. His theory is thus able to differentiate the various feelings, and he works out an elaborate account of the idea that emotions are feelings, going from simple homeostatic regulations to acquired, social emotions. For example, he gives a much more detailed account of the feeling of sadness than the one we find in James who focuses on the physiological machinery of sorrow: 'each fit of sobbing makes the sorrow acute, and calls forth another fit still stronger' (James 1884, p. 197). Damasio claims that alongside perception of our bodily state there is the perception of certain thoughts that might just contribute to the feeling of sadness. These thoughts are meta-representations of our own mental processes that allow the mind to represent other parts of the mind (mental images and long-term memory) together with the perception of bodily states. In this way, Damasio argues for the variety of emotional experience by emphasising the complexity of our perception: 'a feeling is the perception of a certain state of the body along with the perception of a certain mode of thinking and of thoughts with certain themes' (Damasio 2003, p. 86).

To develop this detailed version of the feeling theory, Damasio has continued, for more than a decade now, to investigate the subjectivity of emotional experience, but since he never ceases to insist on the fundamental importance of the homeostasis, i.e. the ebbs and floods of 'the bodily landscape', his notion of subjectivity remains somewhat simplistic. And this simplicity affects his theory of emotion. A subject is what it is, and nothing else. It is a core self that, throughout our existence, develops into an autobiographical self, shaped by education, culture, and unique and contingent personal events. These factors create, in a sort of orchestration, the person that we are. Naturally, he does not exclude our capacity to perform imaginative variations on our actual being, but he seems certain that, in the end, each of us is the self that he or she is constituted to be: 'We can be Hamlet for a week, or Falstaff for an evening, but we tend to return to home base' (1999, p. 225). This idea of a biologically rooted 'home base' underestimates, in our view, the reflective aspect of subjectivity that is clearly manifested in our capacity to question, evaluate, and critically revise our actually being the person that we are.

A more philosophically solid and refined defence of the feeling theory has recently been proposed by Jesse Prinz. Prinz develops what he calls a perceptual theory of emotions as 'gut reactions'. He clearly subscribes to the James–Lange theory of emotions, and in a large part also to Damasio's upgraded version of this theory. He argues that emotions are indeed perceptions of bodily changes, but then goes on to develop Damasio's neuroscientific account in a more philosophical direction by observing that:

> Emotions clearly 'register' changes in the body, but there still is a further question about what such states represent. By analogy one might say that a state in the visual system *registers* a particular luminance discontinuity, but it *represents* an edge. On the theory of representation under consideration, reliable causation is not sufficient for representation. A representation must also have a function. Visual states have the function of representing shapes. The claim that emotions represent bodily changes requires a further premise. If anger represents dilated blood vessels, it must have the function of detecting them.
>
> (Prinz 2004, p. 58)

What makes Prinz's perceptual theory of emotions different from earlier versions is that he furnishes the feeling theory with philosophical scaffolding to explain the complex relation between our immediate perception of bodily changes and the representational function of those perceptions. He intends to curb biological reductionism without recoiling into a cognitive or judgemental understanding of emotions. Emotions are without any cognitive content and the mere function of our bodily constitution, but that does not entail that we are simply helpless puppets under the sway of our bodily constitution. In other words, emotional reactions have both active and passive dimensions (Prinz 2004, p. 240). Prinz does believe, though, that emotions are primarily informed by the anonymous workings of evolutionary forces such as survival and reproduction, and he develops a view that he calls 'integrative compatibilist position' by means of which he differentiates between basic emotions unaffected by cultural and personal influences, and more context-sensitive emotions. Central to this position is the so-called 'core relational themes':

> Emotions track bodily states that reliably cooccur with important organism-environment relations, so emotions reliably cooccur with important organism-environment relations. Each emotion is both an internal body monitor and a detector of dangers, threats, losses, or other matters of concern.
>
> (Prinz 2004, p. 69)

Prinz's theory is of particular interest for our own account in two respects. First, he evidences the fundamental role of the sub-personal character of our emotions. We have learned much from his sustained attempt to develop an account of emotions squarely set in an evolutionary framework and articulated in terms of the physiological constitution of the human body without committing himself to the usual reductionist explanations. Secondly, his subsequent development of his theory with regard to the normative dimension of emotions (Prinz 2007) provides a clear alternative to our own insistence on the normative character of emotional experience. We shall return to Damasio's account later in this chapter, and in Chapter 7 we shall discuss the evolutionary framework for the normative character of emotions developed by Prinz.

For the present, though, we shall look at two explicitly philosophical theories of emotion that, each in its own way, criticise the reduction of emotions to pure bodily feelings. Both theories focus on the role that emotions play in our judgements and evaluations, and insist that this evaluative role cannot be reduced to feelings of bodily changes. Our emotions have intentional or narrative structures that for obvious reasons are ignored by investigations into the unruly feelings of body states. It is the neglect of the intentional (propositional or rational) structure of emotions that the cognitive theories have taken issue with in their criticism of the feeling theories.

Cognitive Theories

Most philosophical theories of emotion are, in some way or another, cognitive theories. The basic claim is that emotions involve propositional attitudes. When I am angry, I am normally angry at someone because of something. When I am happy or sad it is most of the time due to something that I am aware about. Emotions are rational (Solomon

1976), or at least have a rational structure (Gordon 1987) that goes beyond the perception of bodily changes. They are judgements about the world and my situation in it, involving a more global stance towards my existence as a thinking and responsible person. Feelings may occur together with emotions, but as one of the most enduring defenders of the cognitive theory, Robert C. Solomon, writes:

> However predictable the association of feelings and emotions, the feelings no more constitute or define the emotion than an army of fleas constitute a homeless dog. They are always there, take shape of the emotion, but just as easily move from one emotion to the other (love to hate, fear to anger, jealousy to resentment). Feeling is the ornamentation of emotion, not its essence. (1976, p. 159)[1]

Solomon insists that emotions reveal our intimate relation to the world and to ourselves, not only as organisms constituted by a highly developed primate brain and a sensitive nervous system, but as persons with certain ideas, beliefs, and commitments not reducible to the internal feel of bodily states. Emotions are crucial for our personal engagement with the world. We commit ourselves to the world and to other people through and by our emotions. The thrust of his argument is the stout rejection of the common idea that we are helplessly subjected to our emotions. He insists throughout his innumerable works that we are indeed responsible for our emotions, arguing that:

> [T]he idea that responsibility can be an ingredient in our emotional judgments enriches the sophistication of our emotional lives enormously and is unintelligible on any more primitive conception of emotions. It also suggests that these emotions are deeply dependent on cultural as well as ethical presumptions, and whether the prevailing emotion of self-blame is shame or guilt depends in particular on the ethical structure of the society.
>
> (Solomon 2007, p. 210)

Most cognitive theories consider emotions as judgements that have a specific logic or rationality (Nussbaum 2001, pp. 19–85; Sartre 1971). This logic or rationality is sometimes identified with the notion of intentionality in the sense that emotions are expressions of certain beliefs and desires. When I feel irritated in a specific situation, it is because of something going on in this situation. I am irritated at the woman in front of me because of something she said or did. Perhaps her statement makes my opinion look ridiculous, or perhaps she just moves in a stupid way. Or I might be envious because my neighbour has an expensive car or because his kid is better at soccer than my own kid. The combinations are endless, but it is basically a question of structure. The emotion is characterised by an object or a propositional content. In order

---

[1] Solomon is mainly inspired by Nietzsche, Sartre, and the existentialist tradition. He wrote his first seminal work on emotions as a harsh critique of the feeling theory (1976). But in the last years up to his death in 2007, he came to moderate the critique and ended up considering bodily feelings as a significant part of emotional experience. Although he still insisted on the primary importance of the cognitive, evaluative stance (2003, pp. 189–92), he changed his view on bodily feelings and accepted that emotions do not necessarily involve an explicit articulation or propositional attitude, but could also be manifested as 'bodily "kinesthetic" judgments' (2007, p. 205).

to understand different emotions, we must try to sort out the different structures or complexes of this object relation. This may entail feelings, but feelings remain secondary. What is primary is the propositional attitude, belief, desire, thought, or evaluation expressed in the emotion. The emotion can only be understood through an analysis of the propositional attitude, whatever this may imply: beliefs, judgements, convictions, desires, or complexes of these. Martha Nussbaum, who argues along the same lines as Solomon, writes:

> In order to have fear—as Aristotle already saw—I must believe that bad events are impending; that they are not trivially, but seriously bad; and that I am not entirely in control of warding them off. In order to have anger, I must have an even more complex set of beliefs; that some damage has occurred to me or to something or someone close to me; that the damage is not trivial but significant; that it was done by someone; probably, that it was done willingly. It seems plausible to suppose that every member of this family of beliefs is necessary in order for anger to be present.
>
> (Nussbaum 2001, pp. 28–9)

Nussbaum here argues for the complexity at work in fairly straightforward emotions such as fear and anger. To understand the *what* and *why* of our emotions we need to understand how we think and how we cognitively evaluate the situation in which we feel what we feel. In other words, emotions are embodied judgements about the world and ourselves.

On this account, feelings are reduced to 'add-ons' (to use an expression from Peter Goldie 2000, pp. 40–1). We explain an emotion as we would explain any other mental state, that is, in term of some kind of rational structure, and then only afterwards do we add the particular feelings that are coincidental with this emotion. Feelings are not a necessary part of the explanation of emotions. They are either reduced to some other cognitive state with a propositional content (perception or judgement) or left out of the definition of a given emotion (Nussbaum 2001, p. 60). This may sound familiar. Actually, on the cognitive account, feelings seem to suffer from the same over-intellectualisation that for a long time excluded emotions from serious philosophical investigation. As we saw in the introduction, Russell makes a somewhat peculiar distinction between emotions in our life and emotions in philosophy. They are what makes life interesting and important, but in philosophy they are more of an obstacle if we are to secure a philosophical understanding of what human life is about. It is the same distinction that is at play in the cognitive theory of emotion. Feelings are what make emotions interesting and what make us feel that emotions are important, but they are really just obnoxious when we try to understand our emotional life.

It is obvious that such theories have been met with much scepticism (de Sousa 1987, pp. 40–1, 165–6; Goldie 2000, pp. 74–8; Pugmire 1998, pp. 18–40; Robinson 2005, pp. 5–27; Stocker 1996, pp. 38–51). How can one explain emotions without taking the feeling aspect seriously? When we are in the throes of an emotional experience, the felt nature of that experience seems to dominate it almost completely. When I wake up in the middle of the night by some noise down in the kitchen, I feel my body freeze and my heartbeat racing wildly so that I have difficulty to focus my listening on what is going on and rationally sort out the subdued sounds. 'Do we suddenly have a cat? Is it the kids? My wife is sound asleep besides me, so it is not her. Now it stopped. Was that voices? Where did I put that baseball bat? Should I get up and lock the door? We have insurance, but what about the kids? I must get to the kids. There it was again. There is definitely someone down there. How did they get past the alarm?' All these thoughts race through my mind in a matter of seconds in a confused and rambling order. I do indeed think, but my thinking is very different from when I have to decide on what to buy for dinner. My fear influences my way of thinking in such a way that I come to conclusions and evaluations very different from what I would arrive at in other circumstances. The feelings involved in fear do not seem to be merely 'add-ons' to my way of thinking about something. On the contrary, they appear to permeate and change the very structure and workings of my rationality. One of the classic arguments against the cognitive approach is Michael Stocker's 'fear of flying' objection (Stocker 1996, pp. 38–9). I know that flying is the safest form of transportation and still I am afraid to fly. This may be explained as an irrational emotion, but my feelings cannot be calmed by arguing that statistics demonstrate the belief to be untrue. The fact that air traffic is safe and my feelings therefore inappropriate will not change the emotion. And we do not consider a person an idiot for being afraid. It is just how airplanes make me feel. It may be an inappropriate feeling but it still causes me to choose other and more tedious forms of transportation in order to avoid travelling in an airplane. Feelings cannot be rejected as part of our emotions, and this is simply because the cognitively impenetrable feeling often causes a person to think and act in a certain way.

Despite the tendency to over-intellectualisation and the pale rendering of bodily intensity, cognitive theories contribute with decisive insights about the complex workings of emotions. The focus on responsibility and evaluation brings to the fore aspects of emotional experience that are not caught by the feeling theories. The personal significance and engaged attitude of our emotions point to the subjective and rational meaning of emotion. The cognitive insistence on our being responsible for our emotional reactions and for the emotional character of our general behaviour towards other persons makes the normative nature of emotions central to our understanding of the feelings that accompany our lives and make up a significant part of our dealings with other people. Moreover, the seemingly different emotional reactions to the same situation suggest that we must take the sociocultural dimension of emotions seriously. For these reasons, our own account will make use of several of the insights gained by the long tradition of cognitive theories, in particular the question of responsibility for our emotions. For the time being, however, we will turn to another philosophical account of emotions that is of even more importance for our own account than the two previous ones.

Narrative Theories

In recent years, a new cluster of theories is taking shape. Or more correctly, an old view on emotions has taken a new form. It is an attempt to combine the feeling theory with some aspects of the cognitive theory, because '[f]eelings are, as we all know, at the heart of emotion' (Goldie 2000, p. 12). Here, however, the feelings considered are different from the feelings that we find in the traditional, more biologically orientated, feeling theory. Feelings are said to have a certain structure of intentionality. Also, emotions cannot be reduced to beliefs, desires, or intrinsic cognitive structures, and still they are caused by more than mere internal body states. The most recent and influential advocate of the narrative theory is Peter Goldie (2000, 2003abc, 2004, 2007b), but important earlier formulations can be found in the seminal works of Ronald de Sousa (1987), Charles Taylor (1985, 1989), and Richard Wollheim (1984, 1999). The general idea is even older, though. It draws on insights from continental thinkers such as Freud, Heidegger, Sartre, and, as we have seen, Ricoeur. Roughly put, it insists on the personal aspect of emotional experience. The following short outline of the narrative theory draws mainly on the work of Peter Goldie. His recent account of a narrative theory is by far the most developed and influential version of this new approach to emotions.

An emotion remains unintelligible if we try to approach it from an impersonal stance (Goldie 2002b, p. 249). Emotions tell us something about how a person experiences the world, him- or herself, and other people. Where a more scientifically inspired philosophy aims at explaining the impersonal aspects of the human self and the world, a philosophy of emotions, unavoidably, has to deal with how the self experiences the 'magical world' of emotional experience, that is, emotions as part of a *personal* consciousness. Sartre, whose cognitive suspicion of the 'debased' and 'sleeping' character of our emotional life we do not share, has however described this personal aspect of emotional consciousness cogently:

> [T]he consciousness leaps into the magical world of emotion [*le monde magique de l'émotion*], plunges wholly into it by debasing itself. It is a new consciousness in front of a new world—a world which it constitutes with its own most intimate quality, with that presence to itself [*cette présence à elle-même*], without distance, of its point of view upon the world.
>
> (Sartre 1971, p. 78 [42]; translation modified)

In the more recent formulations of this approach, this personal stance becomes the focal point of a narrative structure that holds together the different elements of an emotion: past episodes of emotional experience, imagination, desire, belief, character traits, and dispositions to feel, think, and act in certain ways. The narrative theory reacts against the belief–desire explanations of emotion, arguing that, while a belief or a desire can be feelingless, an emotion always involves feelings as a fundamental part of its nature. For example, I may have the belief that the fjords in Norway are freezing cold, but I do not feel it unless I go to Norway and dip my toe in one of them; I may desire to go on a tour around the world without experiencing it as an emotion. This is not to say that beliefs and desires do not have important bearings on our emotions. The theory simply insists that a satisfactory understanding of emotions cannot be reduced to belief–desire explanations. The nature of an emotion is a much more complex affair which requires of a theory of emotions that it should 'be holistic in its overall approach, seeing feelings as embedded in an emotion's narrative, as a part of the person's life' (Goldie 2000, p. 51).

This way of investigating the emotions, which we have chosen to name the narrative theory, considers emotions according to how they are experienced by an embodied person situated in a world shared with other people. The experience of emotions is, phenomenologically speaking, a complex phenomenon constituted by intentional feelings, dispositions to act, and moods. Emotional experience is, furthermore, articulated by language and made intelligible by unfolding the stories in which particular feelings of emotion are embedded. Charles Taylor captures this hermeneutical understanding of emotions succinctly:

> I can describe my emotions by describing my situation, and very often must do so really to give the flavour of what I feel. But then I alter the description of my emotions in altering the description I accept of my situation. But to alter my situation-description will be to alter my feelings, if I am moved by my newly perceived predicament. And even if I am not, the old emotion will now seem to me irrational, which itself constitutes a change in what I experience. So we can understand why, in this domain, our formulations about ourselves can alter what they are about.
>
> (Taylor 1985, p. 101)

The emphasis on the feeling aspect and the narrative structure of emotional experience makes it possible for the narrative theory to consider more comprehensively two interconnected features of emotions which will be of central importance to the development of our own account, and whose interdependence is neglected, or at least to some extent remains problematic, in the two previous theories, namely, the phenomenological and the normative aspect of our emotional life, and their entwinement.

Emotions are experienced by a human person. The way a person experiences the world and him- or herself can be explained by different methods that result in different explanations of what it means to be a person. The methods used in the feeling theory are those generally employed in the natural sciences. These rely on empirical data and adopt a third-person perspective on being human. In this way, we gain important insight into the physiological underpinnings of what we normally understand as emotional experience. We learn about the biological nature of what it means to have an emotion and how knowledge about the endogenous functions of the brain may help us to understand why we feel and act the way we do. The methods employed by the cognitive theory, on the other hand, rely on more traditional philosophical analysis of rationality and logic. They explore the nature and definition of our emotional concepts and how these concepts work in the larger structures that govern our cognitive engagement with the world. But neither of these theories deals sufficiently with the phenomenological dimension of emotions. A human person experiences emotions as multifarious feelings endowed with a subjective quality that cannot be explained from a third-person perspective. We may infer from external observations that a person reacts or behaves in a specific way when she is in a given situation and under the influence of certain observable factors, but we can never get beneath the skin of that person, so to say, and come to know how she actually feels in this situation. Human feelings are enclosed in the subjectivity of emotional experience. The fact that much emotion research is carried out with more or less explicit neglect of the first-person perspective is an obvious obstacle to understanding the nature of emotional experience. The narrative theory reacts against this tendency by emphasising the subjective character of feelings (in particular, but not only, by means of a more thorough analysis of the concept of intentionality), and thus provides a welcomed appreciation of the phenomenological dimension of feelings.[2]

Closely related to the phenomenological dimension is the normative nature of emotions. The feelings involved in our experience of the world, other people, and ourselves reveal that what we experience matters in a certain way and means something to us (Taylor 1985, pp. 48–50). The felt quality of emotions obviously influences our state of mind and thus has a significant impact on how we evaluate our experiences. As we saw in Part I, phenomenological analysis of the experiential structures involved in feelings disclose and may help to illuminate the normative character of the emotional experience. In this sense, the narrative theory develops further the focus on evaluation and responsibility that we noted as central to the cognitive theory.

In fact, the normative character of emotions is also implicit in the feeling theory as well as the cognitive theory, but in either case the assumption rests on an ontological conception of human nature that is shown to be problematic by the narrative theory. Although we shall deal with the question of normativity in more detail in Chapter 7, we will here, for the sake of clarity, briefly introduce these implicit conceptions of human nature and say something about how the narrative approach renders them problematic.

The feeling theory is usually rooted in the theoretical soil of some version of evolutionary theory. We are only a tiny and insignificant part of a larger phylogenetic development, and like our mammalian cousins we are dominated by the anonymous forces of survival and reproduction. That is, human nature is first and foremost to be understood in terms of impersonal biological explanations. From the crude soil of organic impulses and physiological reactions the individual human being is imprinted with the basic values that shape and orient its existence. Human values are to be somehow derived from the general mechanisms of natural selection by means of the direct influence of a limited number of primary or basic emotions (fear, surprise, anger, joy, arousal, and so on) or combinations of these emotions. This results in a rather simplistic understanding of the normative principles that guide and orient human existence. Behind the subjective and cognitive illusions about the irreducible complexity of human values, we supposedly find the hard facts of natural selection that direct and further the survival and propagation of the species, often in spite of personal concerns. On this account, in other words, human nature is to be understood in terms of natural selection and neurobiological explanations, and questions of subjectivity and personhood can therefore only have a secondary bearing on the explanations of emotional life. The narrative approach questions this conception of human nature and human emotions by arguing that we cannot explain the nature or function of our emotions without appreciating the personal aspect of our feelings and paying close attention to the narrative structures that constitute the emotions we live our life by. In short, there is more to our feelings than the raw workings of our biological nature.

---

[2] Besides the work of Wollheim, Goldie, Taylor, and de Sousa, Matthew Ratcliffe has recently argued for the importance of what he calls existential feelings (2008, 2009, 2010). As mentioned above, we return to Ratcliffe's account in Chapter 7.

The cognitive theory, on its part, works out the account of human emotions on the basis of another ontological conception of human nature. Here we find a strong confidence in the powers of human rationality. In direct opposition to the sway of natural instincts and evolutionary forces, the cognitive approach insists on the rational nature of our values. Human emotions are characterised by the structure of responsible judgements. These judgements may well be embodied and clothed with bodily feelings, but beneath the surface of these merely sensible commotions we find the responsible mind that judges and acts according to rational or at least intelligible standards. Thus, the normative impetus of emotions may be judged by the same standards as those we employ in more general ethical deliberation. This close connection between emotions and responsibility results in an ethical take on human emotional life that, as mentioned, tends to over-intellectualise emotional experience. Emotions are not ethical, or better, they express a moral randomness that makes the purported rational ideal problematic, to say the least (de Sousa 2006, pp. 35–8). By appreciating the complexity of feelings and approaching them in terms of narrative structures, the narrative theory is able to articulate the normative nature of emotional experience without invoking an untenable principle of rationality or questionable ethical standards of 'good' and 'wrong' behaviour. Goldie argues that an appreciation of the narrative structure of emotions will help articulate this personal and normative nature of our emotional life:

> Our thought and talk of emotions is embedded in an interpretive (and sometimes predictive) narrative which aims to make sense of an aspect of someone's life. These concepts give us, so to speak, the equipment with which to understand, explain, and predict what people think, feel, and do: a personal and thoroughly normative approach; thus the normative force of something *meriting* an emotional response, as opposed to, say, merely causing a response.
>
> (Goldie 2000, p. 103)

Moreover, narrative structures expose the problematic relation between voluntary and involuntary aspects of emotions. Narratives allow for a more nuanced analysis of what we can be held responsible for in our emotional life and what is out of our hand, so to speak; because, as Ricoeur remarked, '[w]hat sedimentation has contracted, the narrative [*le récit*] can redeploy' (1992, p. 122 [148]; translation slightly modified). In this way, the narrative theory argues for a less ethical approach to emotion by emphasising the complex, often ambiguous, normative feature of emotions. It also argues for a less rationalistic approach to emotions. The raw structure of a given emotion can be completely irrational, even a-rational, although I may try to make sense of it and superimpose a rational narrative structure on it. Also, the rationality of an emotion can be (and often is) unconscious. My understanding of the rationality (or belief–desire structure) of my fear of flying is an *après-coup*; the reason(s) why I am afraid of flying are probably presupposed, but do not belong to the phenomenal structure of my fear. Put differently, the intentional structure of my beliefs may well be present, but it is present as the skeleton is present in movement: when I move, my skeleton is obviously there, but I am not aware of it. Emotions are opaque, not transparent. Their 'rational skeleton' is not evident. We need the X-rays of a narrative to make it visible. Emotions require a working-through, an interpretation. *All emotions are opaque*—including affects, as we shall see. As Freud says, in melancholy the person might be 'aware of the loss which has given rise to his melancholy, but only in the sense that he knows *whom* he has lost but not *what* he has lost in him' (Freud 1957, p. 245 [431]; emphases added).

There is no doubt that Goldie's narrative theory is a vital contribution to our understanding of emotion. By considering the intentionality of feelings as essential to emotional experience and using narrative structures in the explanation of emotions, he explores aspects of human emotions that are neglected in both the feeling theory and the cognitive theory. However, in our view, a problem with Goldie's narrative approach is that he does not sufficiently account for the biological dimension of emotions.[3] His focus is elsewhere. His work deals primarily with the intentional and personal aspects of feelings, and he concentrates on narrative explanations of these aspects to such an extent that he leaves aside the fact that emotions are the most profoundly embodied phenomena of human experiences (de Sousa 1987, p. 47).[4]

Therefore, we shall now look more closely at the embodied nature of emotions. As we mentioned earlier, today a theory of human emotion cannot but take into account, at least to a certain degree, the neurobiology of emotions. Thus, the following section will present and discuss two neuroscientific theories of emotions.

Neuroscientific Investigations of Emotions[5]

The embodied nature of emotions is deeply involved in the way emotions and feelings enrich and complicate human life. The phenomenology and conceptual intelligibility of emotions cannot be severed from the biological dimension of these ubiquitous

---

[3] He does, however, provide an insightful discussion about possible evolutionary explanations for the cognitively impenetrable nature of some of our emotions, and argues how these can help us understand certain sorts of *akrasia* (weakness of the will). We will return to the question of the cognitively impenetrable nature of some aspects of our emotional life over the next chapters.

[4] In fact, Goldie argues for 'a profound distinction between the science of human nature and the natural sciences' (2002a, p. 98) in at least three respects. Human nature is characterised by perceptivity, normativity, and historical condition (pp. 106–7), all of which are aspects that cannot be explained by the natural sciences, since they adopt an impersonal perspective (Goldie 2000, pp. 181–2; Goldie 2002b, pp. 249–50). We largely agree to this, but part of our approach to human emotions is to argue that this distinction is less profound, and consequently also more complicated, than Goldie makes it out to be.

[5] Since neither of us is a neuroscientist by training, we have found it wise simply to present the theories without discussing the specific neuroscientific detail involved. Moreover, we have found it necessary to avoid specific neuroanatomical and neurobiological terms as far as possible, since the general ideas of the theories may be described without the technical detail. The anatomy, physiology, and chemistry of the brain are complex matters and require, to be only minimally understood, a long preparatory introduction which cannot be provided here. However, the technical detail is important, and in order to fully understand the scope and argument of the theories presented here one must turn to the references indicated in this section.

phenomena of human life.[6] In other words, the biological nature of emotions is too obviously manifest to be passed over in silence. The fact is that it is often my body which makes me aware that I am experiencing a certain emotion or find myself involved in an emotional episode. I feel a tension in my stomach and uneasiness in my limbs during a conversation with a certain person; I may be drumming my fingers on the desk or moving my feet rapidly under the table. And then, suddenly, I come to realise that I am intensely irritated with something about that person. Bodily feelings are involved in the expression and experience of most emotions.

One way to investigate the role of the bodily feelings in emotions is to look at the neurobiological properties and dynamics involved in emotional experience. Over the last couple of decades, three scientists in particular have set the agenda for the bridging of philosophical and neuroscientific study of emotions: Antonio Damasio, Joseph LeDoux, and Jaak Panksepp. All three have done extensive research on various aspects of the neural underpinnings of emotions. Damasio's most important contribution concerns the critical role of emotions in human decision-making (1994) and the connection between consciousness and emotion (1999, 2010), whereas LeDoux has worked mainly on the basic emotional mechanisms common to humans and other animals (in particular insights on emotional learning and emotional memory derived from the study of fear-conditioning in rats) without including the subjective dimension of emotions (1996). Panksepp, on the contrary, is primarily concerned with the subjective dimension (the feeling) of emotions in the functioning of the mammalian brain. He differs from both Damasio and LeDoux (who both mainly deal with the cortical elaboration of emotions) by stressing the sub-neocortical dynamics of affectivity (1998). In what follows, we shall outline Damasio's and Panksepp's theories of the neurobiological dimension of emotions. We shall then argue that Panksepp's research is more congenial to a philosophical approach to human affectivity because of its emphasis on the subjective experience of emotions.

Damasio's contribution to the philosophical investigation of emotions is undeniable. He has convincingly shown that the feeling aspect of emotion is fundamental to our understanding, not only of emotions, but of all cognitive processes. He concentrates on what he has named the somatic-marker hypothesis. By and large, the somatic marker consists of gut feelings 'that increase the accuracy and efficiency of the decision process' (1994, p. 173). Examining neuropathological cases Damasio comes to the conclusion that 'cool' reasoning is not enough to trigger a decision. A person would never be able to decide on anything without the help of bodily induced emotions. He would be in the undesirable state of infinite possibilities of equal (or no) importance. The bodily induced emotions are what highlights some possibilities and not others. That is, emotions are what qualify our experience as a set of affordances that present themselves to

---

[6] Ricoeur argues that it is the affective dimension of subjectivity that evidences the ontological dimension of subjective experience (1966, p. 88 [84]; 1987, p. 103 [119]). The subject's being in the world is revealed by the feelings; it *is* already in the world before it comes to *know* about its being in the world. The particular nature of subjectivity is determined by our being a subject inexorably rooted in the biological nature of our body, considered as an object among objects.

us as feelings of what is the most convenient, appropriate, or reasonable among different possible choices.

Damasio arrives at this theory from the study of, among others, a young man in his thirties whom he—for the sake of discretion—refers to as Eliot. Eliot was an intelligent man, a good husband and father, who tragically developed a large tumour that ended up covering both frontal lobes. Fortunately, the tumour was benign and successfully removed by surgical intervention. During the intervention, though, much of the frontal tissue that had been damaged was completely removed. This had a critical impact on Eliot's life. He had undergone a radical change of personality, even though his mental skills and memory appeared to be completely intact. He became unrecognisable in the eyes of his friends and nearest family. In other words, 'Eliot was no longer Eliot' (p. 36). He was never happy nor sad, incapable of decision, and unable to focus on longer-term projects. Moreover, he always remained uncommonly controlled and indifferent even when he told about the tragedies of his life (divorces, unemployment, and bankruptcy). As Damasio writes: 'I began to think that the cold-bloodedness of Eliot's reasoning prevented him from assigning different values to different options, and made his decision-making landscape hopelessly flat' (p. 51). Against the background of the dramatic changes in Eliot's character, Damasio formed the hypothesis that reason on its own is not able to make a choice. Experience has to be somatically marked in terms of feelings in order to guide stable conscious choices. In this sense, feelings are what makes our particular life matter to us, and the qualification of our experience springs from our ability to feel the world and ourselves: 'consciousness *feels* like a feeling, and if it feels like a feeling, it may well be a feeling' (1999, p. 312).

On the basis of the somatic-marker hypothesis (i.e. the importance of bodily feelings), Damasio has over the years developed a fine-grained neuroscientific theory of the emotions. On the following pages, we shall present a very rough outline of his main ideas on emotions and feelings, and then we shall give the reasons why we prefer Panksepp's model to his.

Damasio's account is a variant of the James–Lange theory, namely, that emotions are basically feelings of bodily changes. However, it shows two important differences from the earlier theory. The first is the possibility that feelings can be activated endogenously by 'as-if' loops that bypass the body and simply stimulate somatic brain areas. We can experience feelings without actual bodily reactions, which saves both time and energy and provides a more nuanced picture of the feelings (in the sense that not all feelings are directly involved with the body). The second difference is Damasio's emphasis on unconscious emotions. The brain can register alterations in the bodily landscape without this resulting in conscious feelings, because '[e]motions can be induced in a nonconscious manner and thus appear to the conscious self as seemingly unmotivated' (1999, p. 48). For example, we may smile or sob spontaneously without knowing why. We may be at unease in a certain situation without being aware of what bothers us. But, by and large, Damasio sticks to the general idea of emotions as constituted primarily of bodily changes (e.g. visceral, musculoskeletal, and hormone alterations). The body is a 'theatre of the emotions' (1994, p. 155), in that our emotional responses always originate, in some way or the other, in the 'internal milieu' of somatic reactions. These physiological responses, triggered by certain brain systems when the organism represents objects and situations, are part of the bioregulatory devices fundamental for the survival and well-being of the organism. Put simply, our emotional reactions can basically be reduced to regulations of the automatic 'homeostasis machine' that approaches or avoids certain objects (2003, pp. 30–1) in accordance with pleasure and pain (2004, p. 51).

Damasio's model is worked out by means of the methodological distinction between emotions and feelings. Although emotions and feelings are part of the same process, they are nevertheless two separate mechanisms: 'While emotions are actions accompanied by ideas and certain modes of thinking, emotional feelings are mostly perceptions of what our bodies do during the emoting, along with perceptions of our state of mind during that same period of time' (2010, p. 110). On the one side, we have emotions, which are consistent physiological reactions that span from the basic process of metabolism (automatic mechanisms of internal chemical balances) over simple pain and pleasure behaviours (reactions of approach or withdrawal) and drives and motivation (appetites such as hunger, thirst, or curiosity) to emotions-proper (such as happiness, sadness, disgust, surprise). On the other, we have feelings that function as a mere 'readout' of these physiological reactions, that is, mental patterns that map or perceive bodily changes. Sometimes this mapping is a straightforward readout; it can, however, also function by means of the 'as-if-body-loop' that provides a pure neural map of the body state, but, in some way or another, it always functions in reference to the body. Alongside the perception of the bodily changes, feelings also depend on the subjective state of the experiencing organism:

> A feeling about a particular object is based on the subjectivity of the perception of the object, the perception of the body state it engenders, and the perception of modified style and efficiency of the thought process as all of the above happens. (1994, pp. 147–8)

This leaves us with a picture of two separate physiological processes, emotions and feelings, at the core of what we know as emotional experience. Emotions are objective and public, whereas feelings are subjective and hidden. Hence, we are able to observe and investigate the emotions, since these are engendered by measurable and clear biological changes, but the workings of the feelings remain in 'complete privacy' (2000, p. 15). We have to derive our understanding of feelings from what we are able to discover about the emotions. Damasio goes on to produce elaborate accounts of how human beings come around to have the enormous variety of feelings that they actually have, but he always returns to the idea that feelings are strictly bound to the body (even if the body is only virtually present) because of the simple fact that 'the body is the main stage for emotions' (1999, p. 287). Accordingly, he boils the variety of human feelings down to six universal feelings that are coined on the six universal emotions derived from facial expression and recognisability: fear, anger, sadness, disgust, surprise, and happiness (p. 285).[7]

---

[7] Damasio here accepts the distinctions worked out by the renowned research of the psychologist Paul Ekman, who holds these emotions to be universal across cultures and gender. Ekman defined the basic emotions according to several characteristics: distinctive universal signals, presence in other primates, quick onset, brief duration, automatic appraisal, etc. (Ekman 1992, p. 175; see also Ekman 2003 for a systematic and elaborate account of this idea).

Damasio's theory of emotion faces the old question that Cannon addressed to the James–Lange theory in 1927. Can such a theory of feelings as perception or readout of bodily changes account for the subtle and multifarious nature of actual human feelings? We believe not, and this mainly because of the methodological distinction of feelings and emotions. If we operate with such a distinction (private vs public, subjective vs objective), we ironically end up with the same Cartesian distinction that Damasio fights so hard against (the title of his famous 1994 book is *Descartes' Error*). Whereas Descartes maintains a strict distinction between deanimated bodies (*res extensa*) and disembodied spirits (*res cogitans*), Damasio transfers this distinction inside the human skull by talking about feelings as a mental readout of a mindless body. As Shaun Gallagher observes regarding Damasio's problematic conception of the embodied mind: 'the details of this embodiment are worked out in terms that either inflate the body to the level of ideas in a phenomenologically untenable way, or reduce it to neuronal processes' (2005, p. 135). The body thus becomes an entirely depersonalised object rooted so firmly in the theoretical soil of evolution that the conscious person's active, practical, and thoroughly personal relation to his or her body is only seen as a feeble and useless scratching on the harder surface of an objective and anonymous nature. Damasio is right, though, when he observes that the body will have its ways despite the conscious struggle of the person. We have to understand the life of the body in order to understand the life of the person who is that body. He calls attention (as most palaeontologists, neuroscientists, and evolutionary theorists) to the fact that the mind is only a conglomerate of newly developed brain systems deeply embedded in millions and millions of years of evolution (1994, p. 254). We agree with Damasio that one must accept that the body has its reasons, its own intelligibility (the working of the emotions) that is ultimately related to the need for survival (1994, pp. 262–4).

We do not in any way question the importance of emotions as embodied appraisals carried out in terms of registration of physiological responses in the body. On the contrary, we believe that emotions are intrinsically linked with the body. We do have a problem, though, with Damasio's conception of the body and its presumed relation to our cognitive faculties. Ricoeur's analysis of the body disclosed an ambivalence in our conception of the body. The body is both *my* body and *a* body. On the one hand, it is *my* personal body by means of which *I* access the world, that is, a body characterised by the person that I am (when and where I was born, how I was brought up and educated, physical constitution, etc.). On the other hand, it is *a* body by virtue of the fact that it is an object in, and part of, an anonymous nature which determines many of the reactions of that body, that is, it is basically just an organism among other organisms in nature. This ambivalence of the body is missed in Damasio's account of emotions, and the cognitive element (judgement and intentionality) is therefore reduced to a somewhat strange, artificial elaboration of the real, basic emotions. We believe that Peter Goldie is right to question the use of the notion 'basic emotions' to explain the (neuro)physiological workings in our instinctive responses to the environment. The evolutionary explanations of our emotional experiences and reactions cannot take the place of the way we ordinarily explain our emotions. Our explanations always involve personal and social interpretations that formulate and thus determine our understanding of why we feel the way we feel. The supposed elimination of commonsense psychology in evolutionary explanations of complex emotions as derived from context-free and timeless basic emotions tends to peel away all the personal and narrative layers that normally clothe our emotional experience. We cannot explain a person's enduring feelings and actions by appealing to basic emotions as universal and timeless reactions to environmental factors. There may be some general, perhaps even universal, features that characterise, for example, anger, joy, or surprise, but the attempt to derive all the various feelings involved in our anger, joy, or surprise from a more or less specific set of basic emotions will necessarily impair our understanding of how human persons experience, reflect on, and cope with such emotions. Thus, instead of talking about 'basic emotions', Goldie suggests that we use the term 'affect programs' that influence and condition our specifically human emotions. By doing so, we avoid reducing the variety of human feelings to a specific number of so-called evolutionary basic emotions, while still acknowledging that evolutionary factors play a significant part in our emotional life (Goldie 2000, pp. 105–6). As we shall see in a moment, this is exactly the strategy of Jaak Panksepp.

The body has its reasons, but we cannot isolate these reasons from the person who feels and acts through that body. In the course of a life, the body becomes a part of the subject in such a way that the individual person is shaped by the body, but the body is also shaped by the subjectivity that it expresses (Gallagher 2005). For example, on a pure neurobiological level, the body of a skilled athlete differs only minimally from that of an immobile academic, and yet the two persons have completely different bodily expressions and different experiences of those expressions. Their bodies are, at least in this sense, radically different from one another. A neuroscientific investigation of the emotions that operates with such a methodological distinction between emotions (body) and feelings (mind) will not be able to interact with a more phenomenologically based account. We mentioned earlier that Damasio's account of the emotions suffers from the simplicity of his view on human subjectivity, and this becomes obvious in his reduction of feelings to perceptions of anonymous physiological reactions.

We have therefore chosen another neuroscientific theory of emotions as the background for our own account. Strangely enough, since we argue for the personal aspect of emotions, this theory comes from a scientist who insists on the necessity of cross-species animal research for understanding human emotions.

Over the last thirty years, Panksepp has argued for the need for more basic cross-species neuroscientific research if we are to understand the neural underpinnings of human emotional experience:

> [T]he best we can presently achieve is the identification of essential neural components shared by all mammals, some of which may suffice to generate raw affective experiences—ancient experiential capacities I call *affective consciousness*. (2004a, p. 48)

Panksepp argues that emotional experience at the cortical level is not merely a result of more recently developed neocortical cognitive capacities such as memory, attention, and cognition, and thus he persistently criticises the cognitive and behavioural neurosciences for ignoring the affective nature of human consciousness (e.g. 2001, p. 136; 2003, pp. 11–12; 2004b; 2005c, pp. 166–8). The picture of the human brain presented by the cognitive and behavioural neurosciences is envisaged on the ground of a neodualism that is even stronger than the old Cartesian one—at least Descartes allows animals to have various passions (1998, p. 340). This neodualism (which he believes to be at work in both LeDoux and Damasio) assumes that emotional experience did not exist before the development of higher brain functions (the human neocortex, in particular). Other animals do not have conscious experience and thus cannot feel emotions, but merely react with instinctive emotional behaviour, enabled by a combination of working memory and specific emotional systems concentrated in the limbic system. Emotional experience is therefore particularly human and must be explained by way of the cognitive elaboration of bodily reactions. Accepting this presupposition, we end up with Damasio's sharp distinction between objective emotions and subjective (human) feelings as the only viable approach to the nature of human emotion (2005a, p. 25). On the one side, we have the ancient emotions developed and refined throughout the eons of evolution, and on the other, the cognitive skills as newly evolved capacities (language, symbols, long-term memory, etc.) that in humans have given rise to much more complex and elaborate emotional experiences (feelings) and the ensuing sophisticated behaviour.[8]

As a reaction to this traditional view, some twenty years ago Panksepp established what he calls affective neuroscience. Contrary to the other branches of neuroscience, affective neuroscience aims at explaining 'the existential reality of our deepest moods and emotions' (1998, p. 14). The central working hypothesis is that emotional experience, including subjectively experienced feelings, plays a vital role in the chain of causation that determines the actions of both humans and other animals. And, more importantly, the subjective nature of feelings does not exclude the possibility of scientific investigation. Panksepp argues that we have to begin emotion research by investigating the neurophysiology of the various sub-neocortical emotional systems that are homologous in all mammalian brains. These systems generate different 'raw affects' or 'raw feels' that instantiate intrinsic emotional values which, on their part, inform and basically orient the animal in the environment. Human and other mammal behaviour originates from the interplay of different basic affective values. The mammalian brain functions at a basic level as an affective consciousness, and cross-species research can help to clarify the neural underpinning of many basic human behavioural patterns. In short, Panksepp's main claim is that the mammalian brain is primarily affective. The brain interacts with the environment on the basis of certain felt values, and the higher brain functions that characterise humans cannot be understood in isolation from these

---

[8] Panksepp does, however, admire and largely agree with the work of both Damasio and LeDoux (1998, p. 340; 2003, p. 7; 2004b, p. 181). What he resists is the methodological watershed between objective and subjective aspects of emotion. While Damasio argues for the importance of feelings, LeDoux is more radical in his approach and considers the conscious affective aspect of emotions (feelings) to be largely epiphenomenal. He concludes his influential book *The Emotional Brain* with a harsh rejection of conscious feelings in the architecture and dynamics of human emotions: 'Emotions evolved not as conscious feelings, linguistically differentiated or otherwise, but as brain states and bodily responses. The brain states and bodily responses are the fundamental facts of an emotion, and the conscious feelings are the frills that have added icing to the emotional cake' (LeDoux 1996, p. 302).

basic affective value systems, or be thought to function as 'top-down' readouts of mere bodily affects (2004b, p. 179). Higher brain functions are themselves immersed in the affective dimension of ethological life, and to understand what is particular about human feelings we have to begin with a 'bottom-up' perspective, that is, with investigations which 'help clarify pre-propositional affective psychodynamics that emerge from sub-neocortical regions of the brain' (2005c, p. 173). Combining the experimental advances of animal study with a phenomenological approach, we get a more refined picture of the emotional brain, where 'emotional affects may be thoroughly embedded within the extended activities of brain operating systems that orchestrate certain instinctual action patterns' (2005b, p. 38).

Panksepp calls this research strategy *dual-aspect monism*, and he considers it to be the only way to challenge the classical behaviourism that is still very much alive in neuroscience. We have to consider the complexities of the brain, both causal and psychological properties, as being of one nature that nonetheless has to be studied from different (or at least two) perspectives. The sub-neocortical affect systems that cause instinctual behaviour and the higher cognitive functions that, by experience and education, develop and refine these instincts are two sides of the same coin and must be linked together in order to identify 'basic dynamic features of brain and mind, such as emotional instinctive expressions and the corresponding affective states, in empirically productive ways' (2005c, p. 163). This approach paves the way for scientific research of the causal foundation of affective consciousness in all mammals, and not only of the neural correlates of human cognitive elaboration of bodily emotions. If we consider cross-species basic affects systems to influence and constrain, with varying intensity, all human cognitions and actions, we obtain a paradigm to study the neuroevolutionary mechanisms involved in the feelings that influence the experience and action of humans. Neuroscience can thereby stick to observable causal dynamics and properties of affective consciousness without simplistic speculations about the far more complex function of the neocortex. We cannot say anything even slightly definitive about the higher brain functions, let alone the way the different basic neocortical systems (e.g. auditory, vestibular, somatic sensory, and visual systems) cooperate to make up what we know as human conscious experience. So, although Panksepp's thesis about core affective consciousness in animals may seem unsubstantiated speculation, since we cannot verify such a seemingly radical presupposition, his strategy is not more invalid or radical than Damasio's elaborate speculations about feelings as mental images about bodily responses. They both presume more than can be empirically verified.[9] In our opinion, however, Panksepp provides a better foundation for an interdisciplinary

---

[9] Panksepp is critical of the enthusiasm generated by the newly acquired brain imaging techniques, since the results are often based on fragile and 'blind' experiential data (what are we looking for? And how do we decipher the images of the living brain?): 'Cross-species, experimental analysis, where key brain variables are evaluated, provides an approach that is not full of false negatives and misleading "neuro-echoes" as is modern fMRI. The interweaving of animal neurobehavioral and human neuropsychological research permits substantive dynamic analyses of the core emotions and their associated feelings' (2005a, p. 26).

approach to human affectivity because of his insistence on the feeling aspect of emotions. He does not drive a methodological wedge between emotions and feelings, but insists on the latter as the most viable access to the first. His dual-aspect monism involves an evolutionary account without excluding feelings as being merely subjective 'frills that have added icing to the emotional cake' (LeDoux 1996, p. 302) cooked up by primordial evolutionary processes. Feelings cannot be methodologically separated from emotions. Their burgeoning presence in human life reminds us that emotional processes are to be considered as unified experiential states, and that these states rely on both objectively detectable evolutionary mechanisms shared by all mammals *and* subjective regulation and refinement due to intrinsic differences in brain structure (e.g. the neocortex in humans) and elaborate social interaction. Affective neuroscience does not tie human feelings to the body. On the contrary, it seeks to clarify the neurobiological foundation for 'the full emotional feeling state' that 'ramifies throughout the organism' by considering the core affective systems 'which can be regulated, but not created, by higher cortico-cognitive activities' (2005b, p. 64). Panksepp does not speculate about how humans actually regulate the core affective processes, neither does he pretend that neuroscientific research can effectively clarify the abundant and unique variety of human emotional life (1998, p. 42). He simply suggests that human feelings are tethered to the primary affective consciousness of the mammalian brain, and argues that a neuroscientific elucidation of the systems operating in this affective consciousness will help understand some of the aspects of the human condition, which is, like that of other animals, deeply embedded in affectivity.

Now, what exactly is Panksepp's proposal for a primary affective consciousness that may help explain the affective nature of human consciousness? He operates with the acronym SELF (Simple Ego-type Life Form) which is an affective consciousness deeply embedded within the brain (1998, p. 309; 2004a, p. 50; 2005c, pp. 178–9). This is a kind of primordial 'self-representation' or 'self-schema' that supposedly originated in the brain stem and developed from the organised motor processes in the midbrain. It is primordial in the sense that it is largely independent of higher cortico-cognitive processes, and therefore not able to account for what we know as human consciousness. It operates as an 'archaic SELF-representation network' (1998, p. 309) that generates basic instinctual behaviour in all mammals. The dynamics internal to this network constitutes an affective consciousness that reacts directly to environmental stimuli by initiating endogenous sensory and emotional responses within the subcortical areas of the brain. The reverberations caused by this affective relation to the environment are critical for 'the most crucial biological values that all mammals share' (1998, p. 183). The mammalian brain is genetically geared to respond in certain ways to the environment, and these response-systems influence the more developed behaviour of humans:

> Once the SELF is considered a very basic brain/mind function rather than being just the highest form of human consciousness, it becomes only natural to consider the existence of objective, nomothetic SELF processes in species other than humans, to consider how such processes may subserve the very genesis of consciousness, and thus to develop a neurobiologically-based trans-species model of a core-SELF. We consequently conceptualize the

core-SELF as a coherent affectively anchored brain function and assume evolutionary continuity and progression from ancestral animals to humans.

(Panksepp and Northoff 2009, pp. 195–6)

The instinctual nature of the core-SELF is structured by various emotional and motivational operating systems that encode endogenous neurodynamic value structures. These value structures are experienced by the self as raw feelings of pleasure and pain that provide it with instinctual choices of responding to the stimuli of the environment. It may seem paradoxical to use the term 'experience' when speaking of instinctual behaviour or talking about instinctual choices, but Panksepp's idea is that the core-SELF experiences internal raw feelings about what is the most appropriate choice or response without having to *think* about it. It is an affective consciousness that *feels* the value of certain stimuli and thereby initiates a certain reaction. The behaviour, however, is not reflective but instinctive in nature, that is, the system responds immediately without delay due to cognitive elaboration. In other words, '[o]ur sub-neocortical animalian brain, with its many basic attentional, emotional and motivational systems, may actually lie at the center of our mental universe' (2004a, p. 49). What is important in relating instinctual affective values common to all mammals to the mental universe of humans is the general idea that the mammalian brain has 'a multidimensional conscious sense of self' (1998, p. 300). To understand the complexity of human emotions, we have to take into account that our more humanly refined emotional reactions are rooted in a 'multidimensional' affective sense of self, which is influenced by basic biological values besides the more reflective values that we consider to be properly human. In this sense, one could say that the reason why human emotions are so difficult to handle has to do with the fact that to feel both the need for justice and love and the need for pleasure and sleep is part of being a human self. This is also one of the corollaries of Ricoeur's theory: our sense of selfhood is troubled and often conflictual, because the values we live by are deeply heterogeneous in the sense that they involve both basic, vital desires (e.g. sleep, food, pleasure) and more reflective or spiritual desires (e.g. justice, recognition, and happiness).

For more than a decade now, Panksepp has identified and refined seven distinct endogenous emotional systems in the sub-neocortical structures of the multidimensional nature of the mammalian SELF (1998, pp. 125–298; 2006, pp. 777–80). These systems all exhibit a certain 'affect logic' that prevails in human cognitive deliberations and can also be envisioned in basic instinctual animal behaviour:

> My main point is that affective feelings are, to a substantial degree, distinct neurobiological processes in terms of anatomical, neurochemical, and various functional criteria, including peripheral bodily interactions. Emotional and motivational feelings are unique experientially valenced 'state spaces' that help organisms make cognitive choices—e.g., to find food when hungry, water when thirsty, warmth when cold, and companionship when lonely or lusty. (2003, p. 6)

The enormous variety of human affective feelings has, at its core, raw affective experiences that 'appear to be pre-propositional gifts of nature' (2005c, p. 169).

The seven systems that generate the affective internal 'state space' are: *seeking, fear, rage, lust, care, play,* and *panic*.[10] Affective experience is saturated with intrinsic values that pertain to these basic systems. The systems function without cognitive interference and can therefore be investigated through a cross-species approach. Here we will not explain the mechanisms involved in all the systems, but we shall provide a brief outline of the main dynamics of *seeking*, since the dynamics of the other systems largely reflect those involved in this one. We have chosen *seeking*, because among all the emotional systems Panksepp dedicates most time and detail to this specific system. It constitutes the affective background for appetitive activities and thus influences all motivated mammalian behaviour (1998, p. 146).

Seeking is characterised by a certain feeling tone that 'leads organisms to eagerly pursue the fruits of their environment – from nuts to knowledge, so to speak' (1998, p. 145). It mediates all the appetitive desires that drive and motivate the animal to engage with the environment. Moreover, the system is self-stimulating. That is, the animal is not a passive recipient of stimuli from the environment, but does, on a 'voluntary' basis, regulate the activity that these stimuli produce in the system. When, for example, the appetite for food is satisfied, the system inhibits the intensity of the stimuli regulating nutrition. This view, then, is opposed to the classical behaviourist view on animal behaviour, since it presupposes an evaluative affective experience that does not agree with a 'cold' mechanistic conception of pleasure and reward. The animal actually feels the raw values pertaining to objects or events in the environment and thereby establishes an interactive relationship to the environment based on these felt values. Panksepp can therefore talk of 'state spaces' in primary process consciousness. The system accounts for the animal's interaction with its environment in terms of affective values. The animal orients itself in its engagement with surrounding world by means of affective values generated by the structure and dynamics internal to the system. The same mechanisms are at stake in the other systems, and together the different systems structure the primordial encounter with the world as that of an affective consciousness which registers and reacts to certain biological values. On this account, 'affect is an organically embodied part of subcortical instinctual-emotional systems that arouse basic *action-to-perception* processes' (2001, p. 136). In other words, perception is shaped by the affective states of the animal that perceives.

In humans, the values experienced as raw feelings have a 'profound influence over what we think and do' (2004b, p. 177), largely because the affective values generated in the basic systems shape and influence the perception of ourselves and the environment. The systems of primal affective and motivational processes that we share with other animals may well be foundational in the evolution of many of the cognitive skills that characterise human

---

[10] In his works, Panksepp normally capitalises these seven core affective systems (e.g. SEEKING, CARE) in order to highlight the affective import of these operating systems that govern the respective instinctual urges. He also does so to indicate the primordial nature of these systems, which are common to all mammals, since as such they do not allow for a simple translation into human emotions. They are a rudimentary and basic form of affectivity that characterises all mammalian life and therefore influences and shapes human emotional life, but they do not exhaust the affective nature of human emotions and feelings.

existence (2003, p. 8). We cannot, according to Panksepp, approach the feeling aspect of our mental life with a methodological separation of the neurobiological properties pertaining to bodily states and those pertaining to the particularly human neocortical capacities. Feelings are not more subjective than emotions. Emotions *are* feelings, even though many of these feelings may not be articulated as conscious affordances. The unconscious feelings need not be articulated conceptually in order to influence human behaviour. We may behave or feel in ways that are cognitively impenetrable. On the other hand, not all human feelings are determined by these core emotional systems, although they may find some of their energy or bodily feeling in more raw feeling-states. Therefore, the individuation of sub-neocortical systems of core feelings does not exclude the peculiar and profound character of psychic feelings (1998, pp. 329–30).

It is in connection with psychic feelings, i.e. feelings with no immediate relation to core emotional systems, that we find what we believe to be the most valuable feature of Panksepp's model, namely, his patient attempt to incorporate into his neuroscientific work a more philosophical approach to human subjectivity. His long-standing insistence on a cross-mammalian affective consciousness has recently brought him into touch with contemporary theories of subjectivity, in particular phenomenological accounts. In collaboration with the psychiatrist and philosopher Georg Northoff, he has developed a notion of selfhood that is informed by both neuroscience and phenomenological theories. They distinguish three levels of selfhood:

> First, the foundational relational self—the proto-SELF, which is characterized as pre-phenomenal and pre-conscious since as such it is not yet accessible to subjective experience at this level. Second, the affective core-SELF, that can be described as pre-linguistic, pre-conceptual and pre-reflective but characterized by phenomenal consciousness, and with primitive learning (e.g., classical conditioning), being able to develop object-relationships with the world. Finally, the third, the reflectively aware or cognitive selves that allow organisms to reflect upon the relationship within and to the environment, all of which requires access or reflective consciousness.
>
> (Panksepp and Northoff 2009, p. 200)

Most of Panksepp's work concentrates on the second level, the core-SELF, but the connection with, on the one hand, the more evolutionarily primitive proto-SELF and, on the other, the human-specific, reflective self provides a sophisticated model for understanding why and how human life is rooted in and continuously shaped by subjectively experienced affective values.[11] All mammalian life is endowed with selfhood, or at least

---

[11] Although he recognises the explanatory gap between the neural, sub-personal level of consciousness and the conscious, personal level, Panksepp is quite optimistic about the future possibilities for bringing light to this multidimensional conscious sense of self: 'We can do this systematically if we recognize that there are (1) primary processes (unconditioned aspects of mind), (2) secondary processes (learning and memory), and (3) in some highly cerebrated species, tertiary processes (thought, deliberations, etc.). Even though the latter can only be well studied in humans, we have so far had the most to offer scientifically for understanding the second. We are also well-positioned to tackle the first, the neural nature of primary-process affective experiences (raw consciousness?), which may be the foundation for many higher aspects of the human mind, that so far can only be decoded through language' (2010, p. xxiv).

an affective sense of self. Even before the development of consciousness or experiential feelings, the proto-SELF is functionally structured as self. Organisms at this level are obviously not aware of being a self, but they function as a structurally individuated self. This pre-conscious structure of selfhood characterises most vertebrates that do not have a sufficiently developed brain to actually interact with the environment in terms of affective values. At the second and third level, organisms actively interact with the environment in virtue of a basic *felt* sense of being a self. At all three levels, however, selfhood is characterised as being relational in nature. To be a self is to relate, in some way or other, to the environment, and at the two more complex levels, to relate to oneself as a self that relates itself to the environment. The transition from pre-conscious to conscious relation is marked by affectivity. Panksepp and Northoff describe this affective transition in the following way:

> We suppose the proto-SELF to be relational at its core thus constituting a selective and adaptive relation between the organism's body and its respective environment. The proto-SELF may thus be characterized as a relational self; this implicit relational self may by itself not be accessible to phenomenal consciousness and subjective awareness yet and may therefore be characterized as pre-phenomenal and pre-conscious. However, this archaic relational proto-SELF as pre-phenomenal and pre-conscious, provides the basis and foundation for phenomenal and subjective experience to be possible which, as we assume, occurs once the proto-relational SELF comes to be linked to affective processing and thus to emotions. In this sense the proto-SELF may be said to be constitutive and necessary for the core-SELF to emerge as an affective functional unity with a raw form of phenomenal consciousness and subjective experience, what we would call 'affective consciousness'. What is subjectively experienced here is the relation of one's body to the incentives in the environment as well as internally generated emotional arousals—the core-SELF thus enables the organism to access this relation in terms of subjective experience, e.g., a primitive form of phenomenal consciousness, which at this level is essentially affective.
>
> (Panksepp and Northoff 2009, p. 196)

Panksepp's theory of a multidimensional notion of selfhood will function as the neuroscientific background against which we will unfold the following investigation of the relationship between emotion and personhood. The intricate relation between affectivity, values, and relational selfhood paves the way for an understanding of emotions that considers both the biological and personal dimension of human affectivity. The insistence on the affective nature of subjectivity both supports and challenges views in contemporary phenomenology. On the one hand, Panksepp argues for a basic notion of self, a core-SELF, that comes very close to the kind of pre-reflective, minimal self that phenomenologists argue for (Zahavi 2005, p. 146). On the other hand, his equally persistent claim that this basic notion of self is essentially relational and affective in nature challenges the notion of a minimal self in that it makes the minimal sense of self more unstable than it is usually conceived in phenomenology. In this sense, his notion of selfhood is closer to the hermeneutical understanding of selfhood that we find in Ricoeur's theory. But more about this in the following chapters.

To sum up: Panksepp's neuroscientific model provides a significant alternative to the account developed by Damasio in two regards of particular interest to our hermeneutical approach. First, he insists on the need for cross-species research on the sub-neocortical structures and dynamics of the mammalian brain. Contrary to Damasio's focus on the prefrontal cortex and on sophisticated cognitive reading of somatic changes in the bodily landscape, Panksepp opts for a model of mammalian affectivity, which attempts to envisage basic affective values that control and orient cross-species mammalian behaviour. He does not work with a categorical distinction between rational humans and other non-rational animals. All mammals are endowed with a subjective experience of the world that may not amount to a rational, reflective or conceptual mind, but can be characterised as a basic affective consciousness. He argues for a cross-species notion of affective consciousness that encompasses the variety of mammalian affectivity and provides a neurobiological foundation of our species-specific investigation of human emotional life:

> If other mammals do, in fact, experience subjective emotional states such as fear, then it may be possible to study the underlying brain mechanisms reasonably directly through an analysis of their instinctual emotional behaviors and arrive at credible working hypotheses concerning the evolutionary sources of basic human affective capacities.
>
> (Panksepp 2004c, p. 512)

This insistence on a general mammalian affectivity entails, secondly, that Panksepp prefers to talk about affectivity and affective systems rather than feelings and emotions. It is difficult to apply concepts such as feelings and emotions to non-rational animals, since these concepts are the reflective result of our particularly human way to handle and make sense of our affective nature. Emotions such as love and shame seem inappropriate when talking about rats or dolphins, as is the case with feelings such as anxiety or sadness when it comes to dogs or elephants. We can surely insist on understanding non-rational animals in this way, but it can hardly qualify as anything other than a Disney-like projection of our emotional life onto that of other animals. On the other hand, it is equally difficult to maintain a watershed between humans and other animals when it comes to understanding our emotional life. A majority of our basic instincts and affective reactions are, like many of our anatomical structures and neurobiological mechanisms, too similar to those of other mammalian species to be considered categorically different. Since Darwin it has become gradually less feasible to investigate human biological life in isolation from other mammalian species, and with the astonishing development in our understanding of the evolution of the human brain it seems outright nonsensical to insist on doing so today. Since human emotions and feelings are the most embodied of mental phenomena, and as such shaped and influenced by the biological constitution of human nature, we need a model that takes into account the biological dimension of emotions without neglecting what is particularly human about human emotions.

In our opinion, Panksepp's model is more successful in doing so than that of Damasio. Panksepp insists that human emotional life is deeply rooted in the common soil of mammalian affectivity, but he does not try, as so many evolutionarily inspired accounts do, to wring the colours and subtleties of human emotional life out of a restricted number of basic mammalian emotions. Neither does he conjure up philosophically barren, or at least highly dubious, hypotheses about the interaction between cognition and emotion in terms of sophisticated prefrontal readouts of physiological changes in the bodily landscape. Panksepp's refined model starts from the explicit hypothesis that cognition and emotion are intrinsically interwoven in human consciousness. And what is even more important for the account that we will develop in following chapters, he opposes Damasio's distinction between objective emotions and subjective feelings by arguing for the traditional phenomenological claim that human consciousness is characterised by subjectivity.[12]

Concepts, Phenomenology, and Ontology

There are many ways to approach and make sense of human emotional life. Here we have only outlined some major philosophical and neuroscientific approaches. As we have seen, there are many reasons why emotions and feelings are so difficult to handle conceptually, to name or even explain to ourselves. We believe that most of these difficulties stem from the fact that emotions are the most embodied of our mental states. This embodied character involves two aspects of our emotional life that tend to complicate our conceptual understanding of emotions. Our feelings, desires, impulses, and sensations are all deeply enmeshed in our biological nature. On the other hand, though, the biological roots of our feelings and desires are always influenced and shaped by the cognitive capacities and personal attitudes that characterise a human being. So the fundamental challenge to an account of human emotions is to think these two aspects together without neglecting the paramount importance of either of them.

[12] Recently, in a long interview with the philosopher Shaun Gallagher, Panksepp has given a highly informative overview of his theory in terms of some of his main claims and the difference between him and Damasio. On the delicate question of reductionism and the dialogue between natural sciences (e.g. neuroscience) and the humanistic disciplines (e.g. philosophy), he says: 'I think self-relatedness is deeply built into the neural matrix at all levels. There is a core-self that is necessary for the rich, cognitively aware personal aspect of our lives. Many people who enjoy thinking about the full complexity of self-related processing – with all its artistic and humanistic aspects, full of rich human imagination – find talk about causality and reductionism highly aversive ways of conceptualizing things. I myself take a bit more of the middle ground, namely, that you can't do good science on basic, evolved emotional systems by trying to capture the full complexity of human emotional life in the laboratory, but without working out mechanisms in the brain research laboratory you can't have refined and replicable knowledge about the sources of mentality. Science can never describe "the whole" but only the "parts", but the whole must be constructed from those parts [. . .] Thus, my work is well within a gentle reductionistic tradition and I certainly do not subscribe to any ruthlessly reductionistic variety, where mind is eventually explained away simply by neuronal firings. This is where my Spinozan dual-aspect monism approach—and empirically supported ontology—allows me to put mentality and neural processing of that mentality on an equal epistemological footing [. . .] Ontologically, the neural aspect may have some kind of priority, but not of the kind that has the "right" to marginalize one of its greatest natural products—experience' (Gallagher 2008, pp. 104–5, 106).

A way to avoid the tendency to explain irreducible aspects of human emotions away is to accept the cognitively impenetrable nature of many of our feelings, and use that acceptance in our approach to those feelings and in the ensuing explanations of human emotional life. This is not, in any way, the same as to say that we should renounce explaining our emotions altogether, but such an acceptance encourages us to avoid reductive attempts to master the confusion of our feelings and sensations in the name of some rational, irrational, or even biological ideal of how human nature *should* be. Instead we should use the confusion that our emotional life provokes in our explanations of human nature to take seriously the explanatory problems that feelings do impose on our theories of human nature. In other words, emotions complicate not only everyday life, but also our ideas and theories about that life. This problematic nature of emotions has made them an *enfant terrible* in the history of Western philosophy. This is also, we believe, part of the explanation of why philosophy in the twentieth century, with its painstaking focus on conceptual analysis and language, has often passed over the emotions in silence or attempted to reduce the variety of emotional characteristics to very broad conceptual categories such as 'feelings' and 'emotions'. Fortunately, as remarked earlier, this attitude has changed drastically over the last four decades, and today emotions have climbed to the very top of hot philosophical topics.

A central feature of this renewed appreciation of emotions in philosophy and science in general is the acknowledgement that we cannot disregard the biological dimension if we want to explain and understand human nature and behaviour.

Today it seems difficult, if not impossible, to ignore the biological character of feelings in any philosophical explanation of emotions. Empirical disciplines such as evolutionary psychology, neuroscience, and cognitive science have provided important insights into the mysteries of the mind, which often challenge the more conceptual approach of philosophy. And if philosophy has learned anything from this challenge it is that the study of mind cannot be done in isolation from other, more empirically informed, disciplines. This is perhaps more true of emotions than of any other features of the human mind. The concept of emotion seems to cover a wide spectrum of mental states that range from bodily feelings and sensations such as nausea, hunger, pain, satisfaction, attention, panic, and arousal to more complex states of mind such as love, hatred, pride, shame, jealousy, and happiness. Endeavours to provide a coherent account of such diversified phenomena can neglect neither the biological nor the phenomenological aspect of emotional experience. Ronald de Sousa, who has spent more than twenty years arguing for the integration of empirical research into philosophical accounts of emotions, writes cogently:

> [W]hat emotions feel like cannot give us full access to their nature. Emotions are also characteristically the most obviously embodied of our mental states. Their manifestations are both mental and physical, and theories of emotion over the last century and a half have distributed themselves along the path of a pendulum swinging between the physiological and intentional poles [. . .] It follows that emotions are not altogether knowable on the basis of what is available only in the moment's consciousness. Indeed, emotions are shaped by history on at least two levels: that of the individual development from zygote through

infant to adult, but also on the phylogenetic scale of our evolution into the animals that we are. Consequently it is not surprising that emotions are not entirely transparent to consciousness.

(de Sousa 2010, p. 100)

Needless to say that today only few would dispute that empirical research is necessary for an understanding of human emotions. The principal difficulty, though, is how to integrate the insights from different empirical disciplines with a more comprehensive philosophical theory about human nature. Most of our emotional concepts and affective vocabulary grow out of everyday life, that is, our affective reactions and attitudes to what we experience; and these concepts and words are perfectly legitimate, and indispensable, tools for coping with our emotional life. Nonetheless, our explanations of emotions and feelings are, or at least should be, continuously refined and re-evaluated in the light of the continuously improving scientific understanding of human nature. As we have seen in this chapter, in recent years neuroscience in particular has provided substantial empirical insight into the neurobiological underpinnings of emotional experience. This process of refining and re-evaluating our emotional concepts and our explanations of emotions depends on how we interpret the neuroscientific data, or said differently, into which explanatory framework we choose to integrate the relevant neuroscientific findings. Neuroscience, like most natural sciences, is local and precise in scope and is thus characterised by well-defined methods and experimental strategies designed to affirm or disprove specific research hypotheses. Hence, neuroscientific research can be done, and is certainly on more secure empirical ground, when it disregards more traditional philosophical questions about human nature, values, and norms. This is not to say that neuroscience, and the natural sciences in general, do not have anything important to say about human nature. On the contrary, much of what we know about human nature we have learned from the remarkable progress of the natural sciences over the last two centuries. There exists an obvious tension, though, between what the natural sciences tell us about human nature and what we as human persons experience as central and formative aspects of our peculiar nature. Our subjective experiences about being a human person bring forth aspects of human nature that are deliberately left out of the natural sciences, such as, among many others, personal values and idea(l)s, social norms, memories, prejudices, and affective nuances.

Wilfrid Sellars once famously described this tension as one between the *manifest image* of man and the *scientific image* of man, and he considered it the central task of philosophy to reconcile or integrate those two images of human nature. This integration should be seen 'as a matter of articulating two whole ways of seeing the sum of things, two images of man-in-the-world and attempting to bring them together in a "stereoscopic" view' (Sellars 1963a, p. 19). The task of bringing about such a general integration is, of course, a very complex business that touches upon almost every discipline of contemporary philosophy, from philosophy of science over philosophy of mind to ethics, and it would lead us too far astray to go into the ferociously disputed debate about whether or not such a reconciliation is possible or even desirable. Nonetheless, an integration or reconciliation of the two images of human nature is particularly important for our understanding of human emotions. Our emotional concepts and our explanations of emotions rely heavily on both phenomenological (i.e. subjective) and ontological (i.e. objective) investigations of human nature, and much of the confusion and disagreement about human emotional life derives, as de Sousa points out, from how the integration of these aspects is carried out. The feeling theories tend towards the ontological investigation of the natural sciences, whereas the cognitive and the narrative theories rely more on the conceptual and phenomenological investigation of human intentionality and judgement.

Over the next three chapters, we will attempt an alternative kind of integration against the backdrop of Ricoeur's hermeneutical theory of subjectivity as reformulated in Part I. We propose an approach to human emotions that focuses on the notion of human personhood, and by developing Ricoeur's hermeneutics in the light of the different theories presented in this chapter, we argue that, when brought together, emotions and personhood mutually illuminate and help explain one another. We shall argue that this approach has the advantage of using the explanatory complications provoked by the cognitively impenetrable aspects of many human emotions and feelings to elaborate a hermeneutical framework for understanding human emotions that is responsive to both the ontological and phenomenological conceptions of human nature.

Chapter 5

Ambivalent Personhood

To be a person is a distinctively human characteristic. We think, act, and feel like persons. Our experience of the world and other people is personal. And we understand ourselves as persons. In other words, to be a human being is to be a person. But what does this actually mean? Is being a person somehow different from the mere fact of being an organism that belongs to the Homo sapiens species? Can a human being lose his or her personhood? Does the notion of personhood contribute to our understanding of being human? Do we understand our emotions and feelings better in the light of personhood? These are some of the questions that we will attempt to answer in this and the following two chapters.

Our central argument in this book is that a better understanding of the relationship between emotions and personhood will help us to articulate aspects of human emotional life that are not always unfolded in accounts of emotions. And, inversely, a more nuanced conception of our emotional life may contribute to an appraisal of the complexity of personhood. This obviously requires a preliminary explanation of our approach to human personhood. In the first section, we argue that the comprehensive, and particularly normative, character of the notion of personhood makes it markedly different from cognate notions such as human nature and selfhood. We have already seen that Ricoeur's analysis of subjectivity uncovered the fragile character of personhood. Our identity as individual persons is not a fact, but a persistent normative task of becoming who we are. We care about being the person that we are. Our sense of selfhood is troubled, characterised by tension and conflict, and to reappropriate our sense of selfhood we must become the person that we are through the dialectic of selfhood and otherness. Here we develop these Ricoeurian themes in terms of the ontological ambiguity of personhood. Following this, we look more closely at the biological and personal dimension of personal identity in the light of two influential contemporary theories. Understanding human emotions presupposes an ontological grasp of what a human being is. In other words, to understand why we feel the way we do we need some kind of idea of what we are. As we shall see, an ontological grounding of human nature turns out to be problematic because of the complexities of personal identity. We close the chapter with a consideration of what feelings, in particular feelings of ambivalence, might tell us about our identity as persons who simply are what we are, and are also capable of changing who we are.

Ontological Ambiguity

It might be a help to start out with at least a preliminary idea of what we understand by the notion of personhood. As hinted at in our introduction, the notion of human personhood is markedly more comprehensive than both the notion of human nature and the notion of selfhood. The notion of human nature is descriptive in the sense that it serves, among other things, to distinguish humans from other animals by identifying specifically human characteristics (e.g. cognition, imagination, and speech). The notion of selfhood, on the other hand, serves to define what the minimal conditions for qualifying as a human self are. The notion of selfhood is also descriptive, and investigations of human selfhood normally concentrate on the phenomenological structures of human subjectivity, such as self-awareness and a minimal sense of self (Gallagher and Zahavi 2008; Zahavi 1999, 2005). The notion of personhood differs from these two on various points. First, personhood is a normative notion. As we learned in Part I, to be a person is not a fact, but a continuous task. The problems of fact and value come to the fore with the notion of personhood. Personhood is an ambiguous notion. To be a human being is to be a person, and yet we deeply care about being a (certain kind of) person. Personhood characterises what we all have in common, and still no person is the same as another. Second, personhood makes evident the problem of identity through time. We are the same person throughout our life, but the sameness of our identity as a person is continuously challenged by the changes that all persons undergo through time. How can we talk about being the same person when, more often than not, we change drastically over the span of a lifetime? Finally, the notion of personhood emphasises the otherness at the heart of selfhood. This third feature somehow brings together the two previous ones (normative ambivalence and personal identity) in the question of how to cope with tension, and sometimes conflict, between otherness and selfhood in being a person over time. I am a person in the eyes of other people, and my particular way of being a person is continuously challenged by the gaze of other people. Again, I am who I am, but I might feel that I am not myself, or that the person that others take me to be, is not the person that I truly am. My choices and actions when done leave my control and may result in unexpected, happy or unfortunate, results that in some way or another influence the person that I am. The responsibility for my words and deeds does not end when they are out of my mouth or hands, so to speak. The future can be oppressive (as in shame, obligation, anxiety, or despair) as well as liberating (as in hope, possibility, surprise, or ambition). My body changes, becomes different as the years go by, and I may become alienated by these transformations. I can accept such changes, despair because of them, or fight them ferociously, but every one of those attitudes affects the person that I am. In short, to be a person involves a permanent struggle with the otherness that constitutes the person that I am.

In the following chapters, we will consider this otherness as it manifests itself through our bodily constitution in terms of feelings that reveal our personal relation to the world, other people, and ourselves. We will argue that feelings are particularly suitable means for understanding the tension between otherness and selfhood in being a person. Our feelings reveal the subjective and biological features of human nature in a way that allows for an appreciation of the respective peculiarity of each of these features without isolating the one from the other. Our particularly personal experience of the world is shaped by both subjectivity and biology. We have feelings of being, on the one hand, significantly unique and active, and on the other, of being insignificantly anonymous and passive. Our existence as persons is constituted by a complex interplay of voluntary and involuntary factors that restrict, enable, and form our lives. A human life is never merely a result of pure accident or sheer will. Neither is it a product of determined necessity or amorphous possibility. A human life is lived somewhere in between those extremes. This is obviously a common insight that most people are familiar with, and try to cope with, in their own lives. Then again, most philosophy is about articulating and arguing for or against common insights. Thus, we believe that articulating the interplay of voluntary and involuntary factors in human existence will enable an argument for the intrinsic relationship between emotions and personhood.

A human being cares about being a person, just as she or he cares about so many other things. However, personhood stands out among the things that we care about. Maybe this is not explicitly so in our daily life, but whenever our sense of being a person is injured, threatened, or offended we feel how much we care about being the person that we are. Somehow, the person that we are expresses what we care about, or how we actually care about the things we think we care about. Personhood remains the firm, but obscure, point of reference when we talk about ourselves and other people. A person can be humiliated, lose his or her dignity, meaning of life, respect for other persons, change character, and become a better or worse person. We can treat another human being as if that human being were not a person. We can drain the humanity out of our own conception of personhood. We can choose to exclude some human beings from our understanding of personhood (history has witnessed many tragic examples of this attitude). Nonetheless, personhood is a normative notion, a principle of humanity, which reveals the person that I am myself in my behaviour towards other human beings. As we saw in Chapter 3, despite the normative thrust of the principle of humanity, it is rooted in our (f)actual need for the other person to recognise our own personhood. To be a person involves a need for a mutual recognition of humanity. It is my own personhood that is a stake in the way I treat another person. Not to treat him as a person, to actively exclude him from the realm of persons, is a matter of active choice on my part. It is therefore my own personhood that is involved in such an exclusion, that is, I implicate myself in my act of exclusion. In this sense, we can kill, torture, humiliate, starve, and laugh at a person, but we cannot kill or laugh away the challenge of humanity that the personhood of another human being imposes on our sense of being a person ourselves. Richard Wollheim writes:

> We are persons, and we know persons. We have friends, lovers, enemies, acquaintances, who are persons. All of us, all of them, have something in common, which is membership of a particular biological species, and, since we also know no human beings who are incontestably not persons, it is easy to conclude that to be a person is to be a human being. They are one and the same thing. (1984, p. 3)

This is a perplexing feature about human nature. We care about being something that we already are. However, such an identification of human beings and personhood gives rise to several questions. Among those are two obvious ones: What does it mean, ontologically speaking, to be a human being and what does it mean to be a person? In this section and the next, we will look more closely at both and try to make sense of the identification of the two. These ontological considerations will have a significant bearing on the development of our hermeneutical account of emotions and personhood, since one of our central arguments for this take on human emotions is exactly that it provides an integration of both the biological and personal aspect of human emotions. But why do we need an ontological grounding for a theory of emotions and personhood in the first place? The answer should be obvious by now. As explained in the last chapter, questions about emotions, more significantly than other philosophical topics, involve our biological constitution, and thus serve to encourage ontological considerations about human nature. Emotions are deeply embodied phenomena and as such involve more fleshy matters than the structure and dynamics of our thin notion of rationality. Accordingly, most philosophers today agree that our emotions are in some way or another directly influenced and shaped by our particular biological nature. An understanding of emotion therefore calls for more comprehensive investigation than other philosophical issues.

In the same way, the notion of personhood encompasses several features of our being human that all extend well beyond an investigation of our mental capacities for rational deliberation and judgement. Personhood concerns what it is to be a person. This is naturally a very broad and even amorphous issue that great minds have pondered over since antiquity, and we have no ambition to contribute to this debate with new theory. We will only look at two aspects of this complex notion that we consider to be fundamental to any talk about persons, and especially relevant with respect to human emotions. These aspects can be summed upon in a twofold question: what and who am I? The first part of the question concerns the anonymous, biological aspect of our being human, whereas the latter involves the personal, psychological aspect. Some central problems about the nature of personhood are due to this twofold aspect of being human. Being a human person is characterised by an inherent ambivalence that makes our understanding of what we actually are extremely difficult. There seems to be at least two incontestable facts about being a human person. On the one hand, we are part of the anonymous workings of the natural world, and on the other, we experience and understand our role in the great chain of nature from a personal perspective, that is, we consider ourselves to be unique and irreplaceable persons. The distinguished primatologist, Frans de Waal, describes this inherent ambivalence of human nature eloquently:

> Being both more systematically brutal than chimps and more empathic than bonobos, we are by far the most bipolar ape. Our societies are never completely peaceful, never completely competitive, never ruled by sheer selfishness, and never perfectly moral. Pure states are not nature's way. What's true for human society is also true for human nature. One can find both kindness and cruelty, nobility and vulgarity—sometimes all in the same person. We're full of contradictions, but mostly tamed ones. Talk of 'tamed contradictions' may sound obscure, even mystical, but they're all around us [...] On top of the inherent duality of human nature comes the role of intelligence. Even if we customarily overestimate our rationality, there is no denying that human behavior is a combination of drive and intelligence. We exert little control over ancient urges for power, sex, safety, and food, but we

habitually weigh the pros and cons of our actions before we engage in them. Human behaviour is seriously modified by experience.

(de Waal 2005, p. 221)

De Waal argues that many of the conflictual aspects of human behaviour have their counterparts in the behaviour of other primates, and that this continuity suggests that our affective nature is rooted in the soil of mammalian evolution. However, human nature is, he argues, significantly more complex than that of other animals. Our peculiar experience and highly developed cognitive capacities makes our nature particularly bipolar. Ontological explanations of human personhood are to some extent caught between our evolutionarily inherited drives and our peculiar way of being human *persons*.

A traditional way of handling the problems about human personhood (and human nature in general) is to drive a wedge between the mammalian constitution that we share with other animals and our distinctively human feature of rationality. We are somehow an ontological agglomerate of a material body and an immaterial mind. This has come to be known as substance dualism, but although it has been a key position in the tradition of Western philosophy, and a handful of philosophers still defend it (e.g. Hasker 1999; Swinburne 2007; Unger 2006), it seems to have largely outlived its role on the philosophical scene. It has been reduced from its former glory to a stubbornly isolated position in the landscape of contemporary scientific knowledge, and seems in many cases to draw most of its arguments from religious convictions (e.g. Plantinga 2007). Thus, most philosophers today adopt some kind of monistic and more naturalistic reference for their explanation of human personhood.

The Personal Animal

Two contemporary theories are particularly informative in their handling of the ontological quibbles surrounding the notion of personhood. They agree about the view that a human person is a biological organism; and still, they differ substantially in their interpretation of how to understand the ontological relation between biology and personhood. One takes biology to be the ontological priority, whereas the other grants this honour to the first-person perspective. The biological approach has recently been defended and developed by Eric T. Olson (1997, 2007), while the latter approach has been advocated by Lynne R. Baker (2000, 2007). The two philosophers are, as can be imagined from their opposing standpoints, very different with respect to both style and argument. Olson prefers to argue by means of logic and sophisticated thought experiments, whereas Baker turns to what she calls the metaphysics of everyday life, which is no less sophisticated but characterised by a greater emphasis on our personal experience of the world. Both theories contain valuable insights, and although we are more in agreement with Baker, Olson's patient argument for the biological approach nevertheless remains significant for our understanding of human personhood.

Olson's theory is apparently quite simple. To be a person is basically to be a human animal. He sets about to show that the nature of personal identity, that is, the persistence conditions that allow a person to maintain his or her identity over time, relies not on some abstruse psychological criterion, but on mere biological conditions. This approach makes two central claims, where the second is significantly more controversial than the first. First and foremost, 'you and I are animals: members of the species *Homo sapiens*, to be precise' (1997, p. 17). By itself, this claim does not provoke much controversy today. Most of us would agree that humans are animals, a peculiar kind of animals to be sure, but still animals. When our biological organism shuts down, our existence as an individual person ceases to be. So far so good. But then Olson makes a second claim that goes much further. Our mental states, our ideas, dreams, plans for the future, and memories from the past are neither necessary nor sufficient for our being the same human animal through time. In other words, our psychological continuity does not matter when it comes to the persisting conditions for human identity. He asks us to consider a person who lapses into a persistent vegetative state. The mind is irrevocably destroyed.[1] Our ideas and intentions vanish as if they never existed, but all our vital functions are still functioning as before. We are not able to respond to stimuli or interact with the surroundings, but we are not transformed from being one person to being another. We are still the same person as we were before, simply without all the mental stuff that characterised our particular way of being who we were.

Olson is well aware that this is a radical take on human nature (2007, pp. 44–7). He argues patiently, though, that our psychological peculiarities have nothing to do with our being the organisms that we are. In fact, he believes that questions about personhood are completely unrelated to, ontologically speaking, what kind of thing we human beings are. Thus, '[t]o know what it is to be a person is therefore not to know what we are. Likewise, to know what we are is not to know what it is to be a person' (2007, p. 17). Personhood is not essential to being human. We do not learn anything about human nature by investigating personhood. Accordingly, he divides questions about personal identity into *absolute* and *relative* identity. To be an individual human animal that endures through the changes of time is what constitutes our absolute identity, while the psychological features that make up who we are as individual persons are relative to that fundamental biological identity:

> [W]e can define a sense of 'being a particular person' as a sort of role or office that a human organism (or any other appropriate object) might fill at a particular time. In unusual cases, a single human being such as you or I might be one particular person at one time, in this sense of 'person', and another particular person later on. I might once have been or might later become a different person from the one I am now. (1997, p. 66)

Such a radical view on human identity may, at first sight, seem futile with respect to questions about human personhood and personal identity, but we can draw at least two important insights from Olson's insistence on biological identity. His elaborate defence of the biological approach evidences the many ways in which we are intimately identical with our biological constitution, and shows that any attempt to separate biological

---

[1] Or, at least, this is what we can argue from a third-person observational perspective. The relational mind, our ability to express emotions and communicate thoughts and beliefs is completely destroyed, whereas we know very little about what goes on in the mind of a person in a persistent vegetative state.

identity from human personhood, or simply to downplay it, has just as much explaining to do as the strict biological approach. Secondly, Olson's 'sparse ontology' operates with a 'biological minimalism' (2007, pp. 226–7) that encourages us to take seriously the complexity of what it actually means to be a biological organism. Among other things, this complexity entails that we are constituted by a human organism, and not just a human body. The notion of organism provides a better foundation for discussing the biological nature of human personhood than does the notion of a human body, since by doing so the continuity between humans and other animals is emphasised rather than downplayed.² As de Wall pointed out in the quote above, we may be very particular beasts, but the biological identity of human nature is nonetheless inseparable from the identity criteria that all animals share.

The fact that we appreciate Olson's biological minimalism as an important contribution to the notion of personhood cannot overshadow some problems that we have with his theory. His argument for reducing the notion of personhood to 'a role' or 'an office' that the human animal may enact or not according to choice or circumstances does seem to transform questions about *personal* identity into questions about the structural identity of biological organisms. On this account, the ontological nature of a human person becomes indistinct from that of a vampire bat or even a lime tree. Human identity is of course slightly more complex, but the general ontological conditions are the same. What is *personal* about being a human animal is neither sufficient nor necessary for understanding the nature and identity of that particular organism. By making personhood relative to the biological nature of human beings, that is, *what* a person is biologically speaking, Olson avoids many of the problems that are normally part of the discussions of personhood. He is, in fact, pretty clear about this strategy. His minimalist approach allegedly avoids all the nasty problems that other theories grapple with. The Constitution View that we shall turn to in a moment tries to supply this basic biological tenor with a personal ontology in order to articulate what is particularly human about being a human, that is, the first-person perspective. Olson, on the contrary, is dismissive about such metaphysical worries

---

² In fact, Olson is quite sceptic when it comes to the notion of the human body: 'I think the notion of a human body is best left out of philosophy, or at least out of discussions of personal identity' (1997, p. 150). Part of his criticism of the notion of the human body is concerned with what phenomenologists identify as the experienced body in terms of a sense of agency and ownership. However, Olson argues, justly in our opinion, that our conception of the human body cannot be limited to the lived or experienced body. It must include as fundamental the biological organism that our body basically is. In order to understand this dimension of the human body, 'we ought to wonder what makes my spleen a part of my body, for I cannot move it directly any more than I can move my pencil directly. Had I not been told, I should never have known that I *had* a spleen. I can move my spleen only by willing to move something else – my torso, say, or the entire living thing [. . .] At any rate I can think of no interesting sense in which I can move my spleen but not my pencil merely by willing to do so. For that matter I have no proprioceptive awareness of my spleen either; and some organs even lack pain receptors' (p. 148). As we will see, this insistence on the problematic nature of the notion of the human body will have significant bearing on our argument for the ambivalent nature of human values.

about personhood and specific human characteristics, which he considers irrelevant to human ontology:

> If you've already accepted minimalism, there is no point in adopting constitutionalism as well. That would be paying twice for the same thing. The two views are also fundamentally opposed in spirit. Constitutionalism is a rich ontology; minimalism is an austere one [...] No one will say that the furniture of the earth consists of nothing but simple particles, organisms, and things coinciding with organisms. That would be like recommending a diet of bread, water, and chocolate fudge cake. So animalists can solve all their metaphysical worries at a stroke by adopting biological minimalism. That may seem a high price to pay, but it does the job. And it may not be such a great sacrifice in the end, compared with the other theories of composition.
>
> (Olson 2007, p. 227)

The resilient metaphysical worry that most perturbs Olson is the fact that if we consider the personal features of the human animal as essential, we end up with a seemingly paradoxical picture of human nature—a human animal that is both absolutely a person and absolutely a biological organism. By making personhood a relative or accidental feature, Olson allegedly avoids this paradox. The problem, though, with such an ontological solution is—to remain with Olson's dietary metaphor—that a person on a recommended diet often does end up devouring a chocolate fudge cake, when he or she would have been better off sticking to merely bread and water. Or to put it differently, human animals behave in ways that makes the biological approach, and the ensuing austere or sparse ontology, seem inadequate if we want to understand the peculiar nature of human persons.

Lynne R. Baker is an influential defender of what is called 'The Constitution View', a richer ontological understanding of personhood. Like Olson, she maintains that substance dualism is not an option, and that to understand human persons, first of all we need to acknowledge that human persons are wholly constituted by human bodies (Baker 2000, pp. 95–6). Accordingly, we are subject to the same biological constraints and functions as all other living creatures. We cannot dismiss our biological nature from our account of human personhood. We are essentially biological organisms. However, besides our biological functions we are also essentially human persons endowed with a particular first-person perspective that permeates all aspects of our ontological constitution. Baker describes the two basic propositions that inform her ontology in the following way:

> On the one hand, human persons are material objects, subject to all the natural laws that apply to other kinds of material objects. Human persons are wholly part of nature, the product of natural processes that started eons before the existence of our solar system, and that account for the existence of everything in the natural world—from atoms and molecules to solar systems and galaxies. On the other hand, human persons have evolved to have the capacity to think of themselves in the first-person. A first-person perspective is the defining property of persons and makes possible their characteristic forms of life and experience.
>
> (Baker 2007, p. 86)

So, a human being is constituted by both the biological organism that we call the human body and the particular personal features that we ascribe to the human person. A person is his or her body, but is not identical with that body. The fact that a human person is endowed with self-awareness and a first-person perspective makes the ontology of human persons considerably more complex than that of other living creatures. A person is a primary entity. In this sense, Peter F. Strawson has argued for 'the primitiveness of the concept of a person' (1959, p. 101) owing to the fact that the nature of a person is constituted by several features that cannot be understood in other terms than those derived from personhood. Baker, however, does not limit the constitutional view to human persons or even living creatures; indeed, she argues that the world as we experience and understand it is generally made up of constituted objects. Ordinary things and artefacts such as sushi, government bills, gothic architecture, and software programmes are all constituted ontological beings that enrich and thicken our understanding of the natural world.

The sparse ontology that Olson proposes cannot, and will not, consider such entities as possessing primary ontological status. On this view, human beings are simply the complex and dynamic structure of an individual organism and sushi merely an aggregate of proteins, carbohydrates, and other organic compounds. Human animals are only accidentally personal and the raw fish on the table in front of us is only conventionally called sushi, but both are, ontologically speaking, actually something else, that is, respectively living and dead organic tissue. Personhood and other personal, social, and subjective features of the world are at best secondary, and some of them actually non-existing. The sparse ontological worldview that Olson proposes has a scent of one-sided Cartesianism. The world as we know it, i.e. all the personal and social features that make up our experienced world, melt away and are transformed into an amorphous material piece of wax when brought under the fire of true philosophical thinking.³ We are, when illusions are dispersed and truth comes to light, only a *res extensa*, and all our cognitive and psychological peculiarities are secondary to the extended organism that we are, a mere by-product of our material constitution that cannot be allowed to confuse our sense of ontological security.

Baker, on the contrary, argues that '[r]ather than squeezing the world into a preconceived metaphysical straitjacket, we should let the metaphysics emerge from the reflection on the world as we encounter it' (2007, pp. 47–8). This argument stands and falls with what we consider the job of philosophy to be. Should 'real' philosophy, in the pursuit of a true ontology, disqualify notions and concepts that complicate logical or biologically informed arguments, in this case ordinary notions such as person, self, human body, or sushi? Or should philosophy face the reality of such notions and use

---

³ A moment ago, we saw how Olson's radical approach bans the notion of the human body from philosophical inquiry. He holds the same eliminative attitude towards the notion of the self. He simply argues that there is *no* problem of the self. The concept of self is so diffuse and multifarious that when philosophers discuss the notion and the problems involved, they are actually discussing about nothing, because there are no agreed standards or paradigms when it comes to the notion of selfhood. Olson writes, with his characteristic verve: 'I am not just quibbling about a word. Real philosophy is at stake. Many philosophers assume that there is something properly called the problem or the problems of the self, and write as if everyone knew what they meant by "self". This often leads to obscurity and muddle. If I am right, the muddle arises because those philosophers believe in a concept that doesn't exist' (Olson 1999, p. 49).

the complications that they provoke as an antidote to minimalistic dreams of a clear-cut, but bare skeleton of the world? A minimal, biological ontology of personhood avoids many of the metaphysical problems that pop up with everyday notions such as subjectivity or personhood, but a stripped-down ontological solution is also bereft of answers to ordinary questions about what it is to be and feel like a person.

We will not go further into the details of the particular theoretical debate about the ontological status of personhood, and we will not nail our philosophical colours to either the biological or constitutionalist mast. We have presented the two theories to give an idea about the ontological complications that the notion of personhood elicits when put under the magnifying glass of philosophy. We take with us an important lesson from this metaphysical dispute about what a person is. A person is both a biological organism *and* an entity endowed with personal experience of the world and itself. We are animals through and through, but we are *personal animals*. And this tiny biological difference has an immense impact on how we understand, live, and cope with our animal nature. We are indeed, as far as we know, the most bipolar and ambiguous animal. This ambiguity becomes explicit in our feelings of ambivalence, and so, instead of following in the argumentative footsteps of either Olson or Baker, we shall approach the nature of personhood and personal identity from the affective aspect of being human.

Identity and Feelings of Ambivalence

The ontological ambiguity of human nature comes to the fore in the way we feel. Many of our basic emotional reactions are similar to those of other animals, and they only differ by being experienced as personal emotions, no matter how diffuse or instinct-like they may be. The suggestion that human beings may be characterised as personal animals finds some support in the way that we experience our feelings about being the kind of animal that we are. Our emotions are felt as personal. All that we feel has some kind of significance for the kind of person that we are. Emotions may vary from instinct-like impulses such as lust, momentary surprise, panic or irrational anger to heart-throbbing jealousy, tender parental love, excruciating remorse or empty sadness, but different as such emotions may be they are all related to the identity of an individual person. Emotions and feelings express what a person cares about. We can feign, deny, fight, or try to change what we care about, but some of our care and concerns are not under the sway of our will. What we care about sometimes stems from the involuntary aspects of our being. Our cares and concerns can express themselves as feelings over which we have no control, but as they come to consciousness we can *appropriate* them, to speak with Ricoeur, as a part of our identity. Once appropriated, these cares and concerns become part of who we think ourselves to be, and thus integrated, in part at least, into our voluntary decisions and actions. We are, however, often exposed by and even caught in our care for someone or something. Feelings of love and hate, joy and sorrow, humiliation and power, pleasure and pain are distinct phenomena in our emotional life, but are nevertheless inextricably interwoven in the texture of our care for somebody or something. This conflation of feelings and emotions is responsible for the perplexity and confusion often involved in our sense of who we are and in our sense of belonging to the world, our values and means of orientation, and our attachment to other people. In other words, our cares and concerns are often deeply ambivalent.

Our emotional responses may contribute to our understanding of personal identity, because emotions and feelings express what we care about. And the nature of our cares and concerns expresses normative aspects of our identity as persons that are not accounted for in the biological or the psychological account of personal identity. The feeling of who I am is as important as the explicit, rational understanding of who I am. Or said in another way, to understand who I am I need to understand why I feel the way I feel. This, of course, needs some explaining.

One way to articulate our ambivalent feelings of identity is to look at our very human capacity for remembering our past. Unlike other animals, humans are in possession of a refined and elaborate long-term memory. We are able to retain an impressive amount of detailed information (auditory, visual, palpable, verbal, rational, etc.) about past experiences. Our life in the world and among other people depends on this refined and sensitive memory. And even more important for our discussion, my identity as a person is inextricably wound up with my memories. My sense of being who I am is bound to my memories of who I was. But like most, if not all, human capacities, memory is a tricky thing.

We tend to forget most of the past, either by willingly or unwillingly repressing it, by transforming it or by plain forgetfulness. Memory is a fragile thing, and no matter how meticulously we cultivate the accurateness of our memories, most of them will eventually fade or become transformed into the indistinct haze of time past. We understand ourselves to be the person that we are in the light of our past. But this light is flickering and often the result of our present ideas and prospects for the future. Like historians, we rewrite our past from where and what we are now.[4] What happened the day I met my wife many years ago may be as clear in my memory as the movie that I watched yesterday, but the mass of years that lies between then and now is more like a (re-)collection of distinct and bleary episodes and sentiments that eludes my full comprehension. Moreover, even momentous episodes such as the first encounter with my future wife are only partly remembered. I may not remember anything we talked about, whereas memories of the colour of her dress, the scent of her skin, or the touch of her hand still make my heart soft. The vastness of my memory exceeds my voluntary effort to remember. Indeed, if my past was only made up of what I am able to recollect, it would be as if a large part of my life never happened. Was I to consider my life on the terms of my recollection alone, the continuity of my identity through the passing of

---

[4] We all share a commonsense, linear conception of time: the past influences the present and the future. If something stressful happened in the past, this will affect the present and the future. This linear, unidirectional conception of time has, however, proved to be incomplete. Not only do we make sense of our present through our past experiences; we also understand our past in terms of the present. This was an important insight of early psychoanalysis called *Nachträglichkeit*. An event placed in the past (especially in the remote past of early childhood) may become traumatic when the person develops the capacity to attribute to it a traumatic (in psychoanalysis, often sexual) meaning. The event itself does not contain the traumatic meaning. There is a backward attribution of meaning to the event that becomes traumatic. A present experience gives new meaning to past experiences. The fragments of our past are reorganised in the light of our present experience, mood, and cognition. Once this has happened, the newly attributed meaning becomes fixed and may be lived, rather than as a *post hoc* attribution, as a discovery.

time would barely be held together by the isolated events that I happen to remember. But my past does not work on me merely by means of what I remember. Time leaves traces on a person's identity in a way similar to how years of smiles and frowns furrow the lines of a face. James Joyce captures this fragile tension of memory and identity in his description of Bloom's thoughts as he strays around Dublin looking for a place to lunch in the *Lestrygonians* episode of *Ulysses*:

> I was happier then. Or was that I? Or am I now I? Twentyeight I was. She twentythree. When we left Lombard Street west something changed. Could never like it again after Rudy. Can't bring back time. Like holding water in your hand. Would you go back to then? Just beginning then. Would you?

(Joyce 1986, p. 137)

Bloom is confused about happiness and grief, the remembrance of youth, and identity through time. Was I happier in the past? Am I the same person as before? The sturdy and good-humoured Bloom first firmly proclaims that he was indeed happier back then, but then he becomes insecure and doubts if it was actually really him, or if he is himself now after the painful loss of his and Molly's newborn Rudy. Something changed drastically with that tragic loss. Did it change him, or Molly for that sake, into a different person? Is that the reason why he and Molly seek comfort and excitement in other lovers? Would he go back and relive both happiness and pain again? It is interesting to notice how Bloom switches from first-person to second-person. His questioning leads him to a displacement of his sense of self. As most human thoughts about life, sorrow, and happiness, Bloom ends his ponderings with a lingering question mark. The philosopher Arne Grøn has cogently described this complex relation between history, remembrance, and identity:

> In remembering, we are already affected by what has happened to us in the past. We carry with us a history without which we would not be what we are. This does not mean, however, that we are our history. We relate to it, also when we try to forget or leave our past behind us. We can carry, on the other hand, our history with us, without appropriating it as our own. Thus, we would not be ourselves without our history, which we also can leave behind. Self-appropriation takes place in relation to a history, but it can do so in complex ways. We can seek to remember what is important to us; we can seek to appropriate our past in order to free future possibilities, and we can remember possibilities that were cut off in the past in order to change our future.

(Grøn 2004, pp. 146–7)

The felt complexities of time and identity, possibility and necessity, memory and present are difficult to clarify, let alone cope with, in the explicative language of philosophy. The poetic foregrounding of the intricate relation between feeling and language is far superior in this regard. One of the strongest examples of this is T.S. Eliot's *Burnt Norton*, which opens his *Four Quartets*:

> Time present and time past
> Are both perhaps present in time future,
> And time future contained in time past.

> If all time is eternally present
> All time is unredeemable.
> What might have been is an abstraction
> Remaining a perpetual possibility
> Only in a world of speculation.
> What might have been and what has been
> Point to one end, which is always present.
> Footfalls echo in the memory
> Down the passage which we did not take
> Towards the door we never opened
> Into the rose-garden. My words echo
> Thus, in your mind.
>   But to what purpose
> Disturbing the dust on a bowl of rose-leaves
> I do not know.
>
>   (Eliot 1944, p. 7)

The dust of time past is brimming with deeds done or abandoned, words said or left unsaid, choices, smiles, subdued pain, and all the apparently insignificant events of everyday life. Time makes our identity vulnerable. Time and identity are wrought inextricably into each other, and thus the question of rational or appropriate behaviour grows complicated to the extent that it can be difficult to ascertain whether a certain behaviour is a result of our presently conscious deliberation and choice or has instead been maturing slowly over hours, days, months or even years. Irrespective of how I rationally understand myself as a person, and no matter how fragile my sense of identity is, the identity of who I am works on me in spite of myself, for instance, in the way my body is constantly affected by the passing of years.

What I eat and drink, what I feel and experience, what I say and do all leave their traces on my bodily constitution. In this sense, Eric T. Olson is right to insist on the non-psychological aspect of personal identity. Much of our personal identity is not explicitly personal at all. The development of the biological organism that I am is a fundamental part of who I am. This is obvious in some cases. Say I am a heavy smoker or too enthusiastic about chocolate fudge cake, then these proclivities will leave their traces on my body. In the first case, I damage my lungs and may over time develop respiratory problems and elevate significantly the risk of lung cancer, whereas the second very likely will result in an excess of body fat and may eventually provoke heart diseases and type 2 diabetes. But the biological recording of time is not always inscribed in our identity in such dramatic ways. Most of what is going on in our body completely eludes our conscious assessment. The workings of my kidneys, my spleen or the level of serotonin in my gut are fundamental to how I feel and behave despite the fact that I have no awareness whatsoever of what is going on. These visceral changes are part of what I am, irrespective of who I believe myself to be. Moreover, the history of my body is infinitely longer than my own personal history. Many of my bodily functions are enmeshed in millions of years of mammalian development, and my emotional life bears vestigial traces of this remote past (de Sousa 2007, pp. 49–55). Our instincts and spontaneous emotional reactions are obvious indicators of this past, but it seems untenable to believe that these vestigial traces do not also, to some extent at least, influence and shape our more explicitly personal emotions such as shame, pride, love or anxiety.

There exists an ambiguity between the organism *that* I am and *who* I think I am. This ambiguity seems to be part of the reason why Olson decides to dismiss mental states as valid criteria of personal identity. Our memory is so fraught with inadequacies and blank spots that it seems a very unlikely candidate to fulfil the function as accountant of our identity. The biological constitution of our organism is much more reliable. As already noticed, however, Olson's radical attempt to dissolve the ontological ambiguity of personal identity, *what* I am and *who* I am, by dismissing basic notions such as body and self, goes too far. Most of the problems about personal identity hinge on these notions and do not go away just because we stop talking or thinking about them. Human beings conceive their personal identity as essentially bound to problems about the self and the body. So instead of disposing of subjectivity and embodiment in order to avoid the ambiguity of personal identity, we will use the emotional ambivalence provoked by this ontological ambiguity to argue that the entwinement of self and body plays a vital role in the identity of a human person. We also argue that personal identity and feelings are inseparably connected and can thus illuminate one another.

As we saw in Part I, Ricoeur approaches personal identity in terms of selfhood and otherness. A person is basically constituted by two kinds of identity. On the one hand, a person remains the same person through time simply in virtue of being a structured biological organism (identity *idem*/sameness). This is a passive identity that the person is subjected to involuntarily. Time leaves traces on a person that cannot be changed or undone. On the other hand, a person cannot but actively engage with his or her identity through the changes of time (identity *ipse*/selfhood). In this sense, a person does not remain the same person through time. Our body visibly changes, we lose and gain habits, memories of things we have said and done relentlessly interfere with our understanding of ourselves, we meet other people who may drastically change the way we understand the world, joy and sorrow come uninvited, some dreams are abortive and others are born. I may not recognise the person that I was once. I may not even like who I was, and today I feel like a completely different person. In other words, I have changed, and I am faced with the essentially normative challenge of how to cope with these changes.

Ricoeur's twofold model of personal identity turns on the fundamental distinction inherent in human personhood between involuntary and voluntary aspects of human identity. The fragility of human personhood is, at least in part, rooted in the normative interplay of these two aspects. We are necessarily the same person through time (identity *idem*), and yet we are not simply the same person because *who* we are depends on how we cope with *what* we are (identity *ipse*). A person is able to voluntarily change who he or she is. On the other hand, this ability to change who we are is necessarily bound to what we are. There are aspects of who I am that cannot be undone or changed at will, but have to be integrated in my understanding of the person that I am.

Now, this ambiguous character of personal identity is first and foremost experienced as feelings of ambivalence. Our feelings reveal what we care about, the values by and through which we lead our lives; and the heterogeneous nature of these values is constituted and continuously shaped by the interplay of voluntary and involuntary aspects of who and what I am. Ricoeur developed an ontology on the basis of this fragile nature of human care. The heterogeneous nature of what we care about is rooted in the ambiguous nature of personal identity. We are both what we are (the identity of our biological organism) and who we want to be (the psychological flexibility of that identity in the form of, for example, idea(l)s and dreams). Put more simply, the identity of a person is constituted by the fact that the person is one and the same human person through inevitable changes in and by time. We care about the person that we are, and we are responsible for being that person, but although we are able to assert ourselves as this particular person in the world, we cannot simply decide who we are. Ricoeur argues, as we have seen in Part I, that the person that we are is constituted by selfhood (who we want to be and who we think ourselves to be) and otherness (what we are despite our conscious choices and our self-conception). We experience the otherness at the heart of our personhood primarily through our bodily constitution and our encounter with the world and other people.

We have attempted to corroborate and develop this idea in terms of two contemporary theories of personal identity. My identity as a person depends not just on who I think I am or who I want to be, but also on the biological continuity of my body, my being situated in the world, and my relation with other people. Otherness, in this sense, is what transcends my self in myself. Or said less cryptically, it is the involuntary aspect of being what and who I am. Ricoeur argues that personal identity is a normative question that can be approached only in normative terms. Human personhood is problematic because of this ambiguous character of personal identity. The identity of a person is continuously shattered in its existence through time (one of the reasons for Ricoeur's internally fractured Cogito). My body is slowly transformed and works on and with me in inexplicable ways, the demands of the world continuously change character, and, perhaps most importantly, my relationship with other people never ceases to challenge my understanding of who I am.

Hence, to be a person is both a fact and a task expressed in our care about being the person that we are, embodied and enmeshed in a world shared with other people. This twofold nature of human personhood brings us back to Wollheim's characterisation of the ambivalence of human personhood at the beginning of this chapter. Wollheim claims that we cannot question the fact that to be a person is to be a human being, namely, a member of a particular biological species. We cannot lose our personhood. We remain persons even in the act or suffering of the most atrocious and inhuman deeds. We can make Wollheim's claim even stronger by emphasising that we are not just *a* person. We are *this* individual person whose identity is bound to the persistence of the biological organism that we are, subjected to the changes of the world, and responsible for the demands and the love of other persons. But despite of, or perhaps exactly because of this biological, contextual, and interpersonal foundation of our personhood, to be a person is a very fragile way of being in the world. As Frans de Wahl noticed in his characterisation of human beings as 'by far the most bipolar ape', our existence is characterised by deeply ambivalent values and concerns. What I care about goes beyond my rational scrutiny and is primarily expressed in the *chiaroscuro* of my emotional life. We are personal animals. And the fact that my being is both personal and animal makes my values more heterogeneous than those of other animals, and renders my existence as a personal animal highly problematic.

I am a person, by the simple fact of being human, but still I care about being the person that I am, even while I do all I can to be a different person. Personhood is a normative notion. It is something that I can be in different ways, but I cannot become a different person. As remarked earlier, this is perhaps most obvious from the fact that the identity of the person that I am is inherently rooted in the specific biological organism that I am. And this biological fact influences me in ways that I cannot control. The fact that I am the person that I am is out of my hands, so to speak. This fact, however, is fragile. The fragility inherent in the notion of personhood is linked to our ability to care about the person that we are. Our care for being the person that we are evidences the ambivalence of *what* we are and *how* we are what we are. Even though our identity is bound to what we are, the human self is, as Arne Grøn beautifully writes, 'a self on a journey. Identity is not something fixed, but to be developed' (Grøn 2004, p. 147). In other words, to *be* a person is a normative task of *becoming* a person.

So our claim is that the notion of personhood is inherently related to our feelings and emotions, and that this relationship comes to the fore if we pay sufficient attention to the normative nature of human affectivity. Hence, in the next chapter and the following, we shall argue for a hermeneutical approach to emotions on the basis of the ambiguous character of human personhood as expressed in our ambivalent feelings about being the person that we are.

Chapter 6

Emotions and Personhood

Feelings disclose the ambivalence constitutive of human personhood. Many of our feelings are related to the problems we encounter in our attempt to cope with our fragile identity. As we saw in the previous chapter, our own body is a major factor in the involuntary dimension of our identity. The biological permanence and change that we experience over time influence how we understand our identity as persons. In many ways, we are who we are despite ourselves. Our identity is rooted in circumstances that are out of our hands. We are constituted and continuously influenced by otherness as it is manifested in our body, the world, and other people—in the way they offer resistance to our goals and actions. There is, however, more to personal identity than these involuntary factors. We care about the person that we are, and how we relate ourselves to what and who we are characterises the voluntary dimension of our identity. We are able to relate ourselves to *what* we are by making sense of our care for *who* we are. This is what we understand as human selfhood. In short, the fragile character of our identity, which we experience first and foremost in our feelings, stems from the complex relationship of voluntary selfhood and involuntary otherness inherent in human personhood.

The aim of this chapter is to explicate how emotions and personhood are related, and how we can use this relationship to make sense of a person's emotional life. We begin with a discussion of the current terminology in emotion research, and argue that the concepts of emotions and feelings are too restricted to encompass, let alone make sense of, human emotional life. We therefore propose an alternative approach that begins with a phenomenological analysis of emotional experience. We argue that a better understanding of how an emotion feels for the person who undergoes that emotion provides the most accurate access into our emotional life. To explain the structure of emotional feelings, we single out two broad categories of human feelings that we call moods and affects. We then analyse the intentional and temporal structure of these affective categories in order to make clear the inherent relationship between emotions and personhood. Following this, we argue that the best way to make sense of this relationship is in terms of the narrative structures of our emotional experiences. Here we draw heavily on Ricoeur's account of narrative identity, and develop his hermeneutical theory in accordance with what we learned from our previous discussions of both the contemporary debate of personhood and the different approaches to human emotions, in particular the narrative approach of Peter Goldie. We end the chapter with a discussion of how we are supposed to talk about our emotions. Despite the ineffable character of many of our feelings, we need a language that is able to at least acknowledge this emotional silence and provide us with a means to deal with the limits of language when trying to make sense of our emotions.

The Feeling of Emotion

The first thing to do is to get hold of the terminology. Despite decades of refinement and development, contemporary research on emotions still suffers from serious conceptual confusion. To feel something is a multifarious phenomenon, so it is not particularly clear what is meant when we say that an experience is emotional. As we have seen in Chapter 4, two concepts seem to dominate the contemporary debate, namely, feelings and emotions. Feelings are generally understood as perceptions of bodily changes and affective states such as discomfort, pleasure, nausea, pain, exaltedness, lust, tiredness, dizziness, and sadness. Emotions, on the contrary, are mostly considered as more structured experiences such as anger (with), surprise (at), love (of), pride (in), shame (at), and guilt (about). In addition to these two concepts, the concept of mood is often indicated as constituting a third kind of emotional experience, but is seldom given more than marginal attention. Emotional experience is far more complex than can be expressed within the framework established on the basis of such a conceptual understanding. In fact, we believe that there is something impoverishing, even unhealthy, about the conceptual dominance of feeling and emotion (Dixon 2003, pp. 24–5). Before the end of the nineteenth century, emotional experience was articulated by means of a variety of terms such as sentiments, passions, feelings, affections, appetites, agitations, and emotions. The scientific spring cleaning of the academic vocabulary together with Darwin's and James's writings on emotions put an end to this novel-like variety. Therefore, in the twentieth century, any philosophical investigation that wanted to be taken seriously focused on the concepts of (structured) emotions and (bodily) feelings.

This narrowing of focus has produced an analytically much stronger understanding of some emotional experiences than would have been possible before. This analytical practice, however, also meant the exclusion of significant aspects of our emotional life. The focus on either the rational, propositional structure of emotions (cognitive theories) or the anonymous working of our bodily landscape (feeling theories) tends to disregard the subjective nature of emotional experience. Over the last decade, there have been attempts to change this picture. As remarked earlier, Peter Goldie's narrative theory argues for a more holistic approach that explains emotions in terms of a narrative, as part of a person's life. Goldie still employs the concepts of emotion and feeling, but his theory also finds room for the personal nature of emotional experience such as intentional feelings (feeling towards as opposed to mere bodily feelings), dispositions, moods, and character traits. This focus on the personal aspect of emotions is an important contribution to our understanding of human emotional life, since it softens the sharp conceptual distinction between emotions and feelings. Emotional experience cannot be explained in isolation from how a person feels an emotion, and not all feelings can be reduced to mere bodily changes. In other words, articulating our emotions and feelings in a narrative structure makes it obvious that the phenomenology of emotions and feelings does not respect the traditional conceptual watershed between cognition and bodily physiology.

Matthew Ratcliffe has recently argued for a more radical departure from the traditional distinction between emotions and feelings. In accordance with Goldie, Ratcliffe argues that cognition and bodily affect are inextricably entangled in emotional experience (2008, pp. 35–40). He develops a phenomenological account of what he calls 'existential feelings', which are radically different from what we normally understand as emotions and feelings. Existential feelings constitute the felt background against which we experience emotions and feelings and orient ourselves in the world. Emotions and bodily feelings become secondary to the constitutive structure of our existential feelings, and thus lose some of their explanatory value in our understanding of human emotional life. Ratcliffe wants to dig below our ordinary categorisation and understanding of emotional experience in terms of emotions and feelings to uncover the constitutive feelings that make our experience of the world possible in the first place. We believe that Ratcliffe's theory is indeed a valuable contribution to our understanding of emotions, because it makes clear the affective dimension of human experience in general. Emotions and feelings are not something that are added on to an otherwise feelingless perception of the world and ourselves, but are constitutive of human experience. Ratcliffe's attentive phenomenological investigation of emotional experience brings to the fore the fundamental role played by feelings in human experience and understanding of the world. Nevertheless, his exclusive emphasis on 'existential feelings' is highly problematic. This special kind of feelings are entrusted to carry a very heavy load of significance (no less than the 'meaning of life'), and Ratcliffe digs so deep in order to expose the most fundamental affective structure of human existence that it becomes difficult to reconnect this profound layer with what we ordinarily mean by emotions and feelings. In fact, his phenomenological account explicitly distances itself so drastically from both the cognitive and the physiological dimension of emotions that such a reconnection appears to become irrelevant (2008, pp. 39–40). We shall deal extensively with Ratcliffe's theory in the next chapter. For now, suffice it to say that we appreciate his emphasis on the general affective nature of human experience but we do not agree with the dramatic significance that he ascribes to 'existential feelings' at the expense of diminishing the significance of more mundane and 'superficial' emotions and feelings.

Both Goldie and Ratcliffe argue that our emotional life cannot be understood without taking into account how we feel about our emotions. In Goldie's own words:

> Consider doing these things unemotionally: Striking a blow; making love; seeking safety. Now consider, and contrast, acting when you act out of emotion: *angrily* striking the blow; making love *passionately*; *fearfully* running away. The phenomenology of such actions— what it is like for the agent—is fundamentally different in character. And an action done with feeling can be distinct in its phenomenology not just for the agent, but also for others involved directly or peripherally in the action; one just has to think what it is like to be made love to with feeling for this to be obvious: it is not like being made love to without feeling, plus feeling. Acting out of emotion is not acting without emotion (explained by feelingless beliefs and desires) plus some added-on ingredient or ingredients.

(Goldie 2000, p. 40)

This attention to how a person feels about the emotions that he or she experiences makes explanatorily relevant the subjective nature of emotional experience, and suggests that there are more to our feelings than mere bodily reactions and that our more complex emotions cannot always be explained as evaluative judgements, belief–desire functions, or intentional attitudes. We believe that this is the right way to go about it. A phenomenological analysis of feelings is suitable to give a more fine-grained account of the feelings that are central to our emotional life, in particular impalpable phenomena such as moods. The use of narratives, on the other hand, can help to explain how our different emotional episodes are related as parts of the history of our lives as persons.

So we agree with Goldie and Ratcliffe that it is necessary to soften the traditional distinction between cognitive emotions and bodily feelings. However, although our approach insists on the importance of feelings, it is not as radical as that of Ratcliffe. Like Goldie, we are not interested in a wholesale conflation of cognitive emotions and bodily feelings in a phenomenological account of more fundamental (existential) feelings. We are convinced that it is possible to retain the analytical benefits from the twentieth century's focus on emotions and feelings while enlarging the framework to include the more subjective aspects of emotional experience, particularly moods, that were often left out for the sake of clarity. The role of the body uncovered in the feeling theories, and the notions of evaluative judgement and responsibility in the cognitive theories, remain fundamental to emotional experience, and we shall use insights from both classes of theories in our own account.

We propose a framework for understanding emotional experience that is grounded on a general notion of normative affectivity and is structured in connection with the notion of personhood. Human consciousness is affective besides being cognitive. Our cognitive skills are always embedded in some kind of affectivity. When we experience something, this something *affects* us in a certain way, and the same goes for our perceptions, thoughts, and actions. As Michael Stocker points out: 'without affectivity it is impossible to live a good human life and it may well be impossible to live a human life, to be a person, at all' (1996, p. 17). The affective nature of human experience is basically illustrated by the fact that our experiences *touch* us and *mean* something to us. We feel our existence in the world as well as we (partially) understand it. We register this being affected by means of more or less distinctive and more or less conscious feelings. Instead of insisting on the conceptual distinction between structured emotions and bodily feelings, our approach begins with a phenomenological analysis of the feelings that constitute two very different emotional experiences that we categorise as moods and affects. By doing so, we are able to pay due attention to the variety of affective phenomena that characterise human emotional experience without deciding beforehand which phenomena are important and which are not on the basis of some pre-established ontological position or other. This approach espouses neither the physicalistic ontology expressed in the feeling theories nor the rationalistic ontology at the heart of the cognitive theories. One of the advantages of such a beginning is that the putting aside of ontological and normative questions (What is an emotion? What is a feeling? Why do I feel like this? Is this emotion appropriate?) paves the way for a more phenomenologically sensible notion of human affectivity. The guiding question in this approach is 'how does it feel?'.

Emotions are rooted in and continually shaped by both physiological reactions and psychological phenomena. On the one hand, 'emotions are bioregulatory reactions that aim at promoting, directly or indirectly, the sort of physiological states that secure not just survival but survival regulated into the range that we, conscious and thinking creatures, identify with well-being' (Damasio 2004, p. 50). On the other hand, as Solomon puts it with his characteristic verve:

> Emotions may typically involve feelings. They may even essentially involve feelings. But feelings are never sufficient to identify or to differentiate emotions, and an emotion is never simply a feeling. One can have an emotion without feeling anything, and one can feel anything (including all the 'symptoms' of emotionality, for example, flushing, pulsing) without having any emotion whatever.
>
> (Solomon 1976, p. 161)

Although we do not agree to this radical separation of feelings and emotions,[1] Solomon is right in pointing out the fact that an emotion is not always bound to the ebbs and flows of the bioregulatory reactions of our body.

We understand emotions as kinetic, dynamic forces that drive us in our ongoing interactions with the environment. This definition of emotion insists on the embodied nature of emotions, but rejects the reduction, implicit in the feeling theories, of the body to an objectified physiological mechanism.[2] It obviously also rejects the conceptualisation of emotions as pure 'mental' phenomena, since an emotion is not primarily a cognitive phenomenon affecting the mind, but a phenomenon rooted in one's lived body. The next section is dedicated to a phenomenological description of this kinetic feature of emotions, so we shall not elaborate further on it here. For now suffice it to say that we understand emotions as primarily characterised by their connection to *motivation* and *movement*. We agree with Ricoeur's definition of emotions as functional states which motivate and may produce movements. This view is also held by contemporary evolutionary psychologists (e.g. Ekman 2003; Laird 2007; Plutchik 1980) as well as by other phenomenologists than Ricoeur (e.g. Sheets-Johnstone 1999; Strasser 1977; Thompson 2007). As functional states that motivate movement, emotions are *protentional* states in the sense that they project the person into the future, providing a felt readiness for action.

Few people doubt that feelings are part of emotional experience, but there is strong disagreement as to how important they are for our understanding of emotions. James identifies feeling with emotion; on the contrary, Solomon distinguishes the two by

---

[1] As noticed in Chapter 4, Solomon himself came to revise his position on this radical separation of emotions and feelings to the extent that he finally 'allowed that (in accordance with common usage) emotions are feelings, but only so long as we expand this notion far beyond the limited notion that feelings are essentially sensations. Some of the feelings involved in emotions are straightforward bodily sensations (for instance, feeling flushed), as William James pointed out, but many more involve the body in more interesting ways, reflecting tendencies to act, for example, or a sense of vulnerability or aggressiveness. But among the feelings involved in emotions are also feelings about the world, thus involving intentionality' (Solomon 2007, p. 232). The feelings that involve intentionality come close to what Goldie has named 'feelings towards' (Goldie 2000, pp. 58–62).

[2] We return to the question of the reductive tendencies inherent in feeling theories in the next chapter, where we take a closer look at Jesse Prinz's updated version of the feeling theory.

saying that we can experience an emotion 'without feeling anything in particular'. Still, detaching feeling from emotion we run the risk of over-intellectualising emotion (Goldie 2000, p. 41) and thus turning off the heat of emotions. If we consider an emotion structured as a feelingless judgement about the world, we lose an important criterion of distinction between emotional actions and unemotional actions. For example, a judge should be able to treat a person justly, regardless of how she feels about him. Only thereby can we say that the verdict was built on just causes and not on the personal feelings of the judge. The feeling dimension of emotion is what permits a distinction between emotional thoughts and actions and their unemotional twins.

However, the distinction between emotions and other cognitive functions is often blurred by the fact that it is difficult to ascertain how or if emotions play a motivational role in our actions. Emotions immerse our cognitive functions in their a-rational movement whenever they appear. The judge is perhaps repelled by the appearance of the accused or by his way of speaking. Or she may be in an irritable mood without being able to put her finger on what exactly this is due to. And both of these emotions might influence her final verdict. Of course, a good judge is one who is able to set aside such personal feelings. The fact, though, that it is difficult to be a good judge reveals that the feelings of emotions tend to impose themselves on most of our rational thoughts and actions.

Feelings are an inherent part of all emotional experience, although how an emotion exactly feels may remain vague to the person. In order to differentiate among various emotional experiences, we need to take a closer look at the feelings that they elicit. For now suffice it to say that feeling may be the best way to know when we are in a certain emotional state, and articulating our feelings will eventually help us understand our emotions. This, of course, presupposes that our conception of emotional experience allows an appreciation of the subtle affective states in which our rational thoughts and actions are embedded.

One reason why the feeling dimension of emotion is important is that emotions can be more or less explicitly conscious. Conscious emotions take up, by virtue of their intentional attitude, a substantial part of our attention in a given situation. For example, I choose not to undress myself in front of other people because I feel ashamed. Less conscious emotions, on the contrary, are not direct objects in our attentional field. They manifest themselves through certain feelings. These feelings can be vague and opaque (as in the case of moods). But the feelings that an emotion elicits are an inescapable component of the emotion itself in the sense that we, as persons, need to acknowledge these feelings in order to fully access the emotion. For instance, our judge may be in a bad mood on the day of the trial. This is indeed a very vague constellation of feelings. Her body feels heavier than usual and the sunlight is annoying. The coffee tastes strange, and even the smallest obstacle, such as a binding door, leaves her exasperated. But although the expression 'bad mood' might seem innocent and insignificant, it is difficult, though, to say with certainty whether or not it is 'a fairly superficial subjective state' (Ratcliffe 2005, p. 55). In fact, being in a bad mood sometimes involves significant feelings that reveal the troubling aspects of the person's values and self-understanding, which are often neglected in an analysis of emotions that does not appreciate the informative values of moods.[3]

---

[3] We shall consider bad moods more carefully in the next chapter.

Furthermore, the constellation of feelings involved in an emotional experience may contain more or less explicit cognitive elements. The feelings involved in fear, for example, may tend to block our cognitive skills in order to enable immediate instinctual flight from whatever is causing the emotion. In sadness, however, feelings and cognition are more closely intertwined. The feelings are both subject and object of our reflections. We are sad because we feel sad, but the thought involved in our sadness may enhance or diminish our feeling of sadness.

And finally, time plays a fundamental role in the feelings of an emotional experience. Whereas some feelings are more or less instantaneous (panic, joy, sexual arousal), others are prolonged (grief, hatred, boredom). The temporal dimension of emotions is best clarified if we pay attention to the feelings that constitute our emotional experience.

In what remains of this chapter, we shall attempt to make sense of our emotional experience in two steps: First, in the following three sections, we engage in a phenomenological description of the feeling of emotions. This involves, among other things, establishing two central categories of feelings, namely, moods and affects, which play a constitutive role in our emotional life. And, secondly, we shall use the concluding two sections to develop our fully fledged hermeneutical account of the vital ways that emotions and personhood are related.

A Choreography of Emotions

How are we to approach the phenomenology of emotions? At least some would answer that, first of all, we need a description of the subjective feeling, for example, what it is like to feel sad, or angry, or happy. Not everybody, of course, would agree to the importance of phenomenal descriptions of emotions. Other approaches include observing the behavioural or visceral aspect of the emotion itself. As noted earlier, LeDoux, for example, is very sceptical about the reliability of phenomenology, or what he calls introspection, for defining emotions. Subjective experiences, he holds, are not a reliable source for the classification of emotions, so 'subjective emotional states, like all other states of consciousness, are best viewed as the end result of information processing occurring unconsciously' (1996, p. 37). Fortunately, not all researchers have such a dismissive attitude towards the subjective dimension of emotions. Jon Elster, for instance, opts for a multi-levelled approach including seven criteria (1999, pp. 244–83): qualitative feel (the intrinsic feature of an emotional experience), cognitive antecedents (beliefs that may trigger an emotion), intentional objects (what an emotion is about), arousal (physiological, mainly visceral, changes), physiological expression (observable features, like bodily posture or voice pitch), valence (being pleasant or painful), and action tendencies (states of readiness to execute an action). On Elster's approach, the first criterion is experiential, the second and the third are cognitive, while the rest are 'visceral' or physiological attributes of emotions.

In this and the following two sections we propose a way to further explore the experiential criterion by means of a phenomenological approach. In the concluding sections of this chapter, we show how the subjective dimension may be integrated with what Elster calls the cognitive aspect of emotions by means of a hermeneutical approach involving the narrative structures of emotional experience. In the next chapter, we shall then argue that this approach makes possible a theory of emotion and personhood which also takes seriously the biological, or what Elster calls the 'visceral', dimension of emotional experience.

A phenomenological description of emotional experience focuses on the qualitative feel of an emotion. The kind of description we propose here can be considered as one way to unfold the short definition of emotions given above, namely, that emotions are functional states which both motivate and produce movement.

In contrast to the cognitive theories, which conceive emotions as intentional attitudes or evaluative judgements inherent in the person's conceptual economy and cognitive engagement with the world, the approach that we advocate here views emotions as pre-reflective dynamic forces driving individuals in their ongoing interactions with the world. It can thus be understood as an elaboration of the feeling theories, since it insists on the embodied nature of emotions. Our approach rejects, though, the tendency in the feeling theories to reduce the body to an object, that is, to some underlying physiological mechanism like visceral changes mediated by the autonomic nervous system. As we shall see in details, our approach to emotions as motivation to movement focuses on the whole-body experience of emotion, and on the kinetic–kinaesthetic bodily experience of emotions.

Such a description of emotions in terms of kinetic–kinaesthetic experience has the advantage of avoiding overtly cognitive and normative characterisation of emotions. Emotions are not characterised as mental states, rather they are portrayed as bodily states. If we consider Solomon's characterisation of three kinds of difficult emotions, it becomes obvious how his cognitive approach differs from a phenomenological one:

> Embarrassment, shame, and guilt can all involve three different dimensions of self-evaluation: (1) the felt evaluation of the self by oneself (thus we can be ashamed or embarrassed even when we are entirely alone, knowing that what we have done is shameful or awkward), (2) an evaluation of oneself imposed by others (thus we can be *made* to be ashamed or embarrassed by other's looks, gestures, and words), and (3) the nature of the situation (there are situations that are embarrassing and acts that are shameful, whatever one feels). Being caught with one's pants down is embarrassing. Not pulling one's pants up is shameful, but pulling one's pants down to make a rude gesture *should* make one ashamed, just because in most situations this will be extremely embarrassing to other people.
>
> (Solomon 2007, p. 93)

We do not wish to deny that people who feel embarrassed, ashamed, or guilty understand their emotions in the light of the three dimensions that Solomon points to. We do indeed evaluate emotional experiences in relation to how we understand ourselves and to how others see us, and in the light of the situation in which the emotion is embedded. However, the problem with a cognitive approach to emotional experience is that it starts out with a reflective assessment of our emotions with a particular normative thrust and an understanding of the conceptual distinction between the similar feelings involved in closely associated emotions. Feelings do not respect conceptual distinctions involved in our emotional vocabulary or the normative judgements that emotions infuse and motivate. On the contrary, feelings tend to blur such distinctions or complicate our normative judgements. The feelings involved in what we understand as emotions of embarrassment, shame, and guilt might complicate our understanding of those emotions, and thus challenge the normative outlook in which this understanding is embedded. To elaborate on Solomon's example, I should be ashamed to pull down my pants in front of other people, but nonetheless sometimes I might feel a twitch of excitement by the thought of doing such an outrageous thing. My feelings of embarrassment and shame are often ambivalent, that is, they involve both attraction and repulsion, or sadness and joy, just as I am sometimes attracted to things that are dangerous and to people whom I know will hurt me. Since most cognitive theories are inherently normative, they also run the risk of becoming moralising in their categorisation of our emotional repertoire. As will become clearer later in this chapter, we do appreciate and indeed make use of the normative characterisation of our emotions as developed by the cognitive approach. We are convinced, though, that a phenomenological bracketing of the normative aspect serves to yield a more refined sense of the ambivalent nature of the feelings involved in emotional experience. Feelings of ambivalence are important, because they may help to articulate the more fundamental ambivalence constitutive of personhood that we argued for in the previous chapter. Also Thomas Fuchs elegantly catches this close relation between ambivalent feelings and human nature:

> All things considered there exists a characteristic ambiguity [*Vieldeutigkeit*] or polyvalence in impressions [*Anmutungen*]: The forest expresses shelter and cover, but also attraction, danger and uncanniness. The lonely column is a symbol of timeless duration or perishability. The mother is nourishing, caring, but also overpowering, devouring; the father is role model or rival, protector or also enemy. This polyvalence is a result of the manifold of emotional relations that are developed to a thing or a person. Because of the dependency on the situation and the mood [*Stimmung*] different qualities of expression emerge. In this regard, particularly, the '*ambivalences*' ['*Ambivalenzen*'] of simultaneously attractive and aversive expressions are of central importance to the basically conflictual structure of human beings.
>
> (Fuchs 2000, p. 201; our translation)

In order to fully appreciate how our emotions motivate and complicate our reflective and rational engagement with the world, other people, and ourselves, we have to pay attention to the way the feelings involved in these emotions affect and influence the pre-reflective, bodily aspect of this engagement. In other words, if we want to know *how it feels* to be embarrassed, ashamed, or inflicted with guilt, we need to acknowledge that when most people try to describe how such emotions affect them they often do so in terms of a concrete vocabulary that refers to their bodily sensations.

A very detailed phenomenological description of the bodily sensations, and more specifically of the kind of movements involved in emotions, is provided by Quentin Smith (1986, pp. 41–62). Smith characterises emotions as sensuous feelings of the 'I that sensuously feels', or as 'I's awareness of its feeling-sensations' (1986, p. 41) and of the corresponding sensuously felt world, or as qualitative-flows that permeate the world. This description, it is argued, enables us to recognise and typify the different emotions. Smith characterises the feeling-sensations of each emotion as *qualitative flows* that accompany each feeling-sensation; or in other words, the way an emotion adheres to the 'I', corresponds to an experience of flowing in a certain direction. Each specific feeling-sensation has its own distinctive feeling-flow. For instance, feeling sad is flowing downwards in a sinking movement. Sadness feels like a slow, sagging flow during which the 'I' slumps down under its own weight. In joy, on the other hand, the feeling-sensation flows upwards in a radiated manner. In hilarious laughter, we feel flowing upwards in quick, *staccato* surges. In retaliatory anger, we painfully feel driven forwards, violently attacking. Love makes us flow forwards in a gently binding way. Pride goes upwards as an inflated rising. Humiliation flows downwards in a plummeting manner; it is a quick and violent emotional drop. In repugnance, the feeling-sensation flows backwards. In awe the feeling-sensation flows backwards and downwards in a shuddering way. Fear makes us move backwards in a shrinking and cringing manner, whereas in anxiety we feel suspended in quavering over an inner bottomlessness.

The above described feeling-sensations adhere to the 'I' as a whole, and as such they must be distinguished from other feeling-sensations which merely adhere to the body. This is the case for fatigue, in which we feel flowing downwards, as in sadness, but with the important difference that in fatigue we experience going down in a dragging manner. Fatigue drags the 'I' down from below. There is, so to say, the sensation of a weight external to the 'I', adhering primarily to the body, which weighs it down. The subjective feeling or internal characterisation of an emotion not only entails a feeling-sensation, that is, the experience of oneself moving forwards or backwards, upwards or downwards. It also entails experiencing a *corresponding movement of the environment* that Smith calls 'feeling-tonality':

> [E]very feeling-sensation of the 'I' is experienced as corresponding to a feeling-tonality of the world, such that through my feeling-sensations I am connected to a sensuously felt reality of the world. This world is not a world of causal reasons but a world that tonally flows in a certain direction and manner. By virtue of these correlated tonal and sensational flows, the world and I are joined together in a extrarational and sensuously appreciative way.
>
> (Smith 1986, p. 53)

Feeling-tonalities are not felt to be features of the 'I', but of the world. We perceive the world as imbued with these flows that appear to be sensuous characters of the world and its parts. We have seen that in sadness the feeling-sensation flows downwards in a sinking manner. Likewise, in the (world-related) feeling-tonality things appear to be forlornly sinking and sagging downwards. In joy the feeling-sensation flows upwards in a radiated manner, imbuing things in one's environmental surroundings. In the corresponding feeling-tonality, things are characterised by uplifted momentum. In love I flow forwards in a gentle and binding manner; in a similar way, the feeling-tonality flows forwards, towards me. In fear things flow forwards, towards me in a looming and menacing manner, while I cringe and shrink from them. In repugnance, while I flow backwards, the repugnant thing flows forwards, towards me. And in awe, while I flow backwards and downwards, in a shuddering manner, the awful thing is flowing forwards and upwards—towering above me.

We may call this approach to emotional experience a *choreography of emotions*, since like a choreography it combines the design of the movements of a person (a dancer) with the design of the environment (the scenario) in which these movements are situated. As we have seen in Chapter 4, an issue that has always stirred up debate in philosophy of emotions is the relationship between cognition and emotion, and more in general, the question to what extent we can say that a person is aware of, and in control of, his or her emotion. We can try to rephrase these questions in terms of our choreography and ask whether or not the 'dancer' is aware, or in cognitive control, of her emotional flows and of the scenario in which these take place.

Our dancer, then, may *sense* what she is doing, nonetheless being scarcely (or not at all) aware in a reflective or propositional way of all that is happening on the stage—including her feeling-sensations and the feeling-tonality of the scenario. That is to say that first and foremost we *embody* an emotion, and this embodiment takes place *before* we make explicit the implicit experience of the emotion itself, i.e. the feeling-sensation and feeling-tonality. The sensation is not a reflective appreciation, rather an immediate connection with the emotion itself or self-affection. In the absence of self-affection, an emotion as a bodily event may remain unfelt, or be sensed as an event occurring in an external, objectified body-machine.

Smith describes a three-layered stratification of the awareness of feelings (pp. 25–7). At the lowest level, feelings are intuitively known as a presence of global importance. The world is experienced by the person as an unquestionable, meaningful whole in an immediate way, without being influenced by any sort of discursive or inferential thinking. On the second level, these intuitive feelings begin to dissipate, losing their immediate presence, and the person experiences a lingering afterglow of the feeling, while the sensations immanent in an emotion become at the same time less vivid and more explicit. In the afterglow, we experience a retention through which we re-live in immediate memory the previously intuited feelings. This evokes thoughts and linguistic formations through which we express and signify these feelings. These verbal significations are metaphorical, often vague but also abundant in connotation. When, at the third level, the afterglow burns itself out, we re-appreciate feelings through a concentrative effort that allows us to single out and analyse our feelings, and capture them more or less aptly in language:

> In the intuitive feeling, what explicitly appeared was the unitary phenomenon comprised of the various aspects and structural articulations inherent in the global importance; the various structural contents themselves appeared only in a tacit way. The significations evoked in the afterglow of the intuitive feeling were evoked by this explicitly appearing unitary phenomenon, and were designed to capture this unitary phenomenon rather than its various structural constituents. It is these structural contents, which fell outside of the explicit appreciative focus of the intuitive feeling and its afterglow, that now appear to be of fascinating interest and worthy of being attentionally appreciated in their own right. They inspire me to concentrate upon them, to single out and analyze them in successive acts of attention, and to capture them in linguistically articulated thoughts. (p. 26)

This phenomenology of the way feelings become manifest in time has important bearings on a hermeneutics of emotions, and it may serve as a method to acknowledge one's own feelings in a way that is not infected by cognitive attitudes or normative judgements. It is a diachronic phenomenology of the self-manifestation of emotions. It must also be admitted that, although we may be completely unaware of being in a particular emotional state, we may nonetheless be influenced and moved by those emotions. The self is not always transparent to its own emotions. I may be sad without being aware of being sad, and still behave like a sad person. We have all experienced that sometimes our emotions may be better (or earlier) noticed by other people, from the outside rather than from within, so to speak. I may have a global feeling of uneasiness and be unable to say what it is, while my friend can see—from my facial expression, posture, and movements—that I am enmeshed in sadness.

This intersubjective capacity to recognise the emotions of other people means that my friend may have an access to my emotions which can be both quicker and more accurate than my own. Or to put it differently, there are times when an outside observer may be more precise in assessing another person's emotional state than the person himself. This is possible because here we have a corporeal connection with other persons which does not require either being self-aware of one's emotions, or being capable of articulating them. This intercorporeal link lets emotions pass from one person to another through the simple fact that interpersonal relationships are made possible, for a large part, by our ability to recognise the emotional states of other people. Also, my friend is not only in touch with me because of her capacity to notice my sadness before I myself am aware of being sad. She is also in touch with the linguistic horizon of sadness, that is, with the way people imagine, think, and talk about sadness. Perhaps she would ask me if I feel down, or drowned, or staggering under a burden; or else dark, or cold, and so on. By doing so, she is helping me to recognise my emotion by means of the intersubjectively shared repertoire of its metaphorical expressions and articulations. In this way, she facilitates my appraisal of my feelings through the intermediary of verbal signification, mental imagery, or discursive thought.

These considerations help us envision three broad facets of the phenomenology of emotions. First is their connection with self-affection, that is, their original belonging to the sphere of pre-reflective self-awareness, tacitly imbuing one's self-awareness and perception of the world with emotional sensations and tonalities, and thus pre-reflectively motivating one's actions. This dimension of emotions is partly revealed by psychological introspection, but even more specifically, as we have seen, we recognise an emotion through our own kinetic/tactile–kinaesthetic bodily experience of it. Secondly is the embodied nature of emotions, that is, their corporeal expression. The embodied nature of our emotions is also revealed by the person's kinetic–kinaesthetic bodily experience of a certain emotion. This facet of the phenomenality of an emotion differs from the previous one by being its outward dimension. It is the way an emotion not only feels from the inside, but also appears and can be seen from the outside. This expressive nature of our emotions is also revealed by the bond between emotions and intercorporeality, that is, by their being meaningful for other people through a pre-linguistic, intercorporeal link. Thirdly, the relation between emotions and language through metaphors. This relationship is characterised by a hermeneutical dialectic: emotions are shaped by language conventions which contribute to our conscious understanding and conceptualisation of emotions themselves; on the other hand, emotions, as parts of our intersubjectively shared bodily physiology, provide the basis for mutual understanding among humans by shaping our language with emotion-based metaphors. It goes without saying that in addressing the metaphorical expressions of emotions, we obviously have to be very attentive to transcultural differences.

We will conclude this section with some remarks on the principal metaphorical domains by means of which we articulate and talk about our emotions. When we turn to the most common metaphors of emotions, we soon discover that they do not only include flow metaphors, although these seem to be predominant. The following are only a few examples (most of them taken from Barcelona 1986 and Kövecses 2000a).

Sadness metaphors reflect the down source domain of feeling-flows above: sad is down (he brought me down with his remarks), dark (she is in a dark mood), a burden (she staggered under the pain), a superior (he was ruled by sorrow). Yet, sadness is also lack of vitality (this was disheartening news) and of heat (losing his father put his fire out). Sadness may also be a fluid in a container (I am filled with sorrow). Although this disparity may reflect an over-inclusive conceptualisation of sadness, all these metaphors are relevant to reveal the link between our bodily sensations and our conceptual managing of these sensations.

Happiness metaphors are opposite to sadness metaphors (Kövecses 1991, 2000a; Lakoff and Johnson 1980), and like sadness metaphors they are congruent with (and integrate with) the feeling-flow described above. Happy is up (we had to cheer him up), off the ground (I was so happy that my feet barely touched the ground), bright and light (she brightened up at the news, or he was swept off his feet), warm (that warmed my heart), a rapture (I was drunk with joy). Happiness is also a fluid in a container (he was overflowing with joy) and obviously implies pleasurable physical sensation (I was tickled pink, or he was happy as a pig in the shit).

Anger metaphors are maybe the most studied from a cognitive semantic point of view (Kövecses 1986, 2000a, 2000b; Lakoff and Kövecses 1987). The main source domain of anger metaphors is that anger is a *hot fluid in a container* (boiling with anger, making one's blood boil, simmering down, or blowing your stack). A major attraction of the *pressurised container* metaphor is that it captures a great number of aspects and properties of anger. It allows us to conceptualise intensity (filled with), control (contain), loss of control (could not keep inside), dangerousness (brim with), expression (express/show). The same general *container* metaphor exists in different cultures, meaning that anger is predominantly viewed as some kind of substance (fluid or gas) inside a closed container that is the human body. Kövecses (2000b, p. 165) proposes that conceptualised physiology provides the basis for the metaphorical description of the angry person as a *pressurised container*. This metaphor arises out of the embodied nature of our emotions, since it is actually the case that people's temperature and blood pressure rise in anger.

Just as importantly, though, it can be shown that although the metaphors for anger are informed and shaped by basic human physiology, they nevertheless vary considerably both across cultures and within the same culture: 'The generic or schematic structure of the concepts seems to be shaped by possibly universal aspects of human physiology in anger, which structure is, at the same time, given differentiated specific-level content by particular modes of cultural explanation' (Kövecses 2000b, p. 169).[4] The universal elements derive from human physiology, and culture-specific elements from cultural diversity in terms of cognitive attitudes and moral judgements.

Shame belongs to the group of social emotions, such as anger, pride, and admiration, in the sense that it is triggered by events that make reference to other people (Elster 1999, pp. 139–45). Unlike fear, for instance, a moral judgement is a necessary condition to elicit shame. Holland and Kipnis (1995; quoted in Kövecses 2000a, p. 32) hold that the central metaphor for shame is 'having no clothes on', which is a kind of experience that makes sense only in the presence of other people who share the same beliefs about nakedness. One could argue, as Kövecses partly does (2000a, p. 33), that this is a conceptual metonymy (a metonymy is a 'stand-for' relationship, it provides access to a domain through a part of the same domain, or to a part of a domain through another part of the same domain), more than a true metaphor (a metaphor's purpose being to represent the more abstract in terms of the more concrete). Nonetheless, shame metaphors also reflect bodily-based flow-sensations like moving downwards and inwards. Two major source domains for shame metaphors are hiding away (I wanted to bury my head in the sand) and decrease in size (I felt *this* big).

These concluding remarks on emotional metaphors are meant as an illustration of how the embodied nature of emotional experience influences and to some extent constitutes the way a person experiences and handles emotions in her engagement with the world and other people. This embodied influence operates in terms of both the biological dimension of our body (the anonymous *Körper*, i.e. the body as an object) and the phenomenological dimension (the personal *Leib*, i.e. the lived body). Kövecses's work on emotional metaphors illustrates how this combination of biology and personhood—the subjective experience of an embodied self situated in a cultural context shared with other people—irrupts even into the way we understand our emotions in language. In Chapter 3, we saw how Ricoeur argued that both these dimensions are crucial if we want to understand how our body complicates our identity as persons, and in Chapters 4 and 5 we attempted to substantiate this argument, first with Panksepp's neuroscientific theory of a dual-aspect monism with its insistence on a unified neurobiological and psychological approach to affective consciousness, and subsequently by means of the feelings of ambivalence caused by the ontological ambiguity of biology and psychology constitutive of human personhood. We have called this initial phenomenological approach to the feelings of this ambivalence a choreography of emotions in order to emphasise the way our feelings bind us to our body, the world, and other people (i.e. otherness). Through our feelings we are enmeshed in the world and connected with other people to such an extent that it becomes difficult to distinguish selfhood and otherness.

---

[4] Arguing that anger, and most other human emotions, are both universal and culture-specific, Kövecses opts for a unified approach: 'it seems possible to propose a synthesis that merges the social constructionist and universalist approaches into a unified view of emotions and emotion language. It seems appropriate to call this unified approach "body-based constructionism" and the prototypical cultural models that the approach aims to uncover the "embodied cultural prototype"' (Kövecses 2000a, p. 183).

Moods and Affects

One way to get a hold on the diffuse and dynamic texture of feelings involved in our interaction with the world is to establish phenomenological categories. In particular, two distinctive categories of feelings, moods and affects, provide an effective tool for understanding how the person lives, experiences, and copes with his or her emotions. Both moods and affects are characterised by the constellation of feelings involved in the experience of them, and an analysis of the phenomenology of these feelings makes possible a better understanding of their influence on a person.

Feelings are the most personal aspect of my experience of the world as a set of *affordances*: a set of relevant possibilities that are my own possibilities as a person situated in this particular world. This being situated in a world of possibilities through a certain constellation of feelings is called 'attunement' (*Befindlichkeit*) by Heidegger (2010, pp. 134–40). Heidegger's use of the notion plays on the semantic density of the reflexive verb '*sich befinden*', which can refer to both a person's location (finding oneself somewhere) and the state of mind of that person, that is, being in a certain mood (*Stimmung*). The notion of *Befindlichkeit* goes straight to the heart of our question 'How do you feel?'. How I feel reflects both how I am situated in the world and how I feel about my being situated in a specific way. The relation between my being situated in the world and my feelings about my being thus situated is complex. It is equally wrong to say that a certain thing in the world elicits specific feelings (that seeing a snake causes fear, for example) or that certain feelings colour my perception of the world (for instance, that anxiety causes me to see a stick as a snake). There is not a simple causal relation between perception and feelings, or vice versa. Both feeling and perception find their explicative correlate in the actual and concrete situation of the person. We feel and perceive the world in a certain way because of our being-in-the-world (*In-der-Welt-sein*). While the internalist concept of 'mood'[5] focuses on the (hypothetical) causes of a given *vision* of the world (e.g. the world of a frightened person), the concept of *Befindlichkeit* focuses on the set of affordable *actions* of a person who is located in a certain context and affected by a certain constellation of feelings that allows her to see the things around her as disclosing certain (and not other) possibilities. This view is aimed at putting person, body, and world together again.

The explanatory virtue of Heidegger's concept of *Befindlichkeit* lies in the emphasis on feelings as a disclosure (*Erschlossenheit*) of one's situatedness in the world, as against being an impediment to objectively appreciating a certain state of things. The significance of an event or state of affairs is not merely a matter of its intrinsic properties, but rather of its relation to me and my current engagement. Feelings reveal what the world is like for me, how the world touches me, and what it means to me to be a person embedded in the world. In Heidegger's analysis, the notion of *Befindlichkeit* is closely tied to that of 'understanding' ('*Verstehen*') and 'language' ('*Sprache*'). We can

---

[5] The internalist concept of 'mood' sees it as a state of mind entailing a given *vision* of the world. On this view, it is because of a 'lowered' mood that the world is darkened ('As if you saw things through dark lenses') and action becomes impossible ('What you lack is the vital drive'). The externalist approach also views moods as internal states of mind, but caused by external events.

only understand ourselves and the world in which we are situated through the context of our practical engagement, and this engagement is primordially enveloped in certain feelings. In other words, how we understand and speak of our engagement with the world is always influenced by how we feel about being a person embedded in and engaged with the world. This way of looking at feelings has fundamental implications for the interpretation and understanding of emotional experience. This will be best appreciated if at first we look more carefully at the phenomenological characteristics of two central categories of feelings involved in a person's *Befindlichkeit*.[6] We have chosen to call these two categories 'mood' and 'affect'.

The phenomenological distinction between affects and moods largely overlaps with Ricoeur's distinction *sentiments schematisés/sentiments informés* (Ricoeur 1987, pp. 104–6 [121–2]). Phenomenologists have contributed to explaining this distinction in an explicit and systematic way (for an overview, see Fuchs 2000; Smith 1986; Strasser 1977). The distinction is merely incipient in Husserl's writings and is first made explicit by Scheler (1966, 1976), and then developed further by Fuchs (2000), Heidegger (1995, 2010), Sartre (1971), and Strasser (1977). In short, the distinction can be summed up in the following way: affects are responses to a phenomenon that is perceived as their motivation, whereas moods do not possess such directedness to a motivating object. Although their terminology differs, and often confusingly at that (e.g. Scheler: *Affekte/Gefühle*; Heidegger: *Affekte/Stimmungen*; Sartre: *affects/émotions*), their accounts concur in the general characteristics (see Table 1).

Affects are focused and intentional and possess directedness. Affects are felt as motivated; they are more determinate than moods and more articulated. Affects do not open up a broad horizontal awareness, but occupy all my attentional space. In fear, for example, I am completely absorbed by the phenomenon that terrifies me. When I am affected, a relevant feature of the world captivates me, irrupts into my field of awareness without me having decided to turn my attention to it. I become spellbound to it, and all of my attention is captured by it. Typical examples of captivating affects are grief (in bereavement, for instance, when the loss of a loved one occupies all my attentional space), fear, phobias, surprise, joy, anger, jealousy, and hate.

Moods, on the contrary, are unfocused and not clearly intentional. They do not possess directedness and aboutness. They are felt as unmotivated, and there are no 'felt causes' for them. They are more indefinite and indeterminate than affects and are often inarticulate. Moods have a horizontal absorption in the sense that they attend to the world as a whole, not focusing on any particular object or situation (Ricoeur's 'fundamental feeling'). Moods often manifest themselves as prolonged feelings as opposed to the more instantaneous nature of affects.[7] Whereas most affects fill up the entire

---

[6] For reasons already explained in Chapter 1, and which are to be further developed in the next chapter, we are not going to follow Heidegger's own development of the notion of *Befindlichkeit*. This is not to deny, though, that our analysis is heavily indebted to Heidegger's seminal work on feelings (in particular 1995 and 2010). On the contrary, Heidegger's analyses remain fundamental to the development of our theory, just as they were to Ricoeur's theory of subjectivity.

Table 1 Moods and affects

Mood	Affect
Unfocused	Focused
Non-intentional/covert intentionality	Intentional
Not motivated	Motivated
Inarticulate	Articulate
Horizontal absorption	No horizontal absorption
Emanated from, not by	Emanated from and by
No captivation	Captivation
No 'felt causes'	'Felt causes'
Indefinite and indeterminate	Determinate
No directedness	Directedness
Sustained and subdued intensity	Wax and wane of high intensity

The list is inspired by Quentin Smith's magisterial analysis of the differences between moods and affects (1986, pp. 109–46). See also the interesting empirical investigation of how 106 non-academic people distinguish between emotion and mood (here we would prefer the term 'affect' to 'emotion', but the characteristics coincide), the result is very similar to the table presented here (Beedie et al. 2005).

field of awareness for a brief period (for example, in fear or anger), moods convey a constellation of vague feelings that permeate, and often transform, my whole field of awareness.

Moods are global feeling-states that do not focus on any specific object in my field of awareness. When we are in a certain mood, we relate ourselves to the world and to our own person *through* that mood. In euphoria, for instance, the perception of my body is feeble and may even vanish. I feel absorbed in my concerns; my self-awareness, my body, and the world fuse together in perfect harmony. In sadness, on the other hand, the perception of my body comes to the foreground; I may feel my body as an obstacle, a hindrance separating me from the world and perhaps even from myself. Thus, moods are atmospheric and often corporeal in that they permeate my perception of the environment. They can lead me closer to or farther from the world because they produce a certain atmosphere that becomes the tonality through which I perceive the world and myself. When I am feeling euphoric, the world and other persons appear in a soft light of possibility and openness; when I am irritated, my perception is different. In this case, things appear as unwelcome obstacles, and even the most sincere smile can be perceived as false and annoying.

---

[7] In fact, the psychologist James A. Russell's neuropsychological account of core affect ('the simplest raw (nonreflective) feelings evident in moods and emotions') defines moods as 'prolonged core affect' (2003, pp. 147–8).

An important aspect of moods is that in virtue of being prolonged and pervasive constellations of feelings, they are dispositional in nature and may develop into character traits: 'our traits are shaped by our emotions and moods, just as our emotions and moods are shaped by our traits' (Goldie 2000, p. 141). Goldie here puts forward an interesting dialectical interplay that we will develop further in the closing sections of this chapter.

Table 1 is an attempt to resume the main characteristics of moods and affects in such a way that their oppositional nature becomes clear.

Examples of moods as opposed to affects are anxiety as opposed to fear, sadness (as opposed to) grief, euphoria/joy, dysphoria/anger, tedium/boredom.

As remarked earlier, little work has been done on moods in the tradition of analytical philosophy. The treatment of moods is often reduced to peripheral mention in investigations of emotions. When they are mentioned, though, their main characteristics concur with the phenomenological account of an objectless phenomenon. The fact remains, however, that moods are often treated as opposed to, or are significantly different from, emotions (e.g. Blackburn 1998, p. 130; de Sousa 1987, p. 311) so that the distinction is not mood vs affect, but mood vs emotion. It is our opinion that if we treat both moods and affects as different constellations of feelings within the same continuum of emotional experience, it will enhance our understanding of the dialectical transitions between the two phenomena and their significance for the person.

While affects seem to admit of a robust definition because of their object-directed nature, moods (due to their disorienting and hazy phenomenality) do not enjoy the same privilege. It may therefore be of help to elaborate more thoroughly on some of the principal characteristics of moods and affects in relation to the concept of a person. This will be the topic of the next section.

The categories of moods and affects may help to unfold the complex and heterogeneous phenomenon that we vaguely call an emotion. Emotion is an 'umbrella' term that is used to describe what we understand as emotional experience. This experience is characterised by different constellations of feelings that range from brief, clear affects at one end to longer, more diffuse moods at the other. What we experience as different emotions lies within these two extremes and can be categorised according to the nature of the feelings involved. In the following sections, we propose a way to articulate the interaction between moods and affects in the emotional experience of a person by means of three conceptual tools: first and second, in terms of the phenomenological categories of intentionality and temporality; third, by means of the hermeneutical model of narrative structures. The aim of this approach is to provide the basis for an interpretation of emotional experience that will, hopefully, strengthen our argument for the relationship between emotions and personhood.

Intentionality and Temporality

As we have already seen, the intentionality of a mental state is its property of being 'of' or 'about' something. The standard phenomenological view on moods and affects is more or less clear as to one fundamental difference: moods are unintentional and affects are intentional. Strasser, who has worked out a rich and detailed phenomenological analysis of feelings, writes:

> We must therefore distinguish more carefully than usual between an irritated, angry, happy or anguished mood [*Stimmung*] on the one hand, and being irritated, angry, happy *about something*, being anxious *over something* on the other. In the first case, irritation is 'in the air' without the conscious apprehension of any motive for irritation. In the second case, we are directed, in the mode of feeling irritation, toward something: being-irritated here has an object that is intentionally 'meant' [. . .] we shall understand by mood only the felt attunement [*fühlende Befindlichkeit*], the pure being-in-a-mood [*reines Zumute-sein*].
>
> (Strasser 1977, p. 183 [111]; translation slightly modified)

This view can be further developed by relating the two kinds of feelings to the person. It is correct to say that an affect such as fear is about the particular object of fear and that an anxious mood does not point to any specific intentional object, but manifests itself as an unarticulated background tonality or atmosphere that pervades my whole field of awareness. Nevertheless, my anxious mood seems to affect the way I relate to the world in the sense that it is accompanied by a certain atmosphere in my perceptions. A situation that beforehand would not intimidate me now fills me with an overwhelming feeling of wanting to run away and look for protection. The feelings involved in the intentional attitude of my affects are in this way changed by my current mood. My mood is expressed by how perceptions or thoughts affect me. Moods materialise in affects in the sense that I am affected *through* my mood. This could suggest what we might call a *covert intentionality* in moods. Whereas affects have a direct and clear intentional object (an object of perception or a thought), moods are characterised by multiple objects.[8] While affects point to an explicit experience such as a dangerous situation, a happy smile, a beautiful landscape, or a difficult task, moods, on the contrary, point to my being the person I am in a given situation.

Moods can be compared with what Ricoeur calls 'ontological sentiments' in that '[t]hey denote the fundamental feeling [. . .], namely, man's very openness to being' (1987, p. 105 [121]). Moods reveal one's situatedness in the world. We can say that whereas affects point *outwards* towards a specific object, moods point *inwards* towards my being the person I am. Or even more precisely, one could say that moods reveal a *bipolar intentionality*. That is, they arise as non-intentional feelings but often materialise in a certain affect directed to an explicit object; and moreover, they point to my being the person I am, and thereby they give rise to questions, doubts, considerations, and evaluations about my being the person that I am. Moods pave the way to self-understanding.

---

[8] The psychologist Matthias Siemer has developed a similar theory called the *dispositional theory of moods* which 'holds that moods are, at least in essential part, *temporary dispositions* to have or to generate particular kinds of cognitions, specifically to make particular kinds of emotion-relevant appraisals' (Siemer 2005, pp. 816–7). He argues that moods are '*multiple-object directed*' (p. 818) and contrasts this with the idea that moods are 'intrinsically objectless, raw feelings' (p. 842). Recently, he has explained why moods have normally been conceived as objectless: 'Because, as a consequence, the person's mood experience is directed at *multiple objects*, the person has the subjective impression that no clear object exists' (Siemer 2009, pp. 257–8).

Moods and affects interact and affect one another in the experience of the person who undergoes an emotion. This way of understanding the interaction of moods and affects can be developed further if we consider the temporality of our feelings.

Moods and affects display different temporal patterns. Affects are often briefer than moods. They captivate me, occupy my whole field of awareness and thereby move me to a determinate action within a restricted period of time. Moods, on the contrary, may last for hours, days, or even months, paralysing my thoughts and restraining me from acting (sadness) or throwing me into unbridled actions without any thoughts of the past or the future (euphoria). The heightened intensity of the feelings involved in affects demands a concrete action regarding our present situation such as to express our anger, escape the bear, return the happy smile, and work on the difficult task. Obviously, often we do not act out of the affect but restrain ourselves from acting out of it. Most of the time we are able to dominate the affect by a cognitive effort. For example, my well-nigh irresistible desire to insult or poke a malicious boss may be suppressed by the fear of losing my job. The intensity of the affect then gradually subsides, and I turn my attention to other matters. This does not imply, however, that the affect vanishes altogether. It may remain as a bitter memory that brings forth unpleasant feelings every time it pops up in my mind.

Also, there exists a dialectic between moods and affects that happens in time. This dialectic is quite complex.[9] Affects sometimes transform themselves into moods and may end up becoming a permanent part of our disposition or character, that is, of who and what we are. Moods, on the other hand, can influence affects because they alter the way we are affected by objects and thoughts. Last but not least, a given mood may transform into an affect when in reflection I articulate it and find its motivations and 'felt causes', that is, the way it roots me in a given situation. In other words, I may be able to make my mood explicit by reflecting on the possible reasons why I am in a certain mood.

An affect can transform itself into a mood that imposes itself on me for days or even longer; for example, grief can turn into a general sadness, anger into dysphoria, and boredom into tedium. In a similar way, a mood may develop out of an affect as the affect itself loses its instantaneous, focused, and motivated character. Also, a mood might not be the product of a single affect and the following action or suppression of action, but a constellation of feelings caused by several episodes. Moods (e.g. irritability, sadness, tedium, euphoria) change the way I am affected by the world (and my own thoughts) in the sense that they predispose the way I experience the world, other people, and myself. And, as we have seen, over time moods can, in virtue of being dispositional, transform themselves into an inherent and *permanent* part of the person that I am. As the intensity of an affect subsides, it can turn into a mood, and a mood can grow into an entrenched embodied emotional tonality as the core emotion of a specific physiological constitution. For instance, a dysphoric state can gain such a hold on my person that it turns into a certain character trait such as an irritable, hostile, mean, polemic,

---

[9] Rosfort and Stanghellini (2009) and Stanghellini and Rosfort (2010). Acute and comprehensive phenomenological investigations of affective transitions and alterations have been made by Fuchs (2000, pp. 193–251), Goldie (2000, pp. 141–75), and Strasser (1977, pp. 203–42 [128–60]).

misanthropic, or adverse character. This basic emotional tonality is a permanent (often implicit) protention or readiness to (re)act and be affected in a given way, and probably also to develop certain moods more than others. In this way, our more indeterminate emotional experiences become entrenched in the involuntary dispositional patterns of a person's behaviour. This is akin to what in mainstream psychiatry is called 'temperament' (Akiskal 1996; Akiskal and Akiskal 2005). Temperament types are prolonged, temporally stable dispositions to behaviour particular to an individual with a certain personal history and social context. Although temperament types are commonly viewed to be biologically *determined* in nature (Evans et al. 2005), our model argues for a more careful analysis of the relation between temperament types and character traits, of which the former are more directly characterised by basic, involuntary feeling states, whereas the latter pertain more to contracted emotional habits.

A basic emotional tonality is usually tacit, and often I notice it only when it is not there. It is important here to keep in mind that usually these transformations from affects to moods to character occur pre-reflectively and without a deliberate and thematic involvement of the person in the process. To be able to understand and cope with how affects may turn into moods, and moods into an entrenched part of a person's character, we need a way to articulate these transformations.

Of great importance is the way in which a mood can be transformed into its corresponding affect. As we have already seen in Chapter 3, the concept of temporality can be understood in terms of how the person experiences time and how the existence of the person is inescapably formed and developed through time. Temporality is not time as an exclusively phenomenological (subjective) or pure cosmological (objective) phenomenon. Time can be conceived both as experienced and lived by the person and as time working on the person. A person is firmly rooted in the time of physical nature, and yet her experience of time differs somewhat from the mere experience of the changing of seasons. Objective and subjective time play an important role in understanding human subjectivity, and the one cannot be reduced to the other. We have seen that Ricoeur proposes a third conception of time, namely, time as configured by narratives. Narrated time includes the way time works on the subject, i.e. how the subject is involuntarily affected by time, as well as how the subject actively copes with time. Just as we do not remain passively receptive to the workings of time, we can also take an active stance in front of our moods. Through time, we reflect on our moods and are able to make them an explicit part of our identity, primarily by means of narratives. We may at first remain passively affected by a given mood, but sooner or later we may be able to articulate and understand our mood, that is, we can establish its origin, what it reveals about our present situation, and its meaning in the context of our life story. We can try to tease out its covert intentional horizon, and by doing so we might be able to get a grip on the relation between our mood and its corresponding affects. In other words, we can appropriate a mood by articulating how that mood is part of who we are and how our affects are influenced by our moods.

This brings us to narratives as a way to articulate the interaction of moods and affects. We shall spend considerably more time on narratives, since with the help of narratives we introduce the final, and properly hermeneutical, level in our theory of emotions and personhood. We begin by arguing for the benefits of using Ricoeur's theory of narratives, developed with insights from Ronald de Sousa and Peter Goldie, to explain emotional experience in general. With this in place, we then go on to show how a narrative structure might help clarify the interaction of moods and affects, and how these may help us to better understand the relationship between emotions and personhood.

Narrating Our Emotions

The phenomenological analysis of moods and affects uncovers details about the basic structures of feelings and the subject who experiences them. However, as we argued in accordance with Ricoeur in Chapter 2, the analysis needs to be complemented by a hermeneutical approach in order to clarify the relation between the feelings and the person who experiences them. In the previous chapter, we argued that personhood is characterised by a felt sense of ambivalence between selfhood and otherness. The experience of a person involves a sense of voluntary selfhood, that is, a sense of the fact that I am a self who is always able to relate itself to the person that I am. In other words, the self always cares about the person that he or she is. This voluntary, reflective sense of selfhood is complicated, though, by the involuntary sense of otherness at work in human selfhood, and is made an explicit problem when confronted with the notion of personhood. To be a self is not simply the same as to be a person. On the contrary, the immediate, pre-reflective nature of voluntary selfhood becomes complicated when viewed in relation to the notion of personhood. To insist that a human self is also a person is to emphasise the fragile, often troubled, sense of being an autonomous human self. Hence, personhood makes explicit the problematic interplay of voluntary (selfhood) and involuntary (otherness) aspects of being a person.

One way to approach the problematic relation between the voluntary and involuntary aspects of a person's sense of identity is precisely in terms of an interpretation of our moods and affects. And the narrative structure of personal identity is an important part of this interpretation.

We have already explained Ricoeur's use of narrative to make sense of personal identity. His theory on narratives is elaborate and works on, at least, four interconnected explanatory levels. On one level, narrative identity seeks to explore what is particular about human time by establishing a third, particularly human, category configured by both cosmological (objective, anonymous) and phenomenological (subjective, lived) time. On a second level, it is a tool to approach the diachronic nature of human identity by articulating the historicity of the person (a person finds itself embedded in a concrete human world constituted by values and norms shaped by certain traditions and sociocultural contexts). A third dimension of narrative identity deals with the intrinsic problems of personal identity (selfhood and otherness). And finally, it helps to bridge the descriptive and prescriptive aspects of identity by articulating the normative problems involved in personhood (the axiological dimension or values). We have dealt more thoroughly with these different aspects in Chapters 2 and 3, where we showed how the different aspects are closely interconnected. Here we shall only deal explicitly with the last two, namely, personal identity and normativity.

Ricoeur argues that narratives can help to sort out the voluntary and involuntary aspects of personal identity; or put differently, the problems involved in the fact that we are what we are, and yet can feel that we are different, and want to be different, from what we (f)actually are—in short, the problems that spring from our care about the person that we are. Narratives provide a way into the difficult issue of how we have become what we are (with our particular ideas, dreams, desires, long time dispositions, habits, character), because '[w]hat sedimentation has contracted, narration can redeploy' (1992, p. 122 [148]). And moreover, Ricoeur argues that narratives are '*the first laboratory of moral judgment*' (1992, p. 140 [167]), since they disclose the normative aspect of our actions and their relation to personal identity. These two aspects of narratives unfold the fact that personal identity is not only a descriptive process of reidentification, but also a normative problem about how we relate ourselves to the person that we are.

Now, Ricoeur does not, regrettably, analyse the role of emotional experience in the narrative structure of identity. And even though Ricoeur's theory of subjectivity and his account of personal identity remain the theoretical background, the following analysis of emotional experience and narrative identity will draw much on the work of Ronald de Sousa and Peter Goldie. Although de Sousa does not advocate a narrative approach, he has nevertheless coined a concept that has important implications for narrative theories, namely, the concept of *paradigm scenarios*. Goldie, on the other hand, has developed two helpful concepts that we will use in the following interpretation of moods and affects, namely, *the external perspective* and *emotional resistance*.

De Sousa argues that we 'are made more familiar with the vocabulary of emotions by association with *paradigm scenarios*' (de Sousa 1987, p. 182). These scenarios can largely be explained as an array of different types of more or less uniform emotional responses to different things, people, and events. Few would deny that there exist prototypes of emotional responses, which are paradigmatic for human persons. Since early childhood we exist in a world characterised and qualified by emotional experience. For example, we learn to fear glowing hotplates because they might hurt us, and we learn that a genuine smile expresses joy, compassion, or pleasure, whereas a frown indicates anger; unpleasant screaming, fear or desperation; downcast eyes, sadness or grief. De Sousa explains that our emotional vocabulary is constituted, developed, and continuously refined in much the same way as our verbal vocabulary:

> As adults, we forget the occasions on which we learned our words; but the associations set up then may remain, to influence the connotations and even the sense of the word. Adult emotions are similarly rooted in original episodes, associated with a characteristic feel (including, but not limited to, bodily feelings and impulses), and with a cast of characters who played the original roles. In these little dramas, whose origins are lost behind the veil of childhood amnesia, our own roles are overlearned, as are our expectations of the roles in which others are unwittingly cast. Just as the meaning of common words retain private connotations and implications beyond the settled reference classes on which we can all agree, so paradigm scenarios determine the *meaning* of the emotions of which they constitute the prototypes.

(de Sousa 2011, p. 34)

Our emotional register is continuously refined and revised through our interaction with the world and other persons. In an important sense, paradigm scenarios shape the very character of our emotions, because emotions are understood in relation to meaningful choices and actions, and therefore 'their essential role lies in establishing specific patterns of salience relevant to interference [...] they are perfectly tailored for the role of arbitrators among reasons' (1987, p. 200). When we experience a certain scenario (e.g. a woman hitting her child, a person helping another in need, starving children, the death of a loved one) we respond emotionally to it, and de Sousa argues that the emotions elicited by such a scenario (e.g. contempt, compassion, sadness, grief) are defined by paradigmatic scenarios that are again constituted by experience, culture, and our biological constitution. These scenarios are, of course, highly context-sensitive and furthermore influenced by a multitude of personal and social factors that make the paradigm scenarios very individual. Nonetheless, de Sousa argues for an objective account of emotions:

> [E]motions tell us something about the real world. To be sure, their mode of objectivity is relative to the characteristic inclinations and responses of human and individual nature. The biological function that makes them indispensable to complex intentional organisms—ones unlike either ants or angels in that they are not subject to simple determinisms—is to deal with the philosophers' frame problem: to take up the slack in the rational determination of judgement and desire, by adjusting salience among objects of attention, lines of inquiry, and preferred inference patterns. In this way emotions remain sui generis: the canons of rationality that govern them are not to be identified with those that govern judgement, or perception, or functional desire. Instead, their existence grounds the very possibility of rationality at those more conventional levels.
>
> (de Sousa 1987, p. 203)

Emotions possess a certain rationality that is irreducible to cognitive or strategic kinds of rationality, but is an axiological rationality linked to values and evaluation. Our paradigmatic emotional responses reveal the values constitutive of the normative framework for what we care about, which, in its own turn, informs and orients our thoughts and actions.

There are at least two important insights to be gained from de Sousa's account. First, the paradigm scenarios allow for an understanding of emotions that includes both the biological and personal nature of emotional experience. Individuality and temporal ('biographical') development are kept as constitutive features of our emotional relation to the world without rendering the biological dimension superfluous. On the contrary, emotional responses characterised by strong biological factors, such as fear, anger, panic, lust, 'retain their power even over individuals whose repertoire include the most "refined" emotions' (1987, p. 184). Secondly, the account emphasises the axiological or normative aspect of emotions. Emotional experience provides information about the world and about me as a person. To put it simply, emotions reveal what I care about and what I despise. Paradigm scenarios are important for the understanding of our values, because 'our only access to the level of reality that emotions reveal is through the paradigm scenarios that have shaped our world view' (1987, p. 315).

Now, one way to explore the idea of paradigm scenarios is to dig into the narrative aspect of emotions. De Sousa does not go in this direction himself, although he repeatedly insists on the importance of literature and art for the development and refinement of our emotions (1987, p. 184; 2011, pp. 208–11). Goldie, however, makes narratives the explicit structure of the experience and explanation of emotions. His general idea is very similar to de Sousa's picture of emotional experience:

> For each sort of emotional experience there will be a paradigmatic narrative structure […] learning the paradigmatic narrative structure of an emotion, one can come reliably to judge that someone else is experiencing that emotion.
>
> (Goldie 2002a, p. 105)[10]

Like de Sousa, Goldie insists on the personal and developmental aspects of emotions and still maintains that our emotional responses, despite their individuality, often arise from common, paradigmatic structures.[11] While the phenomenological and neuroscientific accounts provide us with descriptions of the *what* and *how* of emotional experience, the narrative structures help us to close in on the *why*. My feelings sometimes complicate my understanding of myself: I would like to know, for example, why I have this unpleasant feeling of emptiness when I unlock the door to my apartment, although I know that my family is waiting for me in the kitchen. Or why I become angry with my young child even about the most innocent mistake that she makes. When I ask myself troubling questions such as these, entrenched ideas of who I am become destabilised, and I am driven to re-evaluate the person that I am. This re-evaluation normally takes the form of narratives.

Inspired by the work of Richard Wollheim (1984, 1999), Goldie explores the relation between the person and emotional experiences (and actions done out of emotions) by means of what he calls the external perspective, or acentral imagining, involved in the

---

[10] Goldie criticises de Sousa for making the paradigmatic narrative structures constitutive of the different sorts of emotions (Goldie 2000, p. 33). He says, rightly to our mind, that a narrative may involve what is non-paradigmatic, e.g. laugh out of grief or kill out of love (Goldie's examples). We believe, though, that his general interpretation of de Sousa's idea of paradigm scenarios is incorrect. De Sousa does not exclude that such emotional responses might occur, only that they are in contrast to, and somehow parasitic on, what is paradigmatic (normal) of grief or love, that is, tears or kisses. The paradigm scenarios or paradigmatic narrative structures are what tells us that an emotional response is appropriate or inappropriate. In this sense, they are, at least partly, constitutive of an emotion (de Sousa 1987, pp. 185–6).

[11] He writes, for example, 'one cannot grasp the unfolding of a particular emotional sequence without knowing what emotional life is like, and knowing the characteristic ways in which human emotions unfold in response to the vicissitudes of human experience' (Goldie 2003a, p. 308); or 'within very broad parameters, there is a rather moving common humanity of emotional responses, but, as with faces, there are subtle and important differences between individual characterizations' (2002a, p. 109).

narrative structure of emotions. When, in fiction and in real life,[12] we experience the action of another, we immediately connect this action to certain reasons in order to understand the meaning of that action. To use one of Goldie's own examples, when I see a person treating a child roughly in the street, yelling and pulling the little one's arm, I immediately experience an *emotional resistance* to that action and to the person doing it. I may try to find all imaginable kinds of reasons that excuse such a harsh treatment of the child (a tough day at work, an exasperating divorce, the kid's obnoxious character, financial desperation, and so on), but somehow I judge the parent to be a questionable person. I may possibly identify myself with her feelings, but I feel a resistance toward her action ('I would never treat a child like that'). Goldie argues that I do not understand the feelings and actions of another person (e.g. anger, profound grief, charity, loving, or cold indifference) merely by means of empathy or 'in-his-shoes imagining' (2000, pp. 194–204), both of which are central imaginative processes where I imagine myself as part of the action. On the contrary, I employ an *external* perspective on the action and judge according to certain values.

Now, the interesting move in Goldie's account is that he applies this sort of reasoning to a person's *own* feelings and actions. When I think of my actions (past and future ones), I engage in a narrative process that resembles the one we experience when reading literature. I find both general *causal* relations between my separate actions, and more individually 'thick' explanations which are often person-specific and include an evaluative stance towards actions and events. As discussed in the previous chapter, there are many of my actions that I do not think about (or even remember), but there are also some that I do think about, and these often tell me something about the kind of person that I am. That is, they involve an evaluative and a normative reflection. Those are the ones that I normally understand by means of narrative structures. For example, if I bump into a table so that the coffee cup turns over and ruins my newspaper, it might be a combination of bad luck and an instant distraction. However, if I repeatedly bump into things and other people, this might, on the other hand, tell something about my person or, more specifically, my character (clumsy, confused, absorbed in my own thoughts, inconsiderate, and so on). Or to use a more serious example, if I do not look people in the eyes when I am talking to them, this also tells me something about my person, or more precisely about the emotional structure of my character, for instance, arrogance, shyness, or embarrassment. It can inform me about the involuntary aspects

---

[12] Goldie argues that 'there is no systematic divide between fictional and nonfictional narratives' (2003b, p. 66). He is quick to note, though, that this is not to be taken as a straightforward assimilation of the two cases: 'rather, one should say that a life *can be narrated*, so that the narrative is *about the life*, and thus there remains, in the real life case, but not in the fictional case, the possibility of reference and truth' (2003c, p. 216). Elsewhere he writes, along similar lines: 'Reading great literature, then, can remind us of the complexities of diverging perspectives in narratives—perspectives that sometimes only come into view with careful attention. The point applies not only to fictional narratives, but to works of history, to autobiographies, to diaries and contemporary historical documents, and to confessions. But we must not let the tail wag the dog here, for we find the same divergences, and possibilities of divergences, in our engagement with other people in a shared social world' (2007b, p. 78).

of my words and actions. When I think about my experience of the world, other people, and myself, I configure the actions, events, and occurrences according to narrative structures that include both causal and 'thicker' personal explanations. The concept of person-specific thicker explanations is naturally extremely broad and verges on confusion, but if we restrict ourselves (as Ricoeur does) to the explanations that involve the concepts of responsibility and self-esteem, we might see the relevance of this kind of explanations with regard to emotional experience.[13]

How, then, are emotional experience, responsibility, and self-esteem structured in narratives? Following the analysis of Ricoeur, we focus on the concept of personal identity to understand how narratives may help to unfold the emotional dialectic of moods and affects.

The temporal aspect of who we are is what binds together the various aspects of the hermeneutical approach to personhood. We are changing every second of our life, and yet we remain the same person. Our identity remains the same through time, even though our body may alter and our ideas change drastically. But although our identity remains the same, we nevertheless change as persons during our lifespan. Thus, identity, in the sense of *personal* identity, is not mere sameness. Now, as we saw in more detail in Chapter 2, according to Ricoeur personal identity is formed through a dialectic of two forms of identity: character (*idem*/sameness) and selfhood (*ipseity*/keeping one's word). The fundamental trait of character is permanence in time: '[t]he set of distinctive marks which permit the reidentification of a human individual as being the same' (1992, p. 119 [144]). My character is that in which my feeling of remaining the same in time and through changes is rooted, and that by which other people identify and describe me. A person, however, does not coincide with her character traits. Being who she or he is involves another kind of identity, namely, an identity constituted by selfhood.

My character traits are formed, at least for some part, involuntarily. They are developed and shaped by random events, my past actions and reactions, and contingent factors that are now out of my control. The identity of my selfhood, on the contrary, depends on how I voluntarily relate myself to being the person that I am with this body and this particular character, constituted by a certain past and situated in a world made up of anonymous laws of nature and societal existence with other persons. My selfhood is constituted by my *active* relation to the person I am. In other words, it is I who am responsible for my being this kind of person. Here we enter into the question of responsibility involved in being a person. As Dieter Teichert eloquently puts it: 'Identity as selfhood is linked to a realm where actions are ascribed to agents in the light of ethical norms' (2004, pp. 177–8). It is still me who did that terrible thing in the past, even though it would not cross my mind to do anything like that today. This means that selfhood entails a kind of self-continuity that implies responsibility not as a contingent, but as an essential component of personhood. This sense of self-continuity is mainly shaped through narratives.

---

[13] Goldie has written a fine little book, *On Personality* (2004), that attempts to sort out some of the problems involved in person-specific explanations, where he identifies broad categories of personal characteristics: (a) of acting, (b) habits, (c) temperaments, (d) emotional dispositions, (e) enduring preferences and values, (f) skills, talents, and abilities, and (g) character traits.

Here Goldie's work might shed some light on Ricoeur's more abstract conceptual thinking. The idea of an external perspective hinges on the (Augustinian) idea that 'we sometimes need to see ourselves from the outside' (Goldie 2004, p. 111). Goldie argues for the idea that the narrative sense of self involves a certain detachment from the first-person perspective similar to what we experience when engaged in literary narratives. We experience both the feelings that the author breathes into the lives of the characters and our own emotional response to those feelings. When I engage in Raskolnikov's contempt for Alyona, the pawnbroker, or Emma Bovary's fascination of a street map of Paris or her fatal attraction to Léon Dupuis, I remain somehow external to these feelings in the sense that I do not identify myself with them although completely absorbed in the feelings themselves. This distance opens up a space of evaluation not identical to a space of reason, but somewhat different in that I relate myself to the normative aspect of the feelings. I often experience an emotional resistance to the feelings of the fictional characters, which engenders a normative response that reveals my own values: 'our emotional responses can reveal to us what we value, and what we value might not be epistemically accessible to us if we did not have such responses' (Goldie 2000, pp. 48–9).

Now, if we apply this narrative structure to our own emotional life, we might come to see 'oneself as another' (Goldie 2003a, p. 312), that is, to see ourselves from an external perspective. The fact that what I do and suffer, as my existence in general, is embedded in certain feelings becomes articulated through narratives about myself. We 'loosen' the firm sedimentation of our own character by seeing how the feelings involved in past actions and sufferings have contributed to how we now respond to the humdrum events of our daily life. Through our life, interaction with the world and the other has sedimented into a hierarchical organisation of what Strasser calls our 'pathetic powers' (feelings) that results in 'a certain dispositional comportment of man' (Strasser 1977, p. 325 [224]). Our values are felt in the way we respond to what we experience and do. Some of these values are implicit, since they are dispositions and not clearly formulated but only expressed in the way we engage with the world and other persons. Goldie's central idea is that in trying to understand ourselves as persons in terms of narrative structures, we endorse an external, or acentral, perspective on our own thoughts, actions, and feelings, and sometimes we experience the same sort of emotional resistance to our own feelings as to those of other, fictional or real life, persons. Thus, we always evaluate our feelings according to a kind of external perspective that from time to time provokes an emotional resistance to what we actually feel. The fact that *we can experience an emotional resistance to our own feelings* supports our central argument that our feelings can reveal important aspects about the fragile identity that characterises our life as persons.

We often do and say things that we would not want to do or say. Our self-esteem is interwoven with the responsibility that we have for the person that we are. My ideas, principles, and emotional dispositions are part of what I am, but they can become a burden to me because who I am is deeply intertwined with the existence of other persons. When I feel in a certain way, this feeling is mine and yet I share it with the persons around me. There is always some fraction of my feelings in the actions that I do or the things that I say. My feelings are part of who I am, even though they often motivate my choices silently and unconsciously (the unrequited lover's complaint, 'I cannot choose to feel what I feel'); in fact, they effectively shape my choices and attitudes. Feelings are at the centre of the entanglement of the voluntary and the involuntary aspect of who I am, and if they are articulated, they may help us to better understand the fragility of personhood. The interrelation of self-esteem and responsibility reveals this fragility. Self-esteem draws on my responsibility in relating to others, and yet it also scrutinises my heart's innermost feelings and desires. The unfathomable recesses of my emotional life, my turbid desires as well as my tender love, are intimately entangled with what I do and say, and even though I may not be able to understand what I feel or why I feel the way I do, I always involve other people in the life of my feelings. I may not be responsible for feelings and desires that I am not able to control or even fully comprehend, but in reflection we are able to articulate the opaque dialectic of selfhood and otherness, self-esteem and responsibility, at work in our emotional life.

Jennifer Egan has described this dynamic and intensely normative dialectic superbly in her novel *A Visit from the Goon Squad*:

> [E]ach disappointment Ted felt in his wife, each incremental deflation, was accompanied by a seizure of guilt; many years ago, he had taken the passion he felt for Susan and folded it in half, so he no longer had a drowning, helpless feeling when he glimpsed her beside him in bed: her ropy arms and soft, generous ass. Then he'd folded it in half again, so when he felt desire for Susan, it no longer brought with it an edgy terror of never being satisfied. Then in half again, so that feeling desire entailed no immediate need to act. Then in half again, so he hardly felt it. His desire was so small in the end that Ted could slip it inside his desk or a pocket and forget about it, and this gave him a feeling of safety and accomplishment, of having dismantled a perilous apparatus that might have crushed them both. Susan was baffled at first, then distraught; she'd hit him twice across the face; she'd run from the house in a thunderstorm and slept at a motel; she'd wrestled Ted to the bedroom floor in a pair of crotchless underpants. But eventually a sort of amnesia had overtaken Susan; her rebellion and hurt had melted away, deliquesced into a sweet, eternal sunniness that was terrible in the way that life would be terrible, Ted supposed, without death to give it gravitas and shape. He'd presumed at first that her relentless cheer was mocking, another phase in her rebellion, until it came to him that Susan had forgotten how things were between them before Ted began to fold up his desire; she'd forgotten and was happy—had never not been happy—and while all of this bolstered his awe at the gymnastic adaptability of the human mind, it also made him feel that his wife had been brainwashed. By him.
>
> (Egan 2010, pp. 158–9)

Egan's intense description is an example of how narrative structures may help to make sense of a person's moods and affects. As we have seen, an affect can develop into a mood, which may again grow into an entrenched part of our character and thus become a permanent part of our sense of identity. Inversely, our moods influence and shape the way we react emotionally to our engagement with the world, because affects spring from the background constituted by our moods. Moods and affects are basic categories in the experiential structure of our feelings, and their constant interaction has significant consequences for how we feel, think, and act. This interaction, however, often occurs pre-reflectively and without any deliberate or thematic involvement of the person. The emotional tonality of our existence, our *Befindlichkeit*, is constituted by the ebbs and floods of our feelings, and we can make sense of the affective texture of our experience by articulating our feelings. This articulation involves a two-level approach: first, we must pay attention to the phenomenological characteristics of our feelings ('How do you feel?') and then try to get a grip on the hermeneutical constitution of those feelings ('What do those feelings mean?') by unfolding their inherent narrative structure.

The two central features of the narrative structure of emotions, the personal story involved in our emotions and the normative aspect of what we feel, help us to make sense of our moods and affects by making explicit their relation to the fragile character of human personhood. By embedding our moods and affects in a story of how we have come to feel the way we feel, we pave the way for reflection and evaluation. Our stories can, of course, be more or less accurate. But simply by trying to understand why I react so vehemently to the slightest controversy, find a pleasure letting out sardonic remarks to everything, or feel numbingly drained at the start of a new day, I open up a reflective space in which I can come to see how my feelings reveal something about the person that I am—sometimes in spite of who I think I am. In this sense, moods in particular are connected to self-understanding. I understand who I am in the context of my practical engagement, as embedded in a certain world (private as well as social), and this engagement is enveloped in an array of more or less articulate feelings. My questioning about myself is often elicited by my mood (or by disturbing affects that disclose my mood) before my identity becomes an explicit problem. Moods may disclose to me what words and deeds do not. Feelings are no hindrance to 'dispassionate' rational knowledge, but as Heidegger pointed out, our 'understanding' ('*Verstehen*') is always 'attuned' ('*gestimmt*'), that is, saturated by certain feelings. The possibility of self-disclosure characteristic of moods is fundamental to self-understanding, because a given mood can point to a troubling fracture in the way I, reflectively, understand myself. I can be locked up in my own way of thinking, chained to my thoughts in such a way that my convictions about myself reflect a wrong or at least a problematic understanding of the person that I am. Although our capacity to choose to be who we want to be is a constitutive feature of personhood, these choices are always inescapably tethered to the involuntary aspect of our personhood: 'The normative dimension thus pertains to the self that one already is in relating to others, to a world in between, and to oneself' (Grøn 2004, p. 151). I may find myself to be a kind of person that I do not want to be. The articulation of my feelings in a narrative structure might reveal that my concerns and values are different from what I took them to be. A bad mood or an inappropriately violent or simply immoderate affect might be the expression of a latent emotional resistance to my professed values and concerns, and might thus disclose an emotional fragility at the bottom of my self-esteem and self-proclaimed stability.

This fragile sense of identity exposes the normative nature of personhood: my narrative formulations about myself are constitutive of my person, and yet these formulations can be right or wrong.[14] I can tell a wrong story about myself and therefore

---

[14] As Charles Taylor observes concerning the intimate emotions that are constitutive for the person that we are: 'The peculiarity of these emotions is that it is at one and the same time the case that our formulations are constitutive of the emotion, *and* that these formulations can be right or wrong' (1985, p. 101).

live according to this story, but my mood (and the way it is vented in certain affects) may disclose, through its bipolar intentionality, that something is wrong about this story. Hence, if we take our feelings seriously and seek to interpret them as disclosing something about ourselves and our situation, we gain access into the ambivalence constitutive of personhood, namely, that a person is constituted of both factual features (a particular body, situated in a world shared with other people, tied to a certain past, and endowed with a particular character) and normative ones (I can choose to identify myself with the factual or not, but I somehow have to relate myself to these facts).[15] A narrative articulation of our moods and affects is a way to make sense of feelings by making explicit the voluntary and involuntary factors of my being the person that I am. Emotions uncover this ambiguous nature of personhood and help us cope with it, if we take seriously the complexity of human affectivity.

It is important to note, though, that a narrative approach to moods and affects can only work as part of a more comprehensive hermeneutical theory of emotions and personhood. The two previous chapters paved the way for such an account by discussing first different theories of emotion, philosophical as well as neuroscientific, and then the notion of human personhood. In this chapter, we have proposed an alternative approach to human emotions by means of a phenomenological account of our feelings of emotions and by exploring the narrative structure of these feelings. On the remaining

---

[15] This, however, presupposes that we understand identity and personhood as essentially anchored in a continuity that demands that we take responsibility for our choices, past as future, and that we do not live our lives as 'episodic creatures'. Galen Strawson has attacked this notion of narrative identity quite harshly. The narrative approach expresses 'an ideal of control and self-awareness in human life that is mistaken and potentially pernicious [. . .] the narrative tendency to look for a story or narrative coherence in one's life is, in general, a gross hindrance to self-understanding: to a just, general, practically real sense, implicit or explicit, of one's nature' (2004, p. 447). He builds this claim on a thorough analysis of the concept of a self, where he argues for a distinction between self and personhood: 'there are many short-lived and successive selves (if there are selves at all), in the case of ordinary individual human beings' (1999, p. 100). A self 'is below any cultural variation' (p. 103) and constituted ontologically with a duration of up to three seconds, although the phenomenological experience of selfhood might, wrongly, suggest otherwise. Selves are characterised as 'SESMETs (Subjects of Experience that are Single MEntal Things)' in the sense that each thought involves a self and 'are physical objects, as real as rabbits and atoms' (p. 120). He then uses this ontology to distinguish between episodic and diachronic creatures, where the diachronic creatures (narrative personalities) tend to be stuck with the past and continuous revising, and the episodics (among whom Strawson finds himself) think that '[t]he business of living is, for many, a completely non-Narrative project' (2004, p. 448) and that '[t]he "examined life" is greatly overrated' (1999, p. 100). We naturally disagree with Strawson's understanding of personhood and identity. We do not believe that a person can base his or her identity on Lord Shaftesbury's dictum: 'The *now*, the *now*. Mind this: in this is all' (quoted in Strawson 2004, p. 438). In fact, by emphasising the interconnection between emotions and the normative structure of narratives we see that feelings may disclose the consequences of living as episodic creatures in the magical now; for instance, the feeling of hopelessness emerging when I earnestly try to convince others (and myself) that it was not me who stole the shirt that I am now wearing. It might have been me eons of selves ago, but not the me that I am in this instant (or rather three seconds ago).

pages of this chapter, we will round off our account by gathering together the considerations of the previous chapters in a systematic overview of the key notions and the core structure of our hermeneutical theory of emotions and personhood. We do this by relating what we have said about emotions so far to Ricoeur's theory of subjectivity and to the cognitive and feeling theories in the current philosophy of emotions. Our aim in doing this is twofold. We intend to show that a hermeneutical theory of emotions and personhood must be grounded on a theory of subjectivity and, secondly, that our language of emotions will benefit from the enhanced understanding of the phenomenological characteristics of moods and affects that such a hermeneutical theory provides.

A Hermeneutics of Care

We have argued that, in order to make sense of the complex variety of emotional experience, we need a theoretical approach that does not exclude, or silently pass over, our more inarticulate feelings, as we experience them in our moods and affects. The conceptual framework established by the traditional antagonism between cognitive and feeling theories cannot provide such an approach. Goldie's narrative theory does much better. He puts feelings back into the emotions by means of his 'feeling towards', and his elaborate account of the dialectical development of emotions, moods, and character traits articulates the importance of personhood for understanding emotional experience. Our own account bears many similarities to Goldie's, but we have chosen a different, more traditionally 'continental-style' hermeneutical approach that is meant to bring out more clearly the embodied, biological nature of our emotions, as well as some of the problems that this embodiment generates for how we interpret, understand, and cope with our emotions.[16] Central to our approach is the interplay of voluntary and involuntary aspects of emotional experience. How much are we in control of our emotions? To what extent can we be made responsible for what we feel and for how we act emotionally? And how do emotions affect our sense of identity as individual and unique persons?

In the previous chapter, we argued that human personhood is fragile, and that this fragility, at least in part, stems from the ambivalence constitutive of human personhood. The identity of a human person is characterised by both selfhood and otherness, which creates a continuous tension, varying from incipient to full-blown, between the voluntary and the involuntary aspects of being a person through time. We went on to argue that this tension is first and foremost registered in our emotional life. Among the involuntary aspects of our identity such as the body, the world, and other people, the embodied character of our personhood is primary in the sense that our body upholds and asserts our identity without the need for our conscious appraisal—and sometimes in spite of such an appraisal. This insistent bodily identity entails that an approach to human personhood needs to pay more attention to the biological dimension of being a person than is normally the case in accounts of personhood. The biological

---

[16] The implications of our embodiment will become clearer in the next chapter, where we discuss the complications of the biological dimension of personhood.

constitution of our body influences, conditions, and sometimes directs the values that we live our life by.

In this chapter, then, we developed our argument by means of a phenomenological and hermeneutical analysis of our emotional experience. A phenomenological analysis of human affectivity provides an alternative way into human emotions. Instead of operating with the strict distinction of structured emotions (cognitive theories) and bodily feelings (feeling theories), a phenomenological description of the experiential features of emotional consciousness is able to articulate felt aspects of our emotional life that are often neglected in the traditional insistence on either cognitive structure or bodily sensations. We understand emotions as embodied motivations to move in the sense that emotions situate us in the world in our everyday dealings and pre-reflectively motivate our actions. After a phenomenological choreography of emotions and bodily movements together with a survey of some of the principal metaphors connected with this choreography, we singled out two broad categories of feelings, moods and affects, located at opposed ends of our emotional spectrum. While affect have a direct and explicit intentional structure, moods display a covert intentionality that the person is able to unfold. Articulating the covert intentionality of moods paves the way for a person's self-understanding. A phenomenological approach is a necessary, but not sufficient explanatory tool, though. The phenomenological articulation of emotional experience undoubtedly brings to the fore the different experiential features that allow us to better understand and categorise the array of human emotions. An initial phenomenological approach to our emotional life is particularly valuable, because it enables us to take seriously and articulate the basic question 'how do you feel?', which, though apparently superficial, goes right to the heart of human emotional life. But we do not merely want to articulate *how* we feel, we also want to understand *why* we feel the way we do. In other words, we need comprehensive interpretations in order to understand and cope with our emotions and feelings. One way to secure reflective and critically sound interpretations is to turn to hermeneutics. Thus we have argued, against the backdrop of Ricoeur's investigations, that a phenomenological approach to human emotions must be supplemented with a substantial hermeneutical account of human nature. Contrary to a phenomenological approach, a philosophical hermeneutics does not avoid ontological and normative questions about human nature. By means of the phenomenological analysis of human emotions and feelings, hermeneutics attempts to articulate the ontological and normative dimension of our emotional life and thus provide a philosophically valid account of human nature for tackling questions like 'What are we?' and 'Why do we feel the way we do?'.

In answering these questions, our hermeneutical approach does not draw on phenomenological analysis alone, but argues for the need for a biological understanding as well. A person is not just what he or she experiences. This becomes obvious when we try to understand the problems concerning personal identity. The identity of a person is ambiguous owing to the discrepancies between biological identity and psychological identity. The problems of the voluntary (selfhood) and involuntary (otherness) aspects of personhood stem from this basic ambiguity between the biological (body) and psychological (selfhood) constitution of personal identity. We argued that a sense of ambivalence is a constitutional feature of personhood, mainly because a person is both more and less than what he or she experiences and believes, or wants to believe, to be. And we have argued further that this ambivalence is more often manifested as an emotional fragility than an explicit cognitive issue about ambiguity. The phenomenological analysis of moods and affects unveiled the feelings involved in this ambivalence of selfhood and otherness, but it cannot investigate the ontological and normative implications of such an ambivalence, let alone provide a comprehensive account of how a person copes with the emotional fragility in his or her life. This is the job of the hermeneutics that we have tried to establish here.

We suggested that narratives can be of help in clarifying the dialectical development of moods into affects, and vice versa. If we apply a narrative structure to our emotional experiences, we are enabled to make sense of our emotional experiences in relation to the person that we are. Our emotions are complex precisely because they involve both the personal and the biological aspects of who we are. In fact, we have argued that the embodied nature of our emotions urges us to take seriously the biological nature of human personhood. The fact that our most deeply personal emotions involve involuntary, and apparently anonymous, biological factors such as the vestigial traces of our cross-species evolutionary past, or the sedimentation of previous personal emotional responses into a pre-reflective emotional texture, reveals that to be a person is not merely being a self. There is more to being a person than can be assessed from our explicitly conscious experiences. One way to gain access to the less explicit experiences involved in being a person is to pay attention to the experiential structure of our feelings. Hence, we identified two main categories of feelings, moods and affects, which encompass the experience of human feelings. Our felt experience varies from brief, intense, and clearly intentional feelings to longer, more subdued, and less clearly intentional feelings, and by applying a narrative structure to the interaction of moods and affects we are able to trace the developmental character of this interaction in relation to the person who undergoes these feelings. Moods and affects can reveal the fragile, and often troubled, nature of our sense of identity if we are sufficiently attentive to the ebbs and flows of our feelings and try to make sense of these changes in terms of a narrative structure. Emotional resistances that we often experience in such narratives open up for an external perspective on our feelings which, in turn, enables us to question how and why we feel the way we do.

Now, we said that narratives need to be part of a more comprehensive hermeneutical theory of emotions and personhood to be able to provide sensible answers to the questions that our feelings elicit. Without a secure grip on the nature of personhood and the functions of emotions in the economy of our engagement with the world, other people, and ourselves, we will not be able to provide supportive and helpful answers about how we cope with our emotional fragility. As we have suggested on the previous pages, the relationship between emotions and personhood provokes questions on at least three different levels: 'How do I feel?' (phenomenological), 'What do I feel?' (ontological), 'What do I do about my feelings?' (normative). In facing these questions, we should begin to see the use of our reformulation of Ricoeur's hermeneutical theory of subjectivity. Ricoeur's theory has always lurked in the background of our theory of emotions and personhood, contributing to the methodological and conceptual structuring of our approach. So in pulling together the different strings of our theory it seems appropriate to make this influence more explicit.

Ricoeur's theory is, among other things, an extensive attempt to deal with our emotional fragility and the problems that this fragility brings about in our lives. His detailed diagnosis and subsequent therapy of human fragility, which we distilled and reformulated in Chapters 2 and 3, concluded with a particular ontology constituted on the basis of human care. The conceptual map issued by this peculiar ontology enables us to make sense of our vague and impalpable feelings and integrate these into our common language of emotions without recoiling into either a rationalistic (cognitive theories) or a physicalistic (feeling theories) straitjacket. But more about this in a moment. First, let us try to show how Ricoeur's ontology of care might provide the conceptual buttress for making sense of the narratives about our emotional life. We shall not repeat here what we said about this in Part I, but simply explain how this peculiar ontology may support our theory and enable us to understand and talk about our feelings.

A person is basically constituted by selfhood and otherness. Selfhood is characterised by a persistent conative effort to affirm or assert itself in and through the interaction with the world. In other words, a person wants to be an individual, a unique and irreplaceable self. This is what Ricoeur calls the originating affirmation inherent in human selfhood. The self struggles with the affirmation of itself. Our awareness of being a self is troubled and constantly shattered in our effort to assert ourselves in the world. We are never simply a self. The affirmation of ourselves as a self is fractured through the interaction with that which does not immediately and unproblematically coincide with this affirmation, that is, the otherness that makes up the involuntary part of our existence as an individual self. This otherness is manifested most clearly in three fundamentally involuntary aspects of human selfhood: body, world, and other people. The self can only affirm itself by becoming an embodied person that lives his or her life in a world shared with other people. Our sense of identity is characterised by a constitutional ambivalence, because personal identity is intrinsically ambiguous: it is both a fact and a task of becoming. A self is a person by the sheer fact of existing with and among other people in a world constituted by the characteristically personal interaction of its members. Furthermore, our identity as individual and irreplaceable persons is inscribed in the biological constitution of our personhood that marks us and binds us to who we are. And yet, this facticity of our personhood is fragile because we (and other people) care about the person that we are. Care is the notion that binds together the different aspects of being a person, and the notion that provides a point of orientation for our hermeneutical theory of emotion and personhood.

Our cares and concerns reveal the values that we live our life by. We can articulate what we care about in plans, ideas, hopes, promises, and other reflective considerations (what Ricoeur calls 'the good life'), but first of all our cares and concerns make themselves felt in our emotional life. The pre-reflective and spontaneous nature of our feelings tells us something important about our care, and consequently about who and what we are. We do not always choose what we care about or the values that we live our lives by. Our feelings reveal the involuntary nature of our care, and thus the potential conflict between the voluntary and involuntary aspects of being a person who cares. The fragile nature of personhood is heightened by this heterogeneity of our cares. In our care for being the person that we are, or the person that we want to be, we find the constitutional features of selfhood and otherness. Who I am and what I care about is always interwoven with the otherness of the body, the world, and other people that make up the person that I am. What I want to be and who I strive to become is always disturbed, destabilised, and reshaped by this otherness, whether it be the challenges issued from my body, the world or other people. It is in this sense that our personhood is fragile. I am never simply a person. Who I am is always shattered through my embodied existence in the world and among other people. How, then, can I become the person that I am? I become the person that I am through the appropriation of the otherness that constitutes my personhood. This otherness is that which tackles and menaces my existence since it puts up resistance to my projects and desires; and it is also that which enriches it in terms of possibilities, that is, of love or friendship for another person, of hopes and expectations projected into the future. Otherness, in this sense, constantly challenges the understanding of the person that I consider myself to be and makes self-understanding an infinite appropriation. It is this dialectic between selfhood and otherness in our cares and concerns that is fleshed out in our emotional life. The narratives that we make of our emotional life are attempts to make sense of who we are, who we were, and who we want to be. Narratives are a way to cope with our emotions, to interpret and speak about our feelings about the world, other people, and ourselves. In other words, embedded firmly in a hermeneutics of care, narratives provide us with a language for our emotions, a language through which we can appropriate our feelings about being who and what we are through an articulation of what we care about. This brings us to our final consideration about how the phenomenological categories of moods and affects may improve our language for emotions.

We said that our theory is not meant as a wholesale rejection of other theories of emotion. On the contrary, our approach to emotions and personhood is closely linked to both the feeling theories and the cognitive theories of emotion. Our theory should be considered as an attempt at a conceptual integration of our more indistinct and cognitively impenetrable feelings, moods in particular, into the way we speak about our emotions. We have seen that the conceptual focus of the feelings theories is the changes in our bodily landscape, and the analyses carried out according to these theories normally take place in evolutionary terms and by heavy use of empirical neuroscientific studies. This naturally affects the way such theories speak about emotions. Our emotional life is mostly treated within a third-person perspective, and the multifarious nature of emotions is consequently boiled down to a handful of basic or primary emotions such as anger, joy, surprise, disgust, sadness, pleasure, and fear. The number and character of these emotions vary, but the general, defining conditions for such basic emotions remain more or less the same: they can be registered across different species and are closely linked to the physiological constitution of the mammalian brain. We have argued that the embodied nature of our emotions urges us to take seriously this biological dimension of emotion, and by using Panksepp's theory we have shown how the anonymous, evolutionary nature of our emotional reactions reveals significant detail about the involuntary aspect of our personal emotions. As

William James argued over a century ago, emotions bereft of bodily feelings can hardly be called emotions at all.

There is, however, more to emotions than bodily feelings and sensations. So, on the other side of the emotional divide, we have the cognitive theories that insist on the intentional, judgemental, propositional, and rational structure of emotions. The language of such theories is closely tied to existential, normative, and ethical dimensions of human nature. They normally aim at disclosing the voluntary aspect of our emotional life, that is, how to cope with our emotions, and eventually, how to take responsibility for them. As Solomon writes with the vigour so characteristic of his innumerable writings on emotions:

> I once summed up Sartre's philosophy and existentialism in general with the simple statement, No Excuses! And that is how I would like you to think about the emotions, too. Not that they don't have their causes. Not that they aren't often dictated or circumscribed by circumstances. Not that there are not sometimes passions over which we really do have little control. But instead of shrugging off responsibility, thinking 'I am not responsible for my emotions,' I want to urge you to ask, whenever you can, 'why am I doing this? What am I getting out of this?' And you may well find that by taking responsibility you will no longer feel like the victim of your own emotions.

(Solomon 2007, p. 200)

Emotions are so saturated with our personal thoughts, ideas, strategies, habits, and expectations that it seems obvious to consider to what extent we actually are responsible for what we feel and, even more importantly, for how we act on the basis of our emotions. The way we speak about our emotions must involve considerations on judgement, deliberation, and responsibility. In other words, our language of emotions can be nothing if not personal and normative. Our reflective interpretation and elaboration of emotions in language and narratives plays a fundamental part in how and why we feel the way we do.

Our theory can be seen as a contribution to a better understanding of our emotional life by making sense of those feelings that cannot be accounted for in the language used in either the feeling theories or the cognitive theories. The horizon of our feelings is wider than that of our emotions. One reason for this is that to a given emotion may correspond different feelings for different persons, or to the same person in different periods of her life. Also, usually language has a better grasp on emotions than on feelings. We cannot describe this better than David Pugmire does:

> Because a feeling is a state of a person, rather than a representation of some independent property of an object, it does not have the same kind of fit to the aspects of the world which arouse it that a thought has to the aspect of the world it is about. How one feels may or may not serve to present a state of affairs outside itself; my unease, joy or gloom may but needn't be a reflection on the world beyond (in this, feelings do compare to sensations such as pain, nausea and bitterness). Since a feeling does not just represent, it need not purport to fit. This is why it need not depend on the beliefs that are held. Feelings are causally related to what arouses them, and cognition is one, but only one, of the causal elicitors. Hence the notorious liability of feelings (and hence emotions involving them) to 'blindness'. A rage, a giddy thrill, a trough of depression, a jolt of lust can numb the mind to rational dissuasion.

> Blindness is possible because feeling is responsive to a range of causes which are peripheral to one's thoughts, yet which may enjoy inordinate evocative powers. These include such psychological byways as association, symbolism and even chemistry.
>
> (Pugmire 1998, p. 59)

The complexity of causal elicitors for our feelings is reflected in the fact that feelings can be so difficult to handle by language. Feelings often bind our tongue and leave us without words. They overwhelm us, with intensity or emptiness. They can fill us with boundless energy or drain us to the point of immobility. While we have words for many of the emotions that enrich and frustrate our lives such as love, hate, sorrow, gloom, shame, joy, anger, jealousy, pride, sadness, resentment, affection, ambition, kindness, the multifarious character of our feelings seems hopelessly out of reach of our language. This is why, as we saw on the opening pages of this part, Cordelia says, 'I cannot heave my heart into my mouth'. Her cynical sisters abound with words to reassure their father of their endless love. Their words, though, spring neither from love nor filial affection, but from the expectation of land and power. Cordelia is well aware that words and gestures can distort and mask the nature of feelings, and cannot bring herself to use the word 'love' to describe what she feels. Her most intimate and personal feelings cannot be expressed in a language that allows for deception, sentimentality, and other kinds of feelingless expression of common emotions. Some feelings tend to get lost in translation, even when translated into the colourful language of our emotions.

Poetry, music, and paintings are better at expressing what words and conceptual explanations cannot. We have already drawn upon the poetry of T.S. Eliot, and shall also close this part with his voice. His verses touch at and communicate feelings by dissolving the boundaries of how we normally use words. He communicates the ineffable feelings of time and ageing by evoking feelings that cannot be spoken. Poetry works part of its magic by trying to express in rhythm and atmosphere what cannot be expressed in words. It is a straining of our emotional language in a continually renewed attempt to articulate the feelings involved in our emotions. Eliot foregrounds this perennial problem of finding words for our feelings in *Little Gidding*, the last string of verses in his *Four Quartets*:

> For last year's words belong to last year's language
> And next year's words await another voice.
> But, as the passage now presents no hindrance
>   To the spirit unappeased and peregrine
>   Between two worlds become much like each other,
> So I find words I never thought to speak
>   In streets I never thought I should revisit
>   When I left my body on a distant shore.
>
> (Eliot 1944, p. 39)

How *I* feel what we all understand as anger, love, joy, or sadness, may be significantly different from how another person experiences such emotions. And a better understanding of this subjective difference in the experience of emotions may help us to make sense of what such emotions mean for the person that experiences them.

Our proposal of using the phenomenological categories of moods and affects to access the felt dimension of emotions is precisely such an attempt to better understand these subjective differences inherent in emotional experience. Understanding the phenomenological characteristics of an emotional experience, in terms of moods and affects, enables us to qualify our emotional vocabulary (there are various kinds of anger, joy, jealousy, or sadness), and, by relating moods and affects to the person that experiences them, we can make sense of the developmental dynamics of different emotional episodes that at first glance might seem to have nothing in common. Hence, the general aim of our theory is to enable us to speak about and make sense of those feelings that are part of our emotional life, but are not expressed or articulated by our normal language for emotions. In this sense, our approach acknowledges the language for emotion established by feeling theories and cognitive theories, while attempting to incorporate into that language the feelings that were left out of those theories. We believe that this approach will prove valuable when, in the final part of the book, we try to give an account of the nature and importance of feelings and emotions in psychopathology.

We have now presented the theoretical core of our hermeneutical theory of emotions and personhood. In Part III, we will flesh out the theory in relation to human vulnerability to mental illness. We shall consider two major mental disorders, schizophrenia (Chapter 8) and borderline personality disorder (Chapter 9), and argue that our theory, when applied to psychopathology in terms of vulnerability and care, carries significant therapeutic value (Chapter 10). Before turning to the further development of our theory, though, we shall end the more theoretical part of the book with a chapter concerning the relation between biology and existence in human life. A discussion of the shortcomings of, respectively, an evolutionary and a phenomenological account of the relation between emotions and values will, we believe, strengthen the overall argument for our own theory.

Chapter 7

The Feeling Brain

In Chapter 5, we argued that human beings are personal animals. We are animals because our existence is conditioned and permanently influenced by our mammalian constitution. We share a significant part of our anatomy and physiology with other primates, which is particularly obvious in our emotional life. Many of our emotional characteristics are similar to those of other animals, and we have seen how these cross-species features of our emotional life, in turn, permeate and shape our thoughts and actions. On the face of it, this common mammalian constitution supports the arguments for an evolutionary approach to human emotions. We do indeed espouse an evolutionary tenor in any investigation of human emotional life. We can never hope to unravel the embodied nature of our emotions without a thorough investigation into the mechanisms and dynamics of our mammalian heritage. Nonetheless, we consider our emotional life to be significantly different from that of other animals. The main reason for this is that our emotions are personal. This means that we do not simply feel our emotions, but that we can also take a position so as to face them and relate ourselves to what we feel. Position-taking is a defining feature of being a person. We are passively moved by our emotions, but most of the time we are also able to act upon what we feel, that is, to choose whether to follow passively the movements that our emotions stir up, or to actively resist or transform the ebbs and flows of our emotions. As personal animals we are also intelligent animals. Intelligence derives from the Latin word *intelligentia* (*intus* + *legere*), which basically means 'choose or read inside'. We can go into the pleats of our emotions, look for the right words to name them, make subtle distinctions between one emotion and another, reconstruct the genesis of an emotion as an epiphany of our involuntary biological constitution, understand how it is related to the situation we are in at a given moment, narrate how it belongs to a successive chain of states of mind and life-events, appropriate it as part of our personal identity, and decide what to do with what we feel. To be a person is an undeniable part of what we are, and as such it qualifies our ways of feeling, thinking, and acting in the world. In fact, we have argued that one important key to understanding our emotional life can be found in the ambivalent, and at times conflictual, tension between the biological and personal feelings of being human. In this chapter, we shall look more carefully at this emotional ambivalence and how it influences the values we live our life by. We begin with a consideration of the problem of evolution and intentionality. How do we make sense of the fact that our feelings and actions are, on the one hand, influenced by anonymous evolutionary forces, while, on the other, most of our engagement in the world is so obviously carried out in terms of intentional thoughts, feelings, and actions? To articulate this problem, we then look at the idea of conative forces in human action as it is used by Spinoza and Ricoeur, and in contemporary neuroscience. This discussion is meant to provide us with a background for our subsequent critique of, respectively, an evolutionary and a purely phenomenological approach to human feelings and emotions. We first show the shortcomings of an influential evolutionary theory of emotions by looking briefly at Jesse Prinz's refined development of classic feeling theories. We then turn to deal in more detail with Matthew Ratcliffe's phenomenological account of 'existential feelings', with which our own account has much in common. There are significant differences, though, and our critique of Ratcliffe's account is meant, in part, as a way to make our own account more articulate. We close the chapter, and this part of the book, with an argument for the close relationship between bad moods and personhood.

Considerations on Evolution and Intentionality

Emotional experience is a privileged entry into the scope and limits of naturalistic ambitions. To be sure, cognition is a biological phenomenon as well as emotions and feelings are, but, as argued in Chapter 1, because of their thoroughly embodied nature emotions make the encounter of biological and philosophical investigations of human nature particularly urgent. As we have seen, Damasio and Panksepp present two different perspectives on the neurobiological dimension of emotions, but they both stress the evolutionary importance of emotional experience. And theories of evolution do indeed seem an unavoidable issue when talking about emotions; in fact, we would argue that evolution is not an optional but a necessary factor to take into account (Searle 2000, p. 40). On the other hand, as Solomon writes concerning an emotion that many evolutionary explanations focus on: 'There is no doubt that anger (and some other emotions) are part of our evolutionary heritage and include physiological responses that we share with other animals. But this is surely just a piece of the story' (Solomon 2007, p. 14). Solomon disallows fanciful atavistic tales about our emotional aetiology insisting that emotions are not only caused by distant evolutionary forces. Our relation to the objects or events of our emotions is constituted by more than the ancient 'selfish genes', imparted to us more or less unaltered from the time of our Stone Age ancestors (Dupré 2001, pp. 25–31). Many emotions are intentional in the sense that they express our most personal wishes, desires, and ideas. Our emotional relation to objects or events is therefore often qualified by an individually and socially malleable intentional attitude.

How, then, do we balance the evolutionary and the intentional aspects of emotions? First of all, we have to distinguish between evolution and biology. Functional biological explanations are not identical with evolutionary biological explanations. Whereas functional biology normally disregards historical assumptions while investigating the physiology of all activities of living organisms, historical biology attempts to establish scientifically defensible historical narratives about those organisms. In fact, in the words of the distinguished evolutionary biologist, Ernst Mayr: 'evolutionary biology, as a science, in many respects is more similar to the Geisteswissenschaften than to the exact sciences' (Mayr 2004, p. 33). Biology does not necessarily involve theoretical presumptions about the origin and development of the organisms that it investigates.

It is mainly interested in discovering the diverse laws and mechanisms that govern the manifold biological entities in the world. Naturally, aetiological questions pose themselves more forcibly as we discover more and more about the genome and the fascinating mechanisms of molecular biology. One of the main tasks of evolutionary biology is, in fact, to provide narratives that connect and explain the often disparate research carried out in the diverse branches of contemporary biology. The narrative superiority of Darwin's theory was perhaps one of the fundamental reasons for its immense, and justly enduring, success (Kitcher 1993, pp. 11–57). Evolutionary explanations cannot, however, rely on biology as a simple, let alone obvious, justification for their theories. On the contrary, biology rarely claims to have exhausted the mysteries of the living organism, and the various levels of biological investigation work by means of separate methods that seem to defy any pretension of a unified scientific grasp on the entities of nature, not speak of nature in general (Dupré 1993, pp. 221–43). There are obvious discrepancies between the genotype and the phenotype of biological organisms that do not allow for a simple explanatory reduction of the latter to the former (Dupré 2001, pp. 72–81).

This brings us to a second, far more complex, point about evolution and intentionality, namely, the question of teleology. How do we account for the objects of emotions? If emotions are not to be considered mere epiphenomena, they must have a reason and bring about an actual change in the world. The question is where to look for this reason and change. Do we try to understand the life of the individual person or do we instead scrutinise the general, and highly anonymous, need for survival? Ronald de Sousa has dealt systematically with this problem in terms of the *remote* or *proximate* explanation of emotions. Neuroscientific explanations of emotions are, strictly speaking, proximate in the sense that they aim at uncovering the neurobiological dynamics and properties of emotions. Evolutionary explanations, on the other hand, are explicitly remote, since they seek to expound emotions as mechanisms in a general process of adaptation in terms of survival and reproduction. Now, de Sousa quickly dismisses the simplistic idea of adaptation as survival of the fittest by stressing that 'evolutionary change involves no progress, no inherent direction or "orthogenesis," no built-in drive to mentality or spirituality or group harmony or even complexity' (de Sousa 1987, p. 80). However, if we subscribe to the general idea of evolution, emotions cannot be completely maladaptive, since the creatures that have them remain alive and even flourish. Emotions do have a biological function that we must try to envisage.

So to maintain the complexity of human emotions under the pressure of reductive evolutionary explanations, de Sousa looks at the motivational force of emotions, and more specifically, at the relation between the biological need and the psychological motivation or want. Emotions influence human behaviour at different levels that can be envisaged through the notions of instinct and intentionality. First, he distinguishes between what he calls T-instincts and H-instincts (de Sousa 1987, p. 84).[1] T-instincts are those we find in simple animal behaviour that exhibits predictable stereotyped

---

[1] They are called T-instincts after the Dutch Nobel laureate, ethnologist and ornithologist Nikolaas Tinbergen, who, in his book *A Study of Instinct* (1951), identified this type of basic instincts. H-instincts are particularly human instincts.

responses to precise stimuli. H-instincts are human emotions that are experienced as motivational forces, which do not, however, result in fixed patterns of predictable behaviour. It is not difficult to point out radical differences between the two types of instincts. To explain how they relate to one another is, however, a knotty business. De Sousa solves this issue elegantly by individuating different degrees of intentionality by means of the concept of fungibility. The teleological differences involved in T- and H-instincts are determined by the fact that humans have a capacity for singular reference whereas other animals operate with fungible references. To explain the difference, he uses the example of the dog Fido (de Sousa 1987, pp. 98–100). Fido is fond of its human friend and recognises this individual person by means of his physical qualities (smell, voice tone, characteristic movements, etc.). Because of Fido's ability to recognise its human friend, we tend to believe that Fido actually likes that particular person and not somebody else. This would be a mistake, though. If we imagine that the person died but, miraculously, a perfect clone of that person could be made, then Fido would never be able to tell the difference. It would like the clone just as much and still wag its tail and jump with joy every time they were together. The same would not be the case with humans. We know that if we lose a loved one, nobody can ever fill the place of that person. We know that he is dead, so if we encounter a person completely identical, we still know that this is not our loved one. He is another person in spite of the physical and mental identity. This is due to our particularly human capacity for singular reference. Humans operate with non-fungible references for their emotional states (I like *this* wallet and not another identical one), whereas other animals only refer to the environment in terms of generality. Animals easily transfer the emotion to other objects that have the same general, but not particular, features (e.g. if a dish is empty, the dog immediately turns to another, or the crows mistake a scarecrow for a real person). The transition from one kind of behaviour to another is not due to an ontogenetical difference between humans and other animals. It is due to a difference in intentionality. De Sousa talks about a quasi-intentionality in animals that relies on the general character of the references by which they live their emotional life. Humans are characterised by a 'mental grade of intentionality' (de Sousa 1987, p. 97) that relies on the specifically human logico-linguistic capacities.

The important feature of de Sousa's picture of human emotions is that the mental grade of intentionality particular to human beings is not radically irreducible to the common biological story that we tell about other living creatures. Humans are moved by emotions just like other animals and are therefore restricted by some of the same evolutionary forces. These evolutionary forces are, however, more easily discovered in animals, because their behaviour is restricted by the diffuse generality of T-instincts. The emotional behaviour of animals is more easily explained by the remote explanations of evolution because of the general features of such explanations (food is nutrition and sex is reproduction). And even though the same forces are present in human behaviour, human emotional behaviour is different and more complex, basically due to the fact that 'we *care* about individuals' (de Sousa 1987, p. 100). Evolutionary explanations are central to our understanding of the embodied, physiological nature of human emotions. We are deeply rooted in the processes of primate biology by the particular nature of our emotions, and to fully understand these ubiquitous phenomena in human life we need to clarify the neurobiological processes operating in them. The fact that an evolutionary account cannot provide us with exhaustive explanations of our emotions stems from the singular reference of human emotions. Human emotional behaviour relies on a proximate explanation. As we mentioned above, neuroscientific explanations are carried out at a proximate level. However, such explanations need to be proximate in another sense. Contrary to other organisms, humans have a *biography* and their desires are *time-indexed*, therefore having a causal history is not sufficient. Human emotions cannot be understood if we do not take into account the specific history of the individual person (de Sousa 1987, pp. 104–5). If I wail and cry over having lost an old worthless wallet, it is most certainly because this wallet has some particular personal value to me; it may have accompanied me a long time or be a gift from a person that I care about.[2] The idea of personal history and time will have important bearings on our explanation of bad moods, but before turning to these hazy phenomena, we will briefly position Ricoeur in relation to what we have previously said about the neuroscientific dimension of emotions.

Spinoza, Ricoeur, and Neuroscience on the *Conatus*

Although Damasio and Panksepp both advocate evolutionary explanations of human emotions, it should be clear from our discussion of their respective theories in Chapter 4 that their neuroscientific explorations go in significantly different directions. Damasio considers human feelings to be perceptions of bodily changes that are the real emotions, and as such, feelings are considered to be mere subjective registrations of more fundamental and objective emotions. We have to understand the specifically human feelings by clarifying the neurobiological dynamics of bodily emotions (Damasio 2004, p. 56). Panksepp, on the contrary, resists this methodological separation of feelings and emotions, which, in his opinion, leads to an ontological neglect of basic affectivity (Panksepp 2005c, p. 160). Emotions are feelings, and that already on a pure bodily level. Consciousness is emotional consciousness, in humans as well as in other animals. The cognitive capacities in humans are not, to use Goldie's term, 'added-on' to the body, but deeply immersed in the emotions that characterise the whole organism. It is not the case that we perceive or readout the emotions and *ipso facto* feel in a certain way. On the contrary, emotional feelings shape and influence our perception and cognition in such a way that our higher cognitive brain functions are always embedded in a certain emotional state. Hence, Panksepp writes: 'Descartes's faith in his assertion "I think, therefore I am" may be superseded by a more primitive affirmation that is part of the genetic makeup of all mammals: "I feel, therefore I am"' (1998, p. 309).

Despite their differences, Damasio and Panksepp nevertheless resort to the same thinker as the speculative background for their empirical research, namely, the Dutch seventeenth century philosopher Baruch Spinoza. This is not uncommon among philosophically interested neuroscientists. The renowned neurobiologist Jean-Pierre

---

[2] The temporal and personal aspect of inanimate things is a hotly debated topic in contemporary social psychology, which goes under the name 'endowment effect'. People tend to value things higher once they are actually endowed with them (Goldie 2007a, p. 111).

Changeux confesses, in an extended discussion with Ricoeur, his affection for Spinoza's monism, and that he himself is striving for a new synthesis of objective science and subjective experience (Changeux and Ricoeur 2000, pp. 8 [14], 27 [35–6], 31 [39]). What is interesting here is that Ricoeur himself uses the Spinozist concept of *conatus*[3] as a key concept in his theory of subjectivity, and particularly with regard to human affectivity. We have seen that Ricoeur transcribes *conatus* as the originating affirmation, that is, the subject's basic 'will-to-live' ('*vouloir-vivre*') or original will-to-say-yes. The concept of an originating affirmation is more than just a will to survive and yet even more basic than rationality (2007b, pp. 290–1 [361–2]). It is a primordial energy that drives the subject to affirm its being in the world (1977, p. 46 [53]). At a first glance, it might seem a somewhat dubious metaphysical postulate without any serious grounding or plausible argument in its favour. But if we look at the way in which neuroscientists employ this Spinozist heritage, we might nourish it a bit with some evolutionary arguments.

Damasio is the neuroscientist who has treated the heritage from Spinoza most carefully. In fact, one of his books, *Looking for Spinoza*, is partly an argument for how Spinoza's philosophy could help us make sense of the biology of the mind (2003, p. 13). He is particularly interested in the monistic idea that the mind and the body are two attributes of the same substance, and furthermore, that the human mind is the idea of the human body. But most of all, it is the notion of *conatus* that attracts his attention because, according to him, it can be translated back into current biological terms denoting genetically determined dispositions in the brain that seek both survival and well-being (2003, pp. 36–7). The idea of *conatus* goes well with his somatic-marker hypothesis. The *conatus* renders well the emotional forces present at 'the theatre of the body', i.e. the manifold bodily responses that highlight the positive and negative values in our experience of the world. All living organisms strive to preserve themselves and to optimise pleasure and minimise pain. The conative forces are not the result of conscious efforts but work by means of the anonymous energy of a natural wisdom of aeons of evolutionary development. The conscious, subjective experience of these anonymous forces is described in the following way: 'When the consequences of such natural wisdom are mapped back in the central nervous system, subcortically and cortically, the result is feelings, the foundational component of our minds' (2003, p. 79). This conception of *conatus* as an aggregate of evolutionary forces that non-consciously drive the organism towards bodily self-perseverance and satisfaction, and is later extended with a cognitive brain map and mental ideas of these reactions, the so-called 'machinery of feeling' (2003, p. 80), yields a somewhat distorting and philosophically poor interpretation of Spinoza's use of the notion. The hypothesis that the mind is the idea of the body does not entail that human knowledge is irrevocably tethered to our bodily functions. On the contrary, Spinoza writes clearly in his *Ethics*: 'The Body cannot determine the Mind to thinking, and the Mind cannot determine the Body to motion, to rest or to anything else (if there is anything else)' (Spinoza 1985, p. 494). The mind is indeed the idea of the body, but part of the normative thrust of the *Ethics* is to liberate our cognitive abilities, our reason, from the bondage to our immediate affective

---

[3] Detailed and lucid analyses of the notion of *conatus* in Spinoza can be found in Garrett (2002) and Schrijvers (1999).

nature. Human beings have the capacity to think about their emotional states and by thinking to overcome the passivity of their bodily nature.[4] The multitude of the obscure passive affects that dominate our everyday life must be subdued by the intellective powers of our active mind, i.e. by means of adequate and distinct ideas:

> An affect which is passion is a confused idea. Therefore, if we should form a clear and distinct idea of the affect itself, this idea will only be distinguished by reason from the affect itself, insofar as it is related only to the Mind. Therefore, the affect will cease to be a passion [...] The more an affect is known to us, then, the more it is in our power, and the less the Mind is acted on by it.
>
> (Spinoza 1985, p. 598)

On the one side, we have passions and confused ideas; on the other, affects and distinct ideas. The *intellect* is the means by which we overcome passivity and confusion. Now, this is not the place to go into the interpretive difficulties of Spinoza's thought. We only want to note that Spinozist monism does not necessarily lead to the conclusion that mental ideas always recur only to bodily states. The *conatus* is a general endeavour or will-to-live that is irreducible to the more restricted idea of evolutionary forces. This general will-to-live is surely influenced by the process of evolution, but there is more to the notion of *conatus* if we consider how it is at work in human affectivity.

Ricoeur points to this in his discussion with Changeux. One has to read Spinoza's *Ethics* more carefully to understand the complexity of the *conatus* at work in human affectivity. There is a different teleology at stake in human endeavour to persevere in being, simply because there is more to human life than the absence of death (which is also evident from even a superficial reading of Spinoza's arguments in the fifth and last part of the *Ethics*).[5] Ricoeur agrees to the idea that *conatus* is indeed '[t]he effort to live – the desire to exist' (2000, p. 229 [242]), but maintains that we have to see this effort in relation to Spinoza's idea of 'the good life' (2000, p. 228 [241]). This is somewhat similar to de Sousa's account of remote and proximate explanations. In order to fully understand how the *conatus* works in the human subject, we have to take into account both the evolutionary and personal aspect of the subjective will-to-live. We may all have the same anonymous forces working within us, but these are always experienced in relation to our personal characteristics or biography (Ricoeur would say our 'existential difference'). The *conatus* that drives the human subject relies on, at least, both these factors.

In our opinion, Panksepp's use of Spinozist monism is more congenial to Spinoza's use of the *conatus*. Like Damasio, Panksepp subscribes to the idea that mind and body are two attributes of the same substance, his so-called dual-aspect monism (2005a,

---

[4] Thorough and accessible treatments of the therapeutic nature of Spinoza's philosophical efforts to establish a sustainable argument for his peculiar combination of naturalism and morality can be found in Garrett (2003) and Lebuffe (2010).

[5] Many commentators, though, have found it difficult to reconcile Spinoza's materialism with his arguments for the eternity of the mind in this last part of the *Ethics*. Jonathan Bennett, for instance, in his otherwise magisterial interpretation, contemptuously concludes that 'this material is valueless. Worse, it is dangerous: it is rubbish which causes others to write rubbish' (Bennett 1984, p. 374).

p. 23; 2005c, p. 163), and he himself points to this idea as Spinozist in origin (2005b, pp. 41-2). The neurobiological and psychological properties of the brain are of the same substance, but they have to be understood from different perspectives. The neuroscientific investigation must limit itself to the basic affectivity that is common to all mammals and which results in basic emotional tendencies. Such an investigation might clarify the 'ethological animal brain' and thus 'we should be able to shed light into core human emotional tendencies by studying animal brains' (2006, p. 775). Panksepp focuses on the 'intrinsic value guides for existence' (2005a, p. 22) that characterise all animal affectivity and the consequent behaviour. However, his methodological starting point (all mammals have affective feelings) allows for what he calls 'conative variants' (2005b, p. 40) in mammalian affectivity due to the variation of brain structures in the different animals. The *conatus* is not the same in humans as in other animals. We may share many of the basic instinctual feelings, but there is more to consider in human feelings. Such a neuroscientific approach seems to go better with the philosophical development of the *conatus* in Ricoeur. Ricoeur describes human affectivity in the following manner:

> In a general way, affectivity is the non-transparent aspect of the Cogito. We are right in saying 'of the Cogito.' Affectivity is still a mode of thought in its widest sense. To feel is still to think [*sentir est encore penser*], though feeling no longer represents objectivity, but rather reveals existence [*révélateur d'existence*]. Affectivity uncovers my bodily existence as the other pole of all the dense and heavy existence of the world. We can express it otherwise by saying that through feeling the personal body [*le corps propre*] belongs to the subjectivity of the Cogito. (1966, p. 86 [83]; see also 1987, p. 131 [147])

Feelings are thoughts, insofar as 'thought' is disclosure of existence, rather than a disinterested categorisation of objects. Our thoughts about the world, other people, and ourselves are qualified by feelings in the sense that affectivity 'personalizes reason' (1987, p. 102 [118]). The environment becomes a world *for me*; a world characterised by values, that is, a system of salience and relevance that orients my behaviour. The *conatus*, my will-to-live, drives me to involve myself in my existence in this world, but my affirmation is always influenced by the values that I experience in my affective relation to the world and my own engagement. So, if we consider Panksepp's neuroscientific model of affectivity as the experience of raw emotional values that characterise basic mammalian instinctual behaviour, we might make Ricoeur's notion of *conatus* as originating affirmation more than just a speculative postulate. Panksepp's empirical studies argue for a basic mammalian affectivity that influences human behaviour, because our human feelings are deeply rooted in a common ethological ground. Our behaviour is not qualitatively different from the instinctive conduct of other animals, but as Ricoeur writes:

> It is the instinctive conducts which are decreasing in the case of man. Man has quantitatively more instincts, if we include the new anxieties and new incentives which he invents, but he is less instinctive if we stress his loss of unlearned forms of conduct, spontaneously adapted from the environment. (1966, p. 95 [91]; translation slightly modified)

Ricoeur thus acknowledges the importance of basic instincts in human behaviour, but insists on the increased quantity of 'invented' instincts involved in human life. The human desire or will-to-live is different from that of other animals because of the mediated character of the self's relation to the environment and to itself as a person. The higher cognitive, particularly human, capacities that enable this mediated relation are indeed bound to the biological life of the thinking self. We are tethered to our biological affects, impulses, and desires:

> This reduction of the act of knowing [*connaître comme tel*] attests to the nonautonomy of knowledge, its rootedness in existence, the latter of which being understood as desire and effort. Thereby is discovered not only the unsurpassable character of life [*le caractère indépassable de la vie*], but the interference of desire with intentionality, upon which desire inflicts an invincible obscurity, an ineluctable partiality.
>
> (Ricoeur 1977, p. 458 [442])

In human emotional experience there always remains 'an invincible obscurity' due to, at least partly, the biological roots of human life. We cannot understand human emotions without resorting to general ethological accounts that often include evolutionary explanations. Many of our emotions are driven by vital desires whose immediate satisfaction is rendered impossible by the multiple strata of laws, rules, and customs of conduct instantiated throughout the process of civilisation. I might, for example, feel an intense desire to strike a blow at the idiotic colleague who has just insulted me, instead I yell at him and thump my cup down on the table and leave the room. I have momentarily vented my anger, but I may be left with a feeling that a punch on the nose would have been a more appropriate expression of my anger. It would not, however, be the most appropriate in the given context, since I would probably lose my job and perhaps even face a lawsuit. These immediate reactions might find their explanation in some basic affectivity that generates instinctual mammalian behaviour. Human emotions, though, express more than these basic affective feelings. And we cannot explain them only with an archaeological survey into the mammalian brain systems. Ricoeur therefore calls out for a dialectic of archaeology and teleology as the adequate approach to human emotional experience. The complex nature of human emotions is related to the larger quantity of human instincts generated by the symbolic nature of our interaction with the world and other human subjects. Our emotional behaviour is influenced by the peculiar, proximate teleology that governs human existence, as embedded in a society with other human persons. And, moreover, we do not just want to live among other persons. We want to be recognised as a person by other persons (in our pursuit of 'the good life', of happiness). This *teleology of recognition* is indeed rooted in and, to a certain degree, shaped by our mammalian constitution, but somehow it rebels against our engrained biological dispositions. Ricoeur writes:

> No doubt the passion to achieve recognition goes beyond the animal struggle for self-preservation or domination; the concept of recognition is preeminently a noneconomic concept: the concept of recognition is not a struggle for life; it is a struggle to tear from the other an avowal, an attestation, a proof that I am an autonomous self-consciousness. But this struggle for recognition is a struggle in life against life—by life [*une lutte dans la vie contre la vie, par la vie*] [...] This is the sense in which desire is both surpassed and unsurpassable [*le désir est le dépassé indépassable*]. The positing of desire is mediated, not eradicated; it is not a sphere that we could lay aside, annul, annihilate. (1977, pp. 471–2 [455–6])

Ricoeur's use of the Spinozist concept of *conatus* is not contrary to or hostile towards a neuroscientific approach grounded in an evolutionary theory (Changeaux and Ricoeur 2000, pp. 174–8 [184–8]). On the contrary, Ricoeur insists on the basic mammalian affective feelings present in human emotional experience. What he does reject, however, is the reduction of human emotions to the regulation of physiological responses in the body. There is another kind of teleology at play in human emotional experience that we could call the *desire for recognition*.[6] We want to be part of a human society, to be acknowledged, respected, and loved—as well as simply staying alive. Our emotional behaviour is therefore conditioned and articulated by our existence in that society and by the value of social and personal recognition, alongside with the vital values of our biological life. Furthermore, humans have the capacity for singular reference, which means that the objects of human emotions are often of a non-fungible nature. We care about singular objects and individual persons, and because of this our feelings are much more differentiated and complex than those of other animals. Some of the obscure and seemingly irrational features of emotional experience may very well find their explanation in remote evolutionary forces at work in our basic affective relation to the environment.[7] And a clarification of the neurophysiology of emotions may help us understand why we sometimes feel and act irrationally. By modifying Pascal's famous dictum, one could say that the body has reasons of which reason knows nothing, which nevertheless deeply influence our being in the world, and thus we should not underestimate the embodied nature of emotions. J.M. Coetzee beautifully captures this impenetrable, dark and yet invigorating, dimension of our feelings when he describes the lust and emotional hunger of the aged and sickly Dostoevsky in his novel *The Master of Petersburg*:

> At the core of his hunger is a desire that on the first night did not fully know itself but now seems to have become centred on her smell. As if she and he were animals, he is drawn by something he picks up in the air around her: the smell of autumn, and of walnuts in particular. He has begun to understand how animals live, and young children too, attracted or repelled by mists, auras, atmospheres. He sees himself sprawled over her like a lion, rooting with his muzzle in the hair of her neck, burying his nose in her armpit, rubbing his face in her crotch.
>
> (Coetzee 1994, pp. 128–9)

---

[6] We will see in Chapter 9 that the *need* for recognition is one central feature of the borderline type of existence, characterised by the trauma of non-recognition.

[7] As an example of this, we can refer to all those pathological situations in which we do not behave towards another as if he were himself, but as if he were a replica of someone else. Think of the 'irrational' panic attacks of a traumatised young woman, who in her childhood suffered sexual harassment, when her boyfriend caresses her while she is asleep. She will be terrified and maybe react violently, because she unintentionally generalises her boyfriend's behaviour. She is no more capable of singular reference: an emotion is transferred to a person/situation that has the same general, but not particular, features as another (e.g. both the boyfriend and the harrasser are men, in their thirties, and seductively caress her when she is at her most vulnerable).

But, as Solomon rightly pointed out, this is only part of the story. Although we might be driven by the same *conatus* as other animals, there are important differences ('conative variants' as Panksepp calls them) when it comes to human affectivity. These variants or differences are mainly due to the higher cognitive skills present in humans, which might be characterised by what de Sousa names 'full-fledged mental intentionality' together with the fact that humans have a biography and time-indexed desires (de Sousa 1987, p. 100). Coetzee is perfectly aware of this emotional complexity of primeval lust and sexual hunger when awakened in reflectively frail human beings like us. Immediately after describing Dostoevsky's animal desire for Anna Sergeyevna, he goes further into Dostoevsky's heated mind:

> There is no lock on the door. It is not inconceivable that the child will wander into the room at a time like this and glimpse him in a state of—he approaches the word with distaste, but it is the only right word—lust. And so many children are sleepwalkers too: she could get up in the night and stray into his room without even waking. Are they passed down from mother to daughter, these intimate smells? Loving the mother, is one destined to long for the daughter to? Wandering thoughts, wandering desires! (Coetzee 1994, p. 129)

Evolutionary Well-Being

One reason for our insistence on the subjective aspect of feelings is the basically normative character of affectivity. How something affects us, how it touches us, reveals the values that we hold and ascribe to the world. And our values are a significant part of the persons that we are and central to our relationship with the world. Affectivity and personhood are deeply interwoven phenomena that find expression in the fragility constitutive of human existence. We shall explore this emotional fragility in much more detail in Part III, but for now we can perhaps illustrate what we mean by fragility if we briefly consider how it is disregarded by a contemporary evolutionary account of the relation between feelings and values.

We saw in Chapter 2 that Ricoeur argued for a basic affective generation of values. And throughout the book so far, we have followed his central argument that feelings are what make things matter to us. And it is generally agreed that there exists an intimate relation between emotions and values. The question of the relation between emotions and values is highly complex, though—and indeed vehemently debated.[8]

The philosopher David Pugmire has attempted, we believe successfully, to articulate this complexity in terms of the *epistemic* and *constitutional* relation of emotions to values. Pugmire has no doubts about the intrinsic relationship between emotions and values: 'valuation of some form, at least, is certainly central to emotions. It seems safe to say that there is valuation wherever emotion arises', but he immediately qualifies his statement, '[a]nd yet, not every valuation is emotional' (2005, p. 16). Emotions may reveal values that have nothing whatsoever to do with the emotional experience itself, or with what we ourselves like or dislike. In other words, emotions and values

---

[8] Seminal accounts of the relation between emotions and values can be found in Blackburn (1998), de Sousa (2011), Gibbard (1990), Stocker (1996), and Tappolet (2000).

are not identical. Values can be values without any emotional content or colouring, as for example, principles, laws, or unwritten customs. Emotions do, however, provide a special *epistemic* relation to these impersonal and unemotional values. They express our *personal* relation to these 'rational' values:

> Emotions are also personal in a particular way. They involve the self in a way that judgements need not. To accept something as true is of course to accept it for one's own part (Kant's 'I think' that accompanies all my judgements). But while agreeing dispassionately that *p* is indeed a pity involves one to that extent, it does not involve one's mind as a whole in the way that actually *sorrowing* over *p* and the fact that *p* does. So we could say, borrowing from religion, that having emotions towards something is the bearing of a personal witness to how it matters.
>
> (Pugmire 2005, p. 16)

Besides this epistemic relation of emotions to values, there are also values which are constituted by our emotions:

> [E]motions also *imbues* certain things with value for us, inasmuch as they matter to us specifically for the kind of emotion they arouse in us. This is the emotion's constitutive role in relation to values [. . .] What is important here is that feelings not only register values, they also have or constitute values for us 'primitively'. Where a failure is a personal disaster (as it might not be for a Buddhist), the disaster lies in the anguish it brings. Charm lies less in the eye than in the heart, in the beholder's delight. (p. 18)

Pugmire's distinction is very useful because it introduces two separate ways in which our emotions are related to the values that we live by. Emotions may serve as an epistemic registration of rational and impersonal values, and they may also directly contribute to the, not always rational, constitution of the personal values in our life. What is important to notice here is that both kinds of values find their way into the intimate life of a person by means of emotions and feelings. This tallies well with Ricoeur's central argument, in his analysis of affectivity, that emotions and feeling personalise our otherwise rational judgements and our reflective engagement with the world, other people, and ourselves.

Experience is thus qualified by feelings. My feelings reveal my cares and concerns, which again reflect the person that I am. The thrust of our investigation so far has been to articulate the complex fragility involved in this relationship of feelings and personhood. Most evolutionary explanations, though, operate with a simplistic notion of human personhood and, consequently, with a reductive notion of human values. This view on emotions and personhood basically derives from a restricted evolutionary conception of affectivity. As mentioned in Chapter 4, the philosopher Jesse Prinz has developed the traditional feeling theory into a sophisticated account about the way biological properties control our emotional life, in the form of an 'embodied appraisal theory' where 'emotions are gut reactions: they use our bodies to tell us how we are faring in the world' (Prinz 2004, p. 69). On this account, emotions are bodily appraisals of our conduct in the world and express the values that guide our life and well-being. We fully agree with this picture of emotions as being intimately connected with values, but we strongly disagree with Prinz's understanding of the values that shape and determine our being in the world. He writes, for example:

> To qualify as an appraisal, a state must represent an organism-environment relation that bears on well-being. On the view I have been defending, emotions qualify as appraisals in this strict sense. They represent core relational themes.
>
> (Prinz 2004, p. 77)

This kind of framework basically accepts two forms of influences on human emotional experience: on the one hand, somatic core relational themes of survival, reproduction, and well-being, and on the other hand, the variegated ways culture nurtures these basic themes in different sociocultural contexts. In other words, our emotions reveal biological and cultural values, and our well-being becomes a matter of how we accept and live by these values. In this way, the notion of well-being becomes reductive (to survive is better than not to) and relativistic (just do like the others or isolate yourself from them and do what you like to do) at the same time.[9] Our well-being is constituted by the way we relate ourselves to our 'organism' and our 'environment'. Although Prinz insists that he is against evolutionary reductionism (2004, pp. 117–30) and pleads for an integrative compatibilism between biology and culture (2004, p. 158), his notion of well-being still remains problematic. And it could be argued that this is owing to his simplistic notion of personhood. In fact, his theory (like most other evolutionarily inspired theories) does not discuss the question of personhood at all. This simplistic view on human nature becomes obvious, and trivial, when he tries to account for the complex phenomenology of emotions that are crucial to a human life:

> I think the phenomenology of guilt is often just like the phenomenology of sadness. In some cases, guilt may also share its phenomenology with anxiety, or other more basic emotions. The point is that certain emotions have similar or identical phenomenology. There are many other plausible examples: indignation feels like anger, disappointment feels like sadness, awe has an element of surprise, contempt has an element of disgust, pride feels like a kind of joy, exhilaration feels like a blend of fear and joy, and jealousy feels like a blend of anger, disgust, and fear.
>
> (Prinz 2005, p. 19)

All emotions have 'core relational themes' that are relevant to our needs and interests, that is, our well-being (2004, p. 66); which, in turn, entails that fear, for example, is always somehow rooted in physical danger (2004, p. 219).

However, a person is not simply the product of biology and culture, and well-being is not just a matter of accepting biological needs and following them, or adopting cultural norms and adapting to them. This is not to say that biology and culture do not play inescapably fundamental roles in the constitution of human values. They do. Our feelings reveal that both biological needs (I may be irritated because of lack of sleep or food) and cultural norms (I may be ashamed of myself if I display bad taste or manners) are fundamental to our well-being as persons. Nonetheless, human well-being is more

---

[9] This problematic integration of biological reductionism and cultural relativism is expressed in Prinz's recent isolationist account of moral relativism (Prinz 2007).

fragile than such an account makes it out to be. An appeal to the biological or cultural constitution of our values does not explain, let alone help us live with, the fragile nature of personhood. To be a person is not the same as to be an orchid. We are not what we are simply by being born, growing up, blossoming in our prime years, becoming old, and eventually dying. It may seem ridiculous to point it out, but then again perhaps not, since some evolutionarily inspired philosophers tend to forget that there is more to the human animal than its biological organism and environment. A fundamental feature of human fragility stems from the problematic nature of human identity. As we have seen, a person can want to be different from what he or she actually is, not only with respect to biology or culture, but even different from the very person that he or she is. I may feel that I *am* different from what I *appear* to be. To be a person is not merely a matter of temporal and spatial existence. Rather, a person is 'a projected synthesis that seizes itself in the representation of *a task*, of an ideal of what the person should be' (Ricoeur 1987, p. 69 [86]; emphasis added). Every human being is a person, and yet to be a (certain kind of) person is always *a task of becoming*. The tension between the factual and ideal nature of personhood is primarily experienced in our feelings as an inherent normative feature of being the person that I am.

The normative dimension in which I as a person orient myself is permeated by doubt, hesitation, and questions (even without my being clinically neurotic, but simply humanly fragile) as to what it means to be the person that I am. I know that I am a person with a specific physical constitution and embedded in a given sociocultural context. I have certain character traits, dispositions, desires, ideas, dreams, and habits that shape and express my values, which are again expressed in my *felt* concerns and by what I *care* about. In spite of such cognitive attempts to circumscribe and explain my values, there always remains a kind of non-transparency in human values. Even though I may be a self-confident person, convinced of my values and firm in my actions, doubt, hesitation, and questions are still there, lurking deep inside my seemingly transparent conception of myself as a person. I may be inclined to something that I am not all that clear about. I may honestly believe that I am satisfied with my life, and even try to convince others that I am. And still, there is something that seems to disturb my well-being or scratch the glossy surface of my self-proclaimed stability. Of course, I can ignore this and go on living without paying attention to the supposedly insignificant whims played out by my feelings. But I cannot control many of my feelings, and I may be surprised at my own feelings and, as we have seen with Goldie, even feel a emotional resistance to myself. I may say or do things that I know are wrong, or hurt a person I care about, simply because I am angry, irritated, or annoyed. Human well-being is fragile due to this involuntary nature of many of our feelings and their relation to personhood.

Our fragile well-being becomes particularly evident in our experience of moods. The problematic character of the values through and by which we live our life, and the ambivalence constitutive of personhood, all comes to the fore once we turn to the aspect of our affectivity that concerns our bad moods.

But before we introduce the multifarious phenomena of bad moods, and ask how they may hold a clue to a better understanding of human fragility, we shall first discuss Matthew Ratcliffe's recent account of human feelings. Ratcliffe argues convincingly for a phenomenological approach to human affectivity that provides a theoretical background for appreciating inarticulate phenomena such as moods. As remarked earlier, there are many similarities between our theories, but also significant differences. An account of the differences may be useful for clarifying our own theory, and also for substantiating our argument that a phenomenological account of emotions must be supplemented with a more comprehensive hermeneutical theory of subjectivity. To do this properly, though, we need to present a rough outline of Ratcliffe's sophisticated account.[10]

In this section, we have argued that an evolutionary explanation of human emotions as constituted by a constellation of biological and cultural factors is not adequate for dealing with the fragile nature of human well-being. Ratcliffe's purely phenomenological account is also not up to the task it sets itself—namely, to provide us with the meaning of life.

The Pragmatic Meaning of Life

Ratcliffe's theory starts by breaking down the traditional conceptual barrier between intentional emotions (cognitive theories) and bodily feelings (feeling theories). To get things right we need to suspend our conceptual prejudices and begin with a phenomenological analysis of human emotional experience. Ratcliffe claims that our understanding of emotions always begins in our experience of feelings, and to support this claim he singles out a distinctive phenomenological category that he calls existential feelings:

> I suggest that certain uses of the term 'feeling' do pick out a distinctive phenomenological category. Feelings belong to this category in virtue of two shared characteristics. First of all, they are not directed at specific objects or situations but are background orientations through which experience as a whole is structured. Second, they are *bodily feelings*. As these feelings constitute the basic structure of 'being there', a 'hold on things' that functions as a presupposed context for all intellectual and practical activity, I refer to them as *existential feelings*.
>
> (Ratcliffe 2008, p. 38)

Ratcliffe coins his theory of existential feelings chiefly on Heidegger's concept of mood (*Stimmung*), which plays a fundamental role in Heidegger's early (existentially oriented) works (1995, 2010). Heidegger's analysis of mood is still important today, Ratcliffe rightly points out (2008, pp. 47–50, 56), because it renders the strict conceptual distinction between intentional emotions and bodily feelings highly problematic. Moreover, Heidegger argues that moods are fundamental not only to human emotional experience, but to human experience and existence in general. Hence, if we take Heidegger's arguments seriously, as Ratcliffe suggests we should do, it becomes evident

---

[10] Obviously, here we are only able to account for what we consider to be the gist of Ratcliffe's argument. It would lead us too far afield to expound or discuss all the interesting details of the thorough development of his phenomenological account. One of the merits of Ratcliffe's theory is his patient insistence on enhancing a dialogue between philosophical traditions that normally do not have much to say about each other. Hence, his theory of emotions is developed from his previous discussions of how phenomenology and cognitive science may benefit from one another in the approach to the human mind (Ratcliffe 2007).

that the traditional neglect of moods in contemporary anglophone philosophy of emotions is untenable.[11]

Our moods are fundamental because they express the pre-conceptual and felt source of meaning in human life. To speak with Ratcliffe, 'moods set up the world in which we can have specific object-directed emotions' (2008, p. 50). Ratcliffe distinguishes between what we commonly call emotions (e.g. fear or anger) and moods (e.g. anxiety or boredom) by claiming that the former are directed at something which takes place *in* the world, whereas the latter are that which *constitutes* our being-in-the-world as a whole. Emotions such as love for someone or annoyance over something are only possible on 'the background sense of belonging to a meaningful world' (Ratcliffe 2010, p. 356), which we find expressed in our moods. The gist of Heidegger's meaningful world as revealed by our moods is, according to Ratcliffe, of practical significance. Our existence in the world and our interaction with the objects in that world is not a neutral, speculative relation between a subject and an object. We are *attuned* creatures that always find ourselves in the world in a certain *felt* way. Our attunement (*Befindlichkeit*) characterises how we feel about being in the world. Ratcliffe describes this attuned character of human existence as:

> [T]he way in which moods constitute a sense of belonging to the world. They do so by revealing the world as a realm of practical purposes, values and goals. The world that we take for granted in our activities is a background of significance, a space of potential purposive activities that frames all our experience. (2008, p. 47)

The world matters to us, and the fact that it matters is expressed in our moods. Our other emotions and feelings work on this background of existential significance, which is a fact that makes moods primordial with respect to the other expressions of our emotional life. In other words, emotions and feelings presuppose the existence of moods (2008, p. 49), and Ratcliffe makes his claim even stronger by saying that '[i]t is certain moods, I want to suggest, that constitute the meaning of life' (2010, p. 353; see also 2008, p. 36).

This is all in all a fairly loyal rendering of Heidegger's theory of mood and attunement. And although Ratcliffe suggests that we use the term 'existential feelings' instead of 'moods' and goes on to point out what he considers to be serious shortcomings in Heidegger's theory (2008, pp. 52–6), he is very clear about the Heideggerian heritage of his own theory of existential feelings. But what exactly are these existential feelings, and how do they play the fundamental role that Ratcliffe suggests they do?

Ratcliffe singles them out among the heterogeneous nature of human emotions in the following way:

> Existential feelings, I claim, are not hybrid states. They are non-conceptual *feelings* of the body, which constitute a background sense of belonging to the world and a sense of reality. They are not evaluations of any specific object, they are certainly not propositional attitudes and they are not 'mere affects'. (2008, p. 39)

---

[11] This philosophical *phobia* of moods may have several roots, but one of them is their supposed ineffability. Indeed, moods are ineffable not in the ordinary sense of our lack of words to express them, but rather because of the interminable discourse we can develop around them. There is so much meaning in a mood that it is hard to capture it with an analytical discourse.

Thus, two main features characterise existential feelings: they are bodily feelings, and they constitute a background sense of belonging and reality.

The core of Ratcliffe's argument rests on what he considers to be the inextricable relationship between body and reality. Our sense of belonging to the world is first and foremost constituted through our bodily interaction with that world. This is a traditional phenomenological insight (Gallagher and Zahavi 2008, pp. 141–4; Zahavi 1999, pp. 91–109; Zahavi 2005, pp. 156–9) and Ratcliffe elaborates it to include feelings by emphasising tactile perception. The phenomenology of touch draws attention to the intimate relatedness between bodily feelings and world-experience and thus dissolves an allegedly strict division between body and world (Ratcliffe 2008, p. 106). The world and our body are not two independent entities that are somehow loosely connected through the fact that we are part of the world. On the contrary, the world becomes what it is through our bodily experience of the objects in the world. World and body are interrelated phenomena in the sense that they constitute one another, and this becomes particularly conspicuous in our tactile interaction with the world.

The phenomenon of touch reveals two fundamental aspects of the feeling body: one where the body is the object of our feelings, say, if I hit my thumb with a hammer, and another where it is the body that is doing the feeling, when, for example, I have to find some coins in my pocket. In the first case, it is my body that is in the foreground of my experience, whereas in the latter it fades into the background in order to let the world appear. When I search for coins in my pocket, the focus of my experience is not my fingers but the objects that they touch. In this sense, my body becomes the medium through which my experience of the world is constituted. I use my body to explore and interact with the objects in the world, and through this practical use of my body the world becomes familiar. In our bodily familiarity with the world, the distinction between body and world or between inside (me) and outside (world) is 'not an essential ingredient of tactile experience and the assumption that it is stems from the unwarranted a priori imposition of an internal-external contrast upon it' (2008, p. 92).

So, having established the interdependent phenomenological relationship between body and world, Ratcliffe uses this argument to show how existential feelings constitute our background sense of belonging to the world and our sense of reality:

> There is more than just an analogy between existential feelings and touch—the tactile background contributes to our sense of belonging to the world, structuring more localized tactile experiences and our experiences more generally. Thus it is partly constitutive of existential feelings. (2008, p. 93)

Existential feelings are partly constituted by the way in which our tactile feelings constitute our sense of being in the world. We feel that we are part of the world that we are in touch with. The world becomes real, or gains significance, through our tactile relationship with the objects in the world, and being able to practically interact with the world gives us a sense of belonging to the world. Our existential feeling of the world is, of course, not simply constituted by the solidity of the tactile background. The fact that our feeling of belonging to the world is constituted by our practical interaction with the objects in the world, which thereby becomes familiar, reveals that our existential feelings constitute 'a space of possibilities' (2008, p. 101). Existential feelings thus constitute a sense of belonging to a world that offers us various possibilities to unfold our existence and make it meaningful.

This practical nature of existential feelings is central to Ratcliffe's argument for the fundamental role that existential feelings play in our life:

> A world stripped of *all* tactile possibilities really would look remote and intangible. Similarly, 'losing one's grip' on the world could involve a loss of practical belonging, a failure to connect with things, where nothing appears manipulable anymore. One no longer inhabits a tranquil realm of organized, interrelated practical possibilities that mesh seamlessly with one's activities. Changes in existential feelings are often expressed in terms of an altered bodily relationship with the world. (2008, p. 135)

Existential feelings register changes in our sense of belonging to a world of practical possibilities. Our existence is played out against the background of more or less stable feelings of being-in-a-world which provide the basis for our interaction with the objects in the world. These constitutive feelings are existential because, contrary to other, more object-orientated feelings and emotions, they are not related to any specific objects or events in the world but constitute the general framework (or 'horizon', in the terminology of traditional phenomenology) of orientation that holds together our existence. In this sense, existential feelings are vital to our sense of reality: 'Many if not all existential changes are also subtle or pronounced changes of feelings in the sense of reality. This, I have suggested, consists of a background feeling of practical belonging' (2008, p. 216). Existential feelings therefore play a fundamental role in human life by registering changes in the practical possibilities of human existence, which are first and foremost based on our bodily relationship with the world.[12]

Now, we agree with much of Ratcliffe's careful phenomenological account of human feelings. We believe that his basic claim for a constitutive (felt) sense of belonging to the world is right. We also think that his rejection of the traditional distinction between intentional emotions (cognition) and bodily feelings (affect), on the basis of a phenomenological attention to the felt aspect of human experience, is correct. We disagree, however, with the conclusions that he draws from this phenomenological analysis of human feelings. Our disagreement stems from Ratcliffe's fundamental claim about the constitutive feelings of our belonging to the world, namely, that they are primarily related to bodily practices. The emphasis on these particular aspects of our feelings produces a distorted picture of our emotional life, which, in turn, makes his argument that existential feelings constitute the meaning of life rather diffuse.

---

[12] We should mention that Ratcliffe describes a large variety of existential feelings that are not immediately related to practical possibilities or our bodily relationship with the world. He sums up these variants of existential feelings in the following way: '(a) various kinds of belonging and estrangement, (b) kinds and degrees of bodily conspicuousness or (c) some or all objects of experience appearing a certain way, such as unreal, unfamiliar, contingent and so on. Existential feelings are also describable in terms of different modes of concern, directed at either self or world' (2008, p. 215). However, from the way he analyses and illustrates how these feelings work in both depression and schizophrenia, it remains clear that all kinds of existential feelings rest on the basis of practical belonging to and bodily interaction with the world.

This distorted picture, we believe, has its origin in Ratcliffe's lack of an explicit account of human subjectivity. This conspicuous lack has several problematic consequences for his theory. Here we will discuss only two that are central to our own account. The two are closely interrelated and, we believe, central to human emotional life. The first one is Ratcliffe's notion of the body, whereas the second is his understanding of normative affectivity.

Ratcliffe's theory is, as mentioned, built on a Heideggerian foundation. There is nothing wrong with this. In fact, as we remarked in Chapter 1, Heidegger is indispensable in any phenomenological approach to human feelings. Heidegger's introduction of affectivity into the phenomenological analysis of human subjectivity marked a significant change in the way of doing phenomenology. Whereas Husserl had put aside questions about ontology and metaphysics, Heidegger made these questions the foundation for his investigation of human experience and action. This has been characterised as a shift from reflective to hermeneutical phenomenology: where the former confined itself to clarifying the experiential structures of subjectivity, the latter went a step further (or a step backwards) and asked how we are to understand (i.e. interpret), evaluate, and finally act on what we experience. This ontological shift introduced questions into the phenomenological investigation, which Husserl had done his best to keep out of what he considered to be serious scientific phenomenology, in particular, questions of ontology and normativity. Heidegger does not just ask what and how we experience, but also how we feel about our experiences. And the question of how we feel inevitably entails the further questions about the nature of our feelings (ontology) and what we should do about them (normativity). As suggested earlier, both in Part I and Chapter 6 in this part, phenomenology can make us aware of the ontological and normative implications, but is not able to provide us with answers. To be able to confront and investigate these aspects of our emotional life, we need to combine our phenomenological analysis with a hermeneutical theory of subjectivity.

This is not the place to go into the intricate differences between reflective and hermeneutical phenomenology or the subtleties of Heidegger's theory.[13] What is important for the issue at hand is to make clear that Heidegger's analysis of affectivity is rooted in a strong ontology with problematic normative implications that spill over into Ratcliffe's conception of existential feelings.

First, as Ratcliffe points out himself, Heidegger, despite his unrelenting emphasis on the bodily nature of our practical interaction with the world, does not actually account for the role the body plays in our experience (Ratcliffe 2008, p. 55). Heidegger's famous aversion to natural science, and to empirical understanding of human nature in general, results in a poor account of the human body that intentionally disregards the biological dimension of human embodiment. Ratcliffe's emphasis on existential

---

[13] For a clear and instructive treatment of the important issue about reflective and hermeneutical phenomenology, see Zahavi (2005, pp. 73–98). To get an idea of Heidegger's theory of mood and attunement, and to understand how these are related to his early analysis of human existence, see respectively, Pocai (1996) and Ferreira (2002).

feelings as primarily bodily obviously provides a more thorough account of the role of the body in our feelings. Even so, his account of how the body constitutes our experience of the world remains on a purely phenomenological level. He explicitly dismisses the possibility that non-conscious, bio-regulatory processes play any constitutive role in existential feelings. He concedes that emotions might be a heterogeneous group of feelings, some of which might indeed stem from bio-regulatory processes, but his existential feelings differ from what philosophers normally refer to as emotions or feelings, in that they are not, as we have already seen, 'hybrid states', that is, '[t]hey are not evaluations of any specific object, they are certainly not propositional attitudes and they are not "mere affect"' (2008, p. 39).[14] Thus, existential feelings are not seriously influenced by our biological constitution. We, obviously, believe this to be a mistake and have argued that human affectivity is inseparably connected with our biology, and that to understand our emotional life we need both biology and phenomenology. Now, Ratcliffe goes further than simply dismissing the biological aspect of existential feelings. In fact, he claims that they are radically different from everything that is normally associated with emotions, both philosophically and in everyday life.[15] Since existential feelings are at the heart of the meaning of human life, one is naturally curious to know what exactly makes them so different from other emotional states and, perhaps most importantly, how they play such a fundamental role in the meaning of life. These questions bring us to the issue of normative affectivity.

---

[14] This is not to say that Ratcliffe rejects any significance of a neuroscientific approach to human nature. On the contrary he welcomes the interaction between phenomenology and neuroscience, but he has no doubt about which kind of investigation is more fundamental: 'I reject the goal of naturalization, the reason being that the phenomenological stance reveals a sense of reality that is not accessible to the standpoint of empirical science. The phenomenologist studies aspects of experience that are presupposed by all empirical, scientific investigation into what the world contains. One cannot distinguish between what is and is not the case in the world without having a sense of what it is to be the case. Hence scientific practices do not escape existential backgrounds and then confront them as objects of empirical study. Rather, scientific practices and scientific conceptions of the world arise within the space of possibilities that the phenomenologist describes' (2009, p. 241). As we have attempted to show in the previous chapters, the problem with such a view on the relationship between phenomenology and empirical science is that there may be aspects of our felt relation to the world, other people, and ourselves which cannot be investigated in terms of the 'existential possibilities' revealed by a phenomenological approach. We have therefore opted for a hermeneutic approach that puts phenomenology and the empirical sciences (in our case neuroscience) on a more equal standing that allows a phenomenology of feelings to be informed and extended by our increasing insight into the biological constitution of bodily feelings. To put it differently, there are aspects of our emotional life that escapes the reach of a phenomenologist.

[15] In his endeavour to differentiate existential feelings so radically from what we normally understand as emotions and feelings, Ratcliffe again follows closely in the footsteps of Heidegger, who went to great lengths to separate moods (*Stimmung*) and attunement (*Befindlichkeit*) from other emotional states (Heidegger 1995, pp. 89–103; 2010, pp. 138–42).

As we have seen, Ratcliffe's answer, for all its philosophical subtleties, can be boiled down to the basic argument that existential feelings constitute our sense of practical belonging to the world. In doing so, Ratcliffe once again follows along a Heideggerian path. This time he takes up Heidegger's pragmatic analysis of being-in-the-world and inauthenticity, although he tunes up the former and downplays the latter. Existential feelings are fundamentally different from other feelings and emotions because they do not express our reaction to or concern with anything specific in the world. On the contrary, they constitute the background of basic practical significance which makes our experience of and interaction with the objects of the world possible in the first place. They provide the practical structures of actuality and possibility that shapes our ongoing experience and action by providing a 'horizon' of existential orientation (2008, pp. 131–7). Disturbances or complications of this horizon result in changes of our space of possibilities, which are registered as changes in our existential feelings. Our existential orientation falters, and our bodily dispositions and possibilities become altered or diminished, which may damage our sense of practical belonging and a loss of reality. A phenomenologically conspicuous disturbance of our space of practical possibilities is the existential feeling of 'anxiety' which 'has the role of shaking us out of the disposition to misinterpret ourselves and lose ourselves in idle talk' (2008, p. 262). The world loses all features of meaning, it becomes unreal, and we find ourselves at a loss in our everyday humdrum of sayings and doings.

Although Ratcliffe does not explicitly link such changes to the Heideggerian normative talk of authenticity, the normative aspect of existential feelings cannot but play a role in his account of how these feelings constitute our sense of belonging to the world. Existential feelings are supposed to carry quite a heavy load of significance. In fact, they carry the heaviest of them all, the meaning of life. To be able to do so, though, they have to be intrinsically connected to the values and norms that inform and shape our existence, but this normative aspect is never really articulated in Ratcliffe's account. It seems as if he wants to ground the constitutive values of existential feelings on a diffuse notion of practical possibilities, which can be assessed and accurately described by means of a purely descriptive phenomenological stance that does not involve any normative considerations (2008, p. 278). The normative character of existential feelings is limited to their ability to direct our awareness to the world that a person or a philosophical theory 'obliviously takes for granted' (2008, p. 262). To become aware of the structures of our-being-in-the-world is to free ourselves of our ignorance and our habitual prejudices about the world and human existence and thus find ourselves authentically in the world (as a person as well as a philosopher). Nobody would question the fact that it is a good thing to be aware of the world we belong to. The more interesting question, though, is how the practical values of Ratcliffe's primordial world-structures, his amorphous space of possibilities, are connected to our, often deeply 'impractical', values and concerns, which are expressed in our more intimate feelings such as love, shame, sadness, joy, and hate.

In fact, the abstruse normative character of existential feelings leaves unanswered several questions central to understanding emotional experience, all of them intimately wound up with the normative aspect of our feelings. Why does our existential orientation falter? What is the relation between clearly normative emotions such as anger or guilt and the more diffuse practical background of existential feelings? Why is my sense of practical belonging to the world constitutive of the meaning(s) of life? What is the role of other people in the changes of our existential feelings? Is the other person constitutive of my existential feelings or am I primarily alone in my existential orientation? What is the relationship, if there is any, between the normative features of my biological body (*Körper*), such as drives and impulses, and the practical values pertaining to my lived body (*Leib*)?

As noticed above, we believe the lack of a hermeneutical theory of subjectivity to be the main reason why these questions are not treated in Ratcliffe's account. Like Heidegger before him,[16] Ratcliffe is more interested in clarifying the constitutive, objective structures of the world (what Heidegger called fundamental ontology) that shape and inform human existence, rather than the subjective features of human nature. This results in a flat notion of the human person, whose values and concerns are somehow derived from an allegedly more primary notion of bodily practicality. The normative aspect of human affectivity is guided by an amorphous space of existential possibilities that either obstruct or assist our sense of belonging to the world. But what these possibilities or lack of possibilities actually consist in is not explained in his theory. We only learn that they are so fundamental that they, as they are revealed in certain moods, somehow 'constitute the meaning of life' (2010, p. 353) and are thus so close to the core of human meaning that they are 'presupposed by conceptual judgements' (2010, p. 368). How human meaning and values are generated and conceived by the human subject is not explained either. Hence, both meaning and values remain rather anonymous and inarticulate. This phenomenological understanding supposedly digs so deep into human experience that it goes beyond what can be understood as a psychological or personal stance:

> Personal and psychological understanding, both take the world for granted and so are unable to access this aspect of experience. Phenomenology, in contrast, seeks to describe the structures of our ordinarily presupposed sense of belonging and reality. (2009, p. 226)

Ratcliffe's attempt to ground existential feelings in a practical background of belonging that goes beyond the psychological and personal stance is vulnerable to criticism of the same kind as we saw in Chapter 1, where Jaspers argued against Heidegger's

---

[16] Heidegger was mainly interested in our feelings to the extent that they disclosed the objective structure of human existence. Moreover, Heidegger's aversion to empirical knowledge did not confine itself to the natural sciences. He also disapproved of the philosophical anthropologies that were prominent in the first half of the twentieth century. He considered inane the attempts of Scheler, Jaspers, Gehlen, and Plessner to combine philosophical analysis with the empirical knowledge of the day. These were merely 'regional ontologies' that lacked the a priori strengths of his own 'fundamental ontology' (1990, pp. 224–39; 2010, pp. 13–15). One could argue that it was this obsession with the a priori, objective nature of our existential structures that eventually made him turn away from intricate questions of human beings to the broader, metaphysical question about 'Being in itself' in the mid-1930s (the change in Heidegger's philosophy known as '*die Kehre*').

grounding of human existence in a search of authenticity: basic human feelings such as love and friendship do seem even more fundamental to the meaning of life than our authentic sense of practical belonging to the world. In fact, our sense of belonging to the world is primarily constituted exactly through such subjective feelings, which constitute the personal relationship between people. The fundamental role of the subjectivity of feelings becomes obvious if we consider how a casual joke in a conversation might seem innocent and funny to one person while it is devastating to another, how one person's happiness appears as mere stupidity to another person, or how differently we measure the standards of a 'meaningful life'. To liberate authentic possibilities is not a solution to our existential problems. On the contrary, unqualified possibilities and unspecified authentic freedom is more a problem than a solution. Our freedom is always bound to the obscure desires of our flesh and the love and recognition of other people. The normative character of Ricoeur's theory of subjectivity is grounded in this otherness, these inescapably biological and ethical bounds, which constitute our freedom:

> This liberation in mere thought leads back to absolute otherness [*l'altérité absolue*]; the struggling desires no longer have a self and the self no longer has any flesh; this is the sense in which life is unsurpassable. And the very term 'self'—*Selbst*—proclaims that self-identity continues to be carried by this self-difference by this ever-recurring otherness residing in life [*cette altérité sans cesse renaissante qui réside dans la vie*]. It is life that becomes the other [*la vie qui devient l'autre*], in and through which the self ceaselessly achieves itself.
>
> (Ricoeur 1977, p. 472 [456])

Ratcliffe emphasises that his phenomenological account provides an antidote to the many unwarranted dualisms that still haunt philosophy today, such as body vs world, affect vs cognition, internal vs external (2008, p. 8). Nonetheless, he himself still seems to operate with a strong distinction between objective and subjective feelings. The focus of his investigation is on the inextricable relation between feelings and the (practical) structure of world experience, and *not* on feelings as a disclosure of our state of mind (Ratcliffe 2005, p. 46). He shifts the attention away from the subjective focus of feelings to the objective aspect of feelings that supposedly constitutes our experience of and interaction with reality. We think that this strict distinction between the *subjective* state of mind (internal) and the *objective* world (external) is unwarranted and can, once again, be ascribed to his inarticulate notion of subjectivity.

As suggested in the previous chapter, a phenomenological analysis of human affectivity reveals that our feelings are rooted in our biological needs and in our personal relation to the world, the other, and ourselves. The constitutional aspect of feelings, expressed in the way we find ourselves in the world, involves an affective resonance that discloses the subjective focus of all experiential phenomena. My feelings reveal that the world always affects me in virtue of the person that I am. My experience of the external world is inextricably related to my subjective state of mind, and this complex affective relation between world and personhood is primarily expressed in my feelings. The constitutional feelings of being-in-the-world that Ratcliffe argues for cannot be separated from the subjective aspect of those feelings. Therefore, we believe that

Ratcliffe is mistaken when he dismisses some bad moods as subjective whims without any informative value about our being-in-the-world:

> [S]ome 'moods' seem to be fairly superficial subjective states. For example, one might say 'I'm sorry; I'm just in a bit of a bad mood today', indicating that it is possible to assign a mood to oneself without it enveloping one's whole relationship with the world. (2005, p. 55)

Ratcliffe sometimes uses the terms 'mood' and 'existential feeling' interchangeably, although he argues that the latter remains a better term for the constitutive feelings that he is interested in, because it distinguishes them from the allegedly 'more superficial' feelings that we also call moods (2008, p. 56). Recently, he has coined the term 'deep moods' to distinguish them from mere moods, but still retains 'existential feelings' as a better term (2010, p. 367).

The difficulty Ratcliffe seems to have in maintaining the distinction between the more superficial subjective kind of moods and the (objective) constitutive deep moods or existential feelings might be a telling symptom that the distinction is somewhat artificial and phenomenologically untenable. To make his case convincing, Ratcliffe must be able to show how what we ordinarily call 'moods' are related to his more 'deep moods', and why the former are insignificant and the latter significant when it comes to the meaning of life. Otherwise, deep moods and existential feelings remain diffuse and inarticulate, and it is difficult to see how they are supposed to carry the weight of so thick a notion as the meaning of life, which indeed seems to include these 'fairly subjective states of mind'. As it should be obvious by now, we believe that the only way to sort out the relations between subjective and objective features of emotional experience is through an articulate theory of subjectivity.

Bad moods may be subjective in nature, but it is precisely their subjective tincture that reveals something central about our being human persons. In order to understand why moods are not just subjective whims, and thereby to appreciate the subjective focus of such feelings, we must bring in the notion of personhood in our analysis of moods. Phenomenology remains a fundamental method to disclose the structures of human affective experience, but we need a more comprehensive hermeneutical theory if we are to articulate the values and concerns that are expressed in these feelings, explain how the pre-conceptual and pre-intentional background feelings are related to complex emotions and more intentional feelings, and understand how the anonymous, biological needs of our body are related to our lived body. Strasser, who agrees with Ricoeur's insistence on the combination of phenomenology and hermeneutics, writes about the relation between feelings and meaning in his seminal work on the phenomenology of feelings:

> This illumination of experience from within outwards requires philosophical interpretation. As the process appears [. . .] it is simply incomprehensible. We can descriptively state that, where previously there was formlessness, form now appears; that bluntness [*Dumpfheit*] changes into consciousness; that undirectedness gives way to intentional alignment. But with this we have posed only a riddle. Thus, by means of a philosophical hermeneutics, we must make comprehensible the essential possibility of such transformations.
>
> (Strasser 1977, p. 124; translation slightly modified)

Our critique of Ratcliffe's theory of existential feelings and of the way he connects these to the meaning of life should not overshadow the many merits of his account. His introduction of serious phenomenology into contemporary philosophy remains an important contribution to the present debate. Furthermore, his attention to the intimate connection between moods (or existential feelings, as he names them) and the meaning of life is important too.

As suggested in the previous chapter, we also believe that our moods can tell us something important, if not specifically about the meaning of life, then at least about human meaning and values. On the remaining pages of this chapter, we will look at the experience of bad moods and try to show how the normative character of human feelings, especially visible in these phenomena, makes the questions of the meaning(s) of our life a very complex issue that requires an ongoing interpretation on the part of the person. The complexity, we suggested, is rooted in our ambivalent sense of identity, which is shaped and conditioned by a dynamic conglomerate of personal as well as biological factors. The complexity inherent in our ambivalent feelings of identity, on the other hand, plays a major part in the dynamic fragility constitutive of human personhood. This final section also serves as an introduction to Part III, where we shall attempt to show that this emotional fragility may help us to better understand the peculiar human vulnerability to mental illness.

Bad Moods, Personhood, and Vulnerability

We do not claim that bad moods explain or clarify the notion of a person, but we believe that moods provide valuable information about the complexity of human emotional experience that is involved in the fragile character of personhood. Bad moods are not always superficial whims. If we let them be an integral part of our understanding of human affectivity, they may enable us to shed some light on the particular relation between emotions and personhood.

We saw in the previous chapter that moods are phenomenologically distinguished from other feelings by their lack of clear object(s) and by their relatively long temporal duration. Furthermore, whereas many feelings are characterised by a direct relation to action, moods appear to have a more complicated relation to action. A mood does not prompt me to a specific action, and some (often bad) moods may impede or at least severely complicate action. This is closely related to their lack of object(s). When I am angry, I am normally angry at someone because of something. I have a clear focus for my feelings in the sense that I know to whom I shall direct my attention in order to vent my anger or at least deal with it in some way or other. I may be uncertain about how best to deal with my feelings, but I have a pretty clear idea of what I am feeling and why; in short, I have a more or less uncomplicated grasp of the intentional structure of my feelings when I experience bouts of anger. The same goes for many other emotions, notably those we earlier called affects, such as fear, lust, surprise, shame, resentment, disappointment, and disgust. Moods, however, are different, and bad moods in particular. Moods affect our experience as a whole. Gilbert Ryle describes the enveloping character of moods poignantly:

> [S]omewhat as this morning's weather in a given locality made the same sort of difference to every section of that neighbourhood, so a person's mood during a given period colours all or most of his actions and reactions during that period. His work and his play, his talk

and his grimaces, his appetite and his daydreams, all reflect his touchiness, his joviality or his depression. Any one of them may serve as a barometer for all the others [...] Somewhat as the entire ship is cruising south-east, rolling, or vibrating, so the entire person is nervous, serene or gloomy. His own corresponding inclination will be to describe the whole world as menacing, congenial, or grey.

(Ryle 1949, pp. 99–100)

We are not able to clearly identify an object for our mood, although we may notice that when we are in a certain mood our otherwise heterogeneous feelings are affected by some general attunement or colouring. Moods take a hold of 'the entire person' and affect how this person feels about the world, other people, and herself. Contrary to other constellations of feelings, moods attune or colour our emotional experience as a whole. We often explain our own disparate feelings and emotional reactions and those of others by referring to the generality of moods: 'Normally, he would not react so aggressively, but he has been in a nervous mood for several days now' or 'I am sorry that I yelled at you, but I am just in a bad mood today.' Thus, moods have often been referred to as background feelings, attunement, atmosphere, or, as Ryle does above, as the emotional climate. Such characterisations are accurate and to the point, but they do not say much about what moods are or anything about their informative value. Therefore, we have proposed to understand moods in relation to personhood. This approach is not new. As we have seen above, Ryle emphasises the relation. So do phenomenological philosophers such as Fuchs (2000, pp. 213–17), Heidegger (1995, pp. 78–267; 2010, pp. 134–42, 184–96), Scheler (1966 pp. 344–5), and Strasser (1977, pp. 181–201 [109–27]). However, we believe that contemporary research on emotions can benefit from an even more focused examination of the relation between bad moods and personhood.[17] We choose here to focus on bad moods instead of good moods, or moods in general, not because we believe that bad moods are more frequent or more comprehensive than other kinds of moods, but simply because bad moods have a more disruptive, and at times devastating, effect on our state of mind, our thoughts, feelings, and actions. Whereas good moods normally entice me and make me rejoice in the thoughts, beliefs, emotions, and actions that are characteristic for the person that I am, bad moods have a way of obstructing, or at least somehow making difficult, my customary ways of thinking of and acting in the world. This problematic effect makes bad moods a more conspicuous feature of our emotional life.

The world-direction that characterises many of my feelings is complicated, and sometimes even changed, in bad moods. The way I am touched or moved by certain experiences reveals the values that I hold, reflectively or pre-reflectively. When I feel opposed to someone who treats another person badly it is because this is contrary to my own values—or at least my ideal values; I feel admiration for a person because she stands for something that I cherish and find important; I am ashamed of myself for something I have done or said because it goes against what I believe in—or want to care for; I feel guilty because I have done something wrong. These are all emotions

---

[17] Evan Thompson has recently pointed to something similar: 'Overall there has been regrettably little analysis of emotion at the level of personality in phenomenology' (2007, p. 381).

that disclose my values and often elicit a certain reaction on my part. There exists, we suggested, an intimate relation between my feelings and my values. Feelings are an important part of the constitution of my values because they express the involuntary and pre-reflective aspect of what I value. What I care for is not only those things that I believe or desire to care for. My feelings may be contrary to what I cognitively value or wish to value. But although such feelings may be selfish, mean, stupid, and embarrassing, they are still part of the person that I am. Feelings are often what make me aware of the problematic dissonance between the person that I am and the person that I want to be. And it is exactly with regard to this complicated relationship between feelings and personhood that bad moods may provide some clarification.

A bad mood complicates the relation between feeling and action because it introduces doubt, hesitation, and questions into my emotional coping with the world. The intentional structure that characterises much of human emotional experience is absent, or at least obscured, in moods. Moods do not direct us to anything specific in our relation to the external environment, and we are not able to put our finger on what exactly causes our particular mood. On the contrary, as Strasser notices, a mood 'excludes the thematic prominence of a single object pole; it refers only to the diffuse, undifferentiated totality' (1977, p. 190). This totality is the person that we are. Strasser goes even further to emphasise the intimate relationship between personhood and our most intimate emotional texture, what Strasser like Ricoeur before him calls the heart (*das Gemüt*):

> The most delicate, most vulnerable, most individual aspect of the person is his heart [*Gemüt*]. Everything that has reference to the heart immediately touches that sphere of one's own being [*Eigen-sein*], of intimacy and secrecy which we characteristically call the 'personal'. There is clearly a connection between heart and person.
>
> (Strasser 1977, p. 245 [163]; translation slightly modified)

Personhood, as we have seen, comprises what we (f)actually are (embodied beings with a specific biological constitution and embedded in a certain sociocultural environment, i.e. our physique, character, habits, customs, commitments, etc.) and what we want to be (our plans, dreams, ideals, desires, beliefs, etc.). The tension between what we are and what we want to be can become thematised as an overt problem during our lives, but it often begins and ends as a feeble discomfort in the background of our thoughts and actions; the feeling that I am not present in what I am actually doing or saying; or that I am not at ease and feel that something is not right in my life. I may not be able to articulate what is wrong or understand why I feel the way I feel—I am just in a bad mood. However, a bad mood is not always merely a superficial annoyance during our daily lives, but may carry significant information about the complex emotional dimension of personal identity that we examined in the previous chapter.

A bad mood accompanies me in my everyday doings, and makes my experiences, choices, and actions seem stale and sometimes fatuous. I may feel I cannot connect with the world around me. Things I normally value and cherish lose their attraction and interest, and I feel myself to be somewhat isolated from the world. In this way, a bad mood often plays a secondary role in my relation to the world and other people, in the sense that although I feel enveloped in it I may still be able to disregard it, pull myself together and get through the gloomy days. Nevertheless, it continues to affect the relation to some degree, since it exercises a clear influence on our emotional reactions. As Thomas Fuchs writes:

> Being attuned [*Befinden*] and mood [*Stimmung*] are at first only marginally conscious: They penetrate the field of perception, change the character of expression or work as motivation, without being thematized as such. On the other hand, they tend to concretize and develop into [more explicit] feelings [*Gefühlen*]. Gloom brings about sorrow or feelings of guilt; diffuse anxiety tries to become fear and thus to find a 'point of attack' ['*Angriffsort*'] in space and time. Moods in this way constitute the foundation or ground upon which the more strongly agitated and specifically oriented feelings arise.
>
> (Fuchs 2000, p. 217; our translation)

In contrast to specifically orientated feelings (that is, what we have characterised as affects such as anger, disgust, surprise, shame, and fear), which disclose my locally circumscribed interactions with the environment, moods are expressions of my general faring in the world. The lack of a clear intentional structure in moods does not imply that moods are about nothing (mere atmosphere or raw feelings). On the contrary, moods have a more elaborate structure (what we have called a *covert* or *double intentionality*) that involves my relation to my own emotional experience.

Bad moods disclose a fundamental structure of human emotional experience that is often hidden in the more clear-cut intentional structure of other feelings, namely, that our feelings are both an expression of our relation to the world and of our relation to the persons that we are. Put differently, they inform us both about our relationship to the world (what we value and care about) and about our being the persons that we are. Whereas affects such as anger, love, fear, shame, embarrassment, and joy express my values and concerns, bad moods reveal the problematic—sometimes conflictual, other times opaque, or undefined, unstable or rapidly changing—the nature of those values and my fragile identity as a person who holds and acts upon such values.

The reason why the term 'bad mood' in the sentence 'I am in a bad mood' is so difficult to define (is it a kind of sadness or boredom, anguish, nervousness, emptiness, indifference, staleness or foulness?) is that it expresses an open problem in our relation to ourselves. It undermines my stability by opening access to underlying ambivalences; or to put it differently, a bad mood exposes my emotional fragility by opening up for doubt, hesitation, and questions about my being the person that I am. So, the nature of my values and concerns is often what is at stake in bad moods. My more immediate emotional reactions are complicated and changed by my bad mood in such a way that I am prompted to question why I feel and act the way I do. A bad mood makes me consider the possibility that perhaps there is something wrong with what I care about, with my values and concerns, and that there may be other ways of doing what I am actually doing. It emphasises the problematic relation between what I am and what I want to be in my relationship with the world; in short, by complicating my relation to the world, a bad mood awakens a sense of possibility in my being that may very well feel almost unbearable. Heidegger emphasises this in his treatment of a common kind of bad moods, profound boredom (*tiefe Langeweile*):

> Beings as a whole have become indifferent. Yet not only that, but simultaneously something else shows itself: there occurs the dawning of the possibilities that Dasein could have, but which lie fallow precisely in this 'it is boring for one', and as fallow leave us in the lurch. In any case, we see that in telling refusal there lies a reference to something else. This reference is the *telling announcement of possibilities lying fallow [das Ansagen der brachliegenden Möglichkeiten]*.
>
> (Heidegger 1995, p. 212; translation slightly modified)[18]

A significant part of the fragility of human personhood is due to this 'dawning of possibilities' in bad moods. Our values and concerns are constantly being challenged by the feelings of ambivalence constitutive of our personhood. And this ambivalence between being (*Sein*) and appearing-to-be (*Schein*) is not always clearly experienced as conscious possibilities, that is, as the thematic problem of being something and wanting to be something else. Often we only notice this ambivalence in the form of a diffuse type of emotional experience that we call a bad mood, which colours our relationship with the world and affects our emotional reactions in such a way that things and persons we value and care about may lose some of their interest or even be transformed into something that irritates and annoys us. Bad moods complicate my being the person that I am without providing any answers or solutions. They reveal, however, the complicated nature of human well-being and show that there is more to human values and concerns than is explained by either rational considerations (the structure of emotions) or biological needs (the feelings as vestigial traces of evolution). The feeling of totality experienced in bad moods discloses the precarious relationship between the necessity of being and the possibility of becoming that is at the centre of human personhood. Bad moods, in jeopardising my habitual way of being and being in the world, may disclose a possibility for me: the possibility to apprehend myself as different from what I supposed myself to be. Bad moods may disclose otherness as a possibility, thus kindling the dialectic of identity, the dialectic of selfhood and otherness, that is, the process whereby the person again and again tries to appropriate and live with that which affects him or her. Bad moods, being an open problem in my relation to myself, and opening up for the possibility of doubt, are a main source for self-understanding, and as such for being and becoming, for remaining identical and for changing.

This ends our philosophical exploration of how emotions may help us to better understand the fragile character of human personhood. It is not by chance that we end this part of the book with the phenomena of bad moods. We have attempted to show the informative value of these seemingly inarticulate phenomena based on the previous investigation of the intimate relation of emotions and personhood. It is precisely in the inarticulate character of moods, and bad ones in particular, that we may find what is of most informative value for understanding the human personhood, and why

---

[18] Giorgio Agamben has provided a penetrating analysis of this passage and of the general thought in Heidegger's lectures on the relation between profound boredom and metaphysics (Agamben 2004, pp. 57–70 [60–74]).

being a person is so difficult. Whereas other, more specific, emotional feelings may reveal important aspects of what we care about, our values, our character, our ideas, our dreams, what we fear, what we love, moods are able to, if attended to carefully, disclose what is just as important, namely, how we relate to what we care about, that is, *how* we care about *what* we care about. In this way, moods can help us articulate the complex, and highly fragile, dialectic of selfhood and otherness at the heart of human personhood.

In Part III, we are going to explore how this fragile dialectic of selfhood and otherness at the heart of human personhood plays an important role in human vulnerability to mental illness. We shall concentrate on the phenomenon of mood in the schizophrenic (Chapter 8) and in borderline types of existence (Chapter 9) and argue that our hermeneutical theory of emotions and personhood may substantiate and further develop the insights gained by the traditional accounts of the dialectical model in psychopathology.

In the human condition called 'schizophrenia' at work is not just a special type of bad mood; rather, it is a much more profound and drastic alteration of the biological root of our practical engagement with the world that affects the self involuntarily. We have the almost literal switching off of the force that makes us vitally connected to the world, the primordial energy that drives the person to affirm his or her being in the world. We will try to shed light on this *conative effort*, the basic drive through which factual reality is given to us, which is embodied in nature and experienced through feelings, inspired by Ricoeur's concept of *affirmation originaire*, as well as by Spinoza's concept of *conatus* and Scheler's *Lebensdrang*.

Borderline persons show quite a different emotional profile, characterised by the oscillations between dysphoric moods and angry affects which enact different (and almost antithetical) configurations of the life-world. Dysphoric mood exerts a centrifugal force which contributes to a painful experience of incoherence, emptiness, uncertainty, insignificance. At the same time, however, it also engenders a sense of vitality, although a disorganised, aimless, and explosive one. It is a kind of suicidal adrenaline and excesses of vitality. The protective layers of reflective moderation, the 'inauthentic' discourse of social roles and conventions, are ripped off. Borderline persons feel the strong pulse of naked frailty, of being driven by the force of a painfully extreme vulnerability. They bring themselves in the vicinity of death, but it is dying in a state of ecstasy. The centripetal force of anger restores the cohesion of the self, determines a clear-cut, unambiguous image of the other, and dissipates all doubts and sentiments of absurdity—but at the cost of feeling other persons as insulting, hostile, and persecutory.

We end the book with a consideration of how to understand this vulnerability in view of our previous explorations of the fragile character of personhood, and we propose an outline of how to deal with this vulnerability in terms of a therapy of care.

Part III

Vulnerable Minds

Chapter 8

Schizophrenia as a Disorder of Mood

The aim of this chapter is to portray the kinds of life-world in which persons with schizophrenia live, starting from an analysis of the early stages of this pathological condition and moving to a focus on full-blown schizophrenic pictures where psychotic features, like delusions and hallucinations, are not in the foreground. We will highlight what early and developed schizophrenia have in common, drawing on the phenomenological analysis of emotional experience developed in Part II. We will systematically describe this metamorphosis of the life-world in persons with schizophrenia. Lived space, time, body, the physiognomy of things and of other persons, will be used as the principal descriptors of this transformation. We will try to illuminate the emotional nucleus from which this transformation originates. The kind of mood which brings about this transformation is normally characterised as perplexity (*Ratlosigkeit*), trema, delusional mood (*Wahnstimmung*), loss of vital contact with reality, loss of natural self-evidence, crisis of vital drive (*Lebensdrang*)—or more in general, a disorder of common sense. Each of these concepts sheds light on some aspect of the schizophrenic mood as we understand it here. We will try to grasp its unifying, eidetic core. Persons with schizophrenia are unable to put their finger on what exactly is the content of their particular mood. The intentional structure that characterises much of human emotional experience is absent. The world appears as an undifferentiated totality on which the person has no grasp. In this profound change of the relationship with external reality, the basic structures of subjectivity, like demarcation, unity, continuity, agency, mineness, as well as of personal identity, are challenged. Once we have arrived at a phenomenological characterisation of this emotional core as the nucleus from which the schizophrenic life-worlds originate, we will describe the different types of schizophrenic worlds in the full-blown forms of this disorder. To do this, we shall make use of the hermeneutical account of selfhood and otherness developed in the first two parts of the book, in order to make sense of the dialectic between the schizophrenic person and this experiential, emotion-centred nucleus. The task of clinical phenomenology is to characterise the personal level of experience, whereas the task of clinical hermeneutics is to make sense of how a person understands his own experiences, that is, what they mean to him and how he copes with such experiences. We shall argue that the diversity in the manifestation of schizophrenic full-blown phenomena is a consequence of the ways persons with schizophrenia interpret the schizophrenic mood and the transformation of the life-world that stems from it. The different kinds of personal position-taking in front of the experience of this drastically encroaching type of mood engender the different forms of schizophrenic symptoms, syndromes, and courses. This is the core statement of the dialectical model in the psychopathology of schizophrenia.

The dialectical model draws attention to the active role that the person has in interacting with her basic disorder and in the shaping of full-blown syndromes. This chapter is meant as a contribution to this view on schizophrenia, and draws upon the works of illustrious advocates for this psychopathological approach such as Bleuler, Wyrsch, and de Clérambault. Since the French alienist Philippe Pinel can be considered the founding father of the dialectical model of mental disorders, we also briefly touch upon some of his pioneering ideas about the relationship between personhood and mental disorders as they are distilled through the reception of psychiatrist and historian Gladys Swain. The philosophical background, on the other hand, remains our reformulation of Ricoeur's hermeneutical theory of subjectivity in Part I and our further development of this theory in Part II. In line with the account presented in those two parts, we will be focusing on the interplay between selfhood and otherness, the voluntary and the involuntary, activity and passivity, involved in shaping our identity as persons. We become the person that we are through the confrontation, and sometimes the appropriation, of the otherness that constitutes our personhood and yet disturbs the person that we want to be or consider ourselves to be. The narratives that each person with schizophrenia makes of her emotional life and her awkward experiences are attempts to make sense of what is going on in her life, and establish who she is, who she was, and what she wants to be. As we have seen, a narrative structuring of our feelings is a crucial way for the person to live with her disturbing emotions, and to interpret and speak about the feelings involved in her engagement with the world, other people, and herself.

But before we start to explore the emotional core of schizophrenia and the metamorphoses of the schizophrenic life-world, we will briefly resume some basic aspects of the clinical phenomenology of schizophrenia.

The Clinical Phenomenology of Schizophrenia

Schizophrenia is a paradoxical condition in many respects. One of the paradoxes of schizophrenia becomes evident if we look at the century-long research on this mental illness, especially phenomenologically oriented psychopathological studies. Here we find the basic idea that the manifestations of schizophrenia can be most accurately characterised as being unique, exceptional, and unrepeated phenomena. At this extreme, there is the idea—epitomised by Binswanger's (1960) motto 'Each patient has her own schizophrenia'—that the forms of schizophrenia are as many as the single individuals affected by it. But at the same time there is the search for a common ground, the underlying unitary characteristic modification, or basic vulnerability, for the multifarious manifestations of this disorder. Many, if not all, clinical phenomenologists subscribe to this 'one root-many branches' understanding of the manifold of schizophrenic lived worlds.

The essential disorder, or core-property, underlying schizophrenic phenomena has been searched for in two main domains of the psychopathology of schizophrenia: its initial stages, and its sub-delusional or sub-apophanic manifestations.[1] The ideas of

Conrad (1958) and Blankenburg (1971, 2001) are among the most representative in these two domains. Blankenburg argued that for patients with long-lasting forms of schizophrenia, whose main characteristics were not delusions or hallucinations but more subtle forms of detachment from reality, the core-property was the loss of the natural evidence of commonsensical everyday experience. In particular, this loss is:

> [P]ronounced in the slow and insidious course of hebephrenic schizophrenia or schizophrenia simplex. This frequently begins with a barely noticeable decline in the ability 'to take things in their right light.' This subtle loss or atrophy precedes the emergence of other symptoms. What becomes striking for those around the patient is that there is a withering away of a sense of tact, a feeling for the proper thing to do in situations, a loss of awareness of the current fashion or what is 'in', and a general indifference toward what might be disturbing to others.
>
> (Blankenburg 2001, p. 305)

In our everyday experience, as healthy persons, we feel rooted in our world; the meanings of things we encounter in the world are 'naturally self-evident'; a sense of familiarity accompanies us even when we meet new objects and situations, because we are able to spontaneously refer them to our past experiences and classify them as something meaningful for us. This feeling of rootedness and *at-homeness* in the pre-reflective meanings of our life-world is absent in the experience of these patients. Before Conrad and Blankenburg, Minkowski (1997, pp. 35–68) had described a similar abnormal expressive-perceptual attunement between the subject and the outer world as 'loss of vital contact with reality [*perte de contact vital avec la réalité*]'. Vital contact with reality appears to be linked to 'irrational factors' in life, concerning the intimate dynamics of our existence. It provides a latent awareness of reality that makes us attune with it in a contextually relevant manner but without distorting our overall values, scopes, and identity. It is owing to this irrational feeling that a 'marvellous harmony between ourselves and reality' is instantiated, 'a harmony that allows us to follow the progress of the world while at the same time safeguarding the notion of our own life' (Minkowski 1927, p. 83; our translation).

The concepts employed by both Blankenburg and Minkowski address a pragmatic impairment where what is actually impaired is not just the possession of a reflective knowledge about the governing rules of human sociality. Rather, the fundamental disorder is understood to be in our seemingly immediate, pre-cognitive grip on social situations, a kind of pre-reflective indwelling in the world or attunement to it—a tacit skill that allows us to see things in the right perspective and shapes our behaviour in a contextually and inter-subjectively relevant manner.

---

[1] 'Sub-apophanic' is a term used by Blankenburg (1971) to qualify those forms of schizophrenia in which psychotic symptoms are not in the foreground. By 'psychotic symptoms' we mean those abnormal phenomena that psychopathology also names positive or productive: delusions, hallucinations, and experiences of passivity (e.g. experience of alien control). Sub-apophanic forms of schizophrenia are thus characterised by something that is missing, rather than by something that is exceeding normal experience. Blankenburg's sub-apophanic schizophrenia partly overlaps with Bleuler's 'schizophrenia simplex' and Minkowski's 'autisme pauvre'.

These patients' sense of disentanglement from a commonly shared reality is also the core of the beginning of schizophrenia, as in the '*das Trema*' (Conrad 1958) where behaviours, cognitions, and emotions are markedly inappropriate to the context. Trema is a paradoxical mixture of anguish, hope, despair, and suspicion whereby reality becomes suspended between meaninglessness and the imminent revelation of a new meaningfulness. It characterises the prodromal, pre-delusional stages of schizophrenia where everything feels strange, ominous, uncannily transformed; reality has undergone some inexplicable and ineffable change. The world is pervaded by a kind of latent meaningfulness: it has lost its habitual familiarity, and has not yet acquired a new kind of significance. Understanding reality and acting upon it has an 'achievement character' for patients. The condition of 'perennial beginners' of these patients is the *eidos* of what is considered by phenomenological psychopathology as the matrix of the early stages of schizophrenia as well as its sub-apophanic forms.

Clinical phenomenology is not merely a synonym for the cataloguing and study of mental symptoms; rather, it is at the heart of any attempt to understand individuals and types of human existence. We can understand the type of existence of persons with schizophrenia, but in order to do so we must grasp the profound and hard-to-describe disturbance characteristic of their way of experiencing the world, other people, and themselves. We must pay closer attention to those parts of the life-world of persons with schizophrenia that are usually neglected in diagnostic manuals because of their elusive qualities, like subtle disorders of selfhood and world-experience or of the enmeshed value-structure of such experiences, and acknowledge that insight into mental disorders does not come only from florid symptoms like delusions and hallucinations.

The profound and characteristic modification of schizophrenic existence or being in the world on the phenomenal level is a typical kind of depersonalisation and derealisation. Schizophrenic persons undergo a particular kind of depersonalisation: the living body becomes a functional body, a thing-like mechanism in which feelings, perceptions, and actions take place as if they happened in an outer space. They also endure a special kind of derealisation and desocialisation: the interpersonal scene becomes like a theatre stage, pervaded with a sense of unreality, on which the main actor is unaware of the plot, out of touch with the role he is acting and unable to make sense of the objects he encounters and of what the other people are doing. Persons with schizophrenia experience the world in ways profoundly different to the majority. Typical schizophrenic depersonalisation/derealisation can also be described as a disorder of common sense epitomised by the hendiadys 'deanimated body', i.e. the experience of feeling lifeless and distant from the source of vitality, and 'disembodied spirit', i.e. the sharp awareness of observing from without the behaviour of one's own self, or parts of it, that appears separated from the experience of existing (Stanghellini 2007b, 2008, 2011). This basic disturbance is sometimes experienced by persons with schizophrenia, at other times it may pass unexperienced, but it is manifest in the way they perceive themselves and the world, and in the way they act. In short, we can reconstruct the structures of their life-world by means of an analysis based on the principles of clinical phenomenology. This basic disturbance is a typical emotional state of which the features are described in clinical-phenomenological studies as delusional mood, perplexity, trema, and life-drive reduction. We will go into the details of these in the following sections of this chapter. For now, suffice it to say that this basic disturbance is *typical* of persons with schizophrenia, in that it contributes to a clear-cut differentiation, better than surface signs and symptoms, between schizophrenia and other forms of psychotic existence such as manic-depressive disorder, Asperger's syndrome, or severe borderline personality disorders.

In psychopathological syndromes, we can find 'surface' and 'profound' phenomena. Eugène Minkowski was perhaps the first to make this point clearly: a psychopathological syndrome is the 'expression of a profound and characteristic modification of the human personality in its entirety' (1933, p. 211). Grasping this 'profound and characteristic modification' is to make sense of the intimate transformation of subjectivity underlying the manifold of phenomena of a given psychopathological syndrome. This deep metamorphosis confers to abnormal psychic phenomena their structural unity, that is, the kernel of 'organized living unity' of abnormal psychic phenomena. Thus, phenomenological psychopathology brings to light 'deeper' phenomena compared to the 'surface symptoms' on which contemporary nosology is based. These deeper phenomena, as Kendler and Zachar have recently noticed, are much more informative than surface ones:

> Ironically, although the DSM institutionalizes the approach called *descriptive diagnosis*, it is actually remarkably thin, descriptively. The operationalized criteria for the various disorders have become the phenomenal universe of what is assessed. The actual phenomenal universe of any family of conditions is considerably larger.
>
> (Kendler and Zachar 2008, p. 373)

Clinical phenomenology assumes that the group of phenomena of a given (pathological) existence—or (pathological) *type* of existence—is a meaningful whole, i.e. a *structure*. These phenomena intimately interpenetrate each other, and thus the 'mental syndrome is for us not a simple association of symptoms' (Minkowski 1933, p. 211). In phenomenological psychopathology, a syndrome is conceived as a coherent way of being in the world. The scope of clinical phenomenology is neither just to unfold the phenomena that are present in the experiential field of a specific person, nor to select symptoms in view of a nosographical diagnosis. These are the tasks of descriptive and clinical psychopathologies respectively (Stanghellini 2009). Rather, it aims to recover the underlying characteristic modification that keeps the manifold of phenomena meaningfully interconnected in the life-world of the person. In order to make sense of the internal organisation of this life-world, the clinician must suspend any prejudice concerning the referential dimension of the patient's discourse. She must bracket any question concerning the truthfulness or correspondence to reality of the patient's self-reports, and additionally treat the patient's discourse as a wholly self-encoded entity which she attempts to decipher as a structured totality. The schizophrenic person's own experience remains the principal means of access into this type of existence (as with any kind of existence), in order to reproduce it faithfully and to make sense of it. This is the kind of *empiricism* that characterises the phenomenological approach to psychopathology.

As a pathology of the mind, schizophrenia involves many aspects: an experienced condition, a family of behaviours, feelings, and conscious contents, the peculiar significance of which emerges within a personal history, and a sociocultural context. From this perspective, a pathology is in itself a way of experiencing life. Such kind of pathology therefore only comes fully into view by means of what has been called 'personal level of explanation' (Hornsby 2000, p. 19). In fact, only at this explanatory level can the actual correlates of a psychopathological condition be understood in their *peculiar feel, meaning, and value* for the subjects affected by them (Stanghellini 2007b; Stanghellini and Ballerini 2008). This is the kind of *objectivity* that is needed in the study of mental pathology. Obviously, in line with our previous analysis and our appreciation of a general naturalistic framework, we do not deny the causal relevance of functional sub-personal mechanisms of our brain or the dynamic unconscious. We only reject a definition of mental disorders which is exclusively based on a sub-personal and consciousness-free level. There are, of course, objectively knowable regularities concerning lesions, functional alterations, or unconscious mechanisms which are causally relevant for our mental health, but the comprehension of the pathological significance of a mental state, that is, its meaning in a personal life, also requires a type of analysis which goes beyond the narrow and often reductively exclusive roads of a naturalistic approach (Gabbani and Stanghellini 2008).

The ambivalence constitutive of human personhood is, as suggested in Chapter 5, caused by the ambiguity of biological (anonymous) and psychological (subjective) factors at play in personal identity. A phenomenological approach to human experience brackets this ontological ambivalence by concentrating on the subjective structures of conscious experience. This does not mean, as we have argued throughout the book so far, that a phenomenological approach simply dismisses the biological level of explanation. On the contrary, the initial phenomenological account of subjective experience (first-person experience) provides a solid foundation upon which we can then try to explore the biological level of existence. Any hope of uncovering the biological factors that influence and shape the phenomena of our life-world hinges on an initial description of the experiential features of these phenomena. The biological dimension of schizophrenic existence is encapsulated in the first-person experience persons with schizophrenia have of the involuntary dimension of their existence, namely, the radical experience of otherness that affects the person and thus involuntarily disrupts the basic structures of the self. We have suggested a view of human subjectivity as characterised by non-coincidence: the self does not coincide with itself, and the person does not coincide with her world. Rather, being a self is a task of becoming a person through otherness. This otherness is manifested most clearly in three fundamentally involuntary aspects of human selfhood: my body, the world, and other people. Notwithstanding the fractured nature of the human self, we feel nonetheless engaged with the world, and connected (although not identical) with ourselves and with other persons (although distinct from them). These are basic bodily values in human existence. We consider practical engagement and connectedness as defining features of our biological (i.e. involuntary and anonymous) constitution as human persons.

These values, we argued, are sustained by a basic emotional texture that we tried to grasp using Ricoeur's analyses of the originating affirmation—the conative effort to assert oneself in and through the interaction with otherness. The affirmation of selfhood is troubled by the interaction with that which does not immediately and unproblematically coincide with the self, that is, the otherness that makes up the involuntary part of our existence as an individual self. It is owing to this conative effort, we suggested, that we feel vitally related to our self, other people, and the world.

The subjective experience that persons with schizophrenia have of their basic constitution is radically different from this. After experiencing a breakdown of the usual *Gestalten*—a sense of disconnectedness from themselves and disengagement from the human world—persons with schizophrenia *feel* a kind of existential orientation that is profoundly different from what the majority of persons feel. The analysis of the world(s) persons with schizophrenia live in documents deep experiential differences that reveal, or at least suggest, a radical difference in the ontological conception of these worlds. We have seen that such a phenomenological description also uncovers an unstable, often troubled and conflictual, sense of selfhood. Indeed, persons with schizophrenia may take markedly different personal stances in front of these experiential differences. This serves to reintroduce the ambiguity of the biological and subjective aspects of human identity, primarily by virtue of the ontological question of what kind of being the human self is, namely, a person whose thoughts, feelings, and behaviour are deeply influenced by both the biological and subjective aspects of its being. Persons with schizophrenia may either struggle against their experience of radical difference or uniqueness, or submit to it, or embrace it with enthusiasm.

The introduction of the notion of personhood, as the result of the dialectic between selfhood and otherness, marks the transition from phenomenology to hermeneutics. At the end of this chapter, we will deal with the transitional step from phenomenology to hermeneutics, and in the concluding Chapter 10 we shall argue that accurate understanding of mental illness, and thus a careful therapeutic endeavour, needs both steps. Phenomenology provides a nuanced and rigorous characterisation of the experience of otherness, while hermeneutics helps understand the way persons with schizophrenia try to make sense of it and cope with it.

A phenomenological approach, thus, argues for a third way, in between surface assessment as performed by descriptive and clinical psychopathologies and the kind of profundity explored by 'depth' psychologies. Clinical phenomenology has a concept of 'profundity' in its own right, different from, for instance, the psychodynamic and the cognitive 'unconscious'.

One example of such an approach is to examine schizophrenia as a disorder of common sense. Schizophrenia has long been considered as a disorder of common sense. There are two main interpretations of this: first, schizophrenia as a disorder of coenesthesia, i.e. an impairment of the functional symphony in which all the single sensations are synthesised—the *carrefour* of all senses which is the basis for self-consciousness, including the feeling of agency and of ownership. The second one focuses on the schizophrenic person's difficulty to share with others the axioms of everyday life and sees schizophrenia as an impairment of practical knowledge, i.e. a disorder of our ability to appreciate the rules of the human game. This latter interpretation is, in its own turn, twofold: on the one hand, a lack of *sensus communis* is emphasised, i.e. of the propositional knowledge consisting in a set of rules of inference shared by the members of a social group through which its members conceptualise objects, situations, and the behaviour of other people. On the other hand, the schizophrenic dyssociality is considered a disorder of pre-reflective attunement, i.e. of a kind of non-propositional skill consisting in the ability to perceive the existence of others as similar to one's own, to make emotional contact with them, and thus intuitively to access their mental life.

The philosophical kernel of this proposal is to assume that all these dimensions of common sense (coenesthesia, *sensus communis*, and attunement) and their disorders are related to each other (Stanghellini 2008). A disorder of common sense is related to the 'spatializing-temporalizing vortex' (Merleau-Ponty 1964, p. 297) which imbues all the things that a person with schizophrenia experiences, including himself. It is the existential buttress that engenders the peculiar life-world of a person with schizophrenia; in other words, the deep architecture of his disembodied and deanimated type of existence.

Delusional Mood, Perplexity, and the End-of-the-World Experience

Our analysis of the emotional states which characterise schizophrenia, and especially the early stages of schizophrenia, will begin with a series of essays of the Italian psychopathologist Bruno Callieri (1982, 1999)[2] who attempts to define and distinguish delusional mood, perplexity, and the so-called end-of-the-world experience.

Delusional mood (*Wahnstimmung*) is a constellation of feelings characterising the pre-delusional phase of schizophrenia, which has been extensively studied in phenomenological psychopathology since the beginning of the twentieth century (Berze and Gruhle 1929; Bleuler 1911; Jaspers 1997; Minkowski 1927). Advocates of 'dynamic' theories, as opposed to theories that assume cognitive changes to be the main factor in the genesis of delusions in schizophrenia (Berner 1991), consider delusional mood the matrix from which delusions in schizophrenic persons arise.

In delusional mood, thought contents, and especially the meanings of things and situations, are out of focus, dim, faint (Callieri 1982, p. 74). Its principal character is supposed to be 'the eclipse of meaning' (Callieri 1999, p. 5) or the crisis of the 'quality of familiarity' (*Bekanntheitsqualität*). The 'known quality' of experience, its familiarity, is considered to be the effect of a 'mnemotive' factor. The mnemotive factor (a neologism for the sedimentation of emotional memories) is the effect of various habits that generate an atmosphere of basic trust. The mnemotive factor is the emotional background that makes the world appear familiar. In the delusional mood the mnemotive factor is disrupted, and as a result the sedimentation of emotional memories becomes disturbed. The kind of life-world manifest in the delusional mood is abstract, atmospheric, non-substantial, fugacious, fluid resulting in the transformation of lived time into 'a succession of fragmented moments' (1999, p. 5), or mere presentification. Moreover, the lived space is characterised by the absence of coexistence and reciprocity.

Callieri argues that '[t]he borderline world of perplexity' is very near to that of delusional mood, and both perplexity and delusional mood *are* 'the doorway to delusion'

---

[2] The quotes from Callieri are all our own translations.

as well as 'the cipher of condicio humana' (p. 3). The perplexed schizophrenic is characterised by:

> [E]xtraneousness from the world and from himself, the premonition of something awkward, the tone of mystery: this is the opposite of the taken-for-granted, it is the uncanny [. . .] the object is there, suddenly extraneous or unknown, or charged with menacing and impending valences.
>
> (Callieri 1982, p. 83)

In the life-world of perplexity, space is anonymous, time momentary, the other person is never apperceived as a *socius*, and language is not univocally determined. Most characteristic of perplexity is the configuration of the lived body: 'perplexity is the paralysis of the body as the instrument for the discovery and the organization of experience' (p. 89).

A memorable passage in Callieri's writing on perplexity concerns the 'well known image of the schizophrenic who looks at his empty hands, again and again' (p. 82). This image, with which experienced clinicians are well acquainted, represents someone who does not know what to do with his hands, who does not know how to grasp things and put them to use. Understood this way, the image carries 'a profoundly anthropologic significance, beyond the significance of a mere symptom' (p. 82). The anthropological significance of this gesture is the profound relationship between manipulability and meaning, embodiment, and familiarity of the world.

Callieri follows the German psychopathologist Gustav E. Störring (1939) by defining perplexity as a disturbance of the lived body, and more exactly of motility. Störring, who was a pioneer in the study of perplexity, understood this phenomenon (*Ratlosigkeit*) as a disorder of movement.[3] Postures and motor disorders of perplexed patients, including gesturing and wide-eyed faces, were compared by Störring to the Darwinian descriptions of states of surprise and stupefaction. Perplexity is a mood wherein the patient's empathic capacity is declining, his activity is lessening, and he is gradually becoming detached from external reality. He undergoes a kind of withdrawal in which uncanny experiences dominate the whole perceptual world. Perplexity engenders feelings of strangeness and acute anxiety (Berrios 1996, p. 123), colouring the world with alien qualities that bewilder and unsettle the patient. Perplexity is not present in schizophrenia only, but in other psychopathological conditions it has a significantly different qualitative feel. In manic-depressive patients, for instance, the feature of strangeness is absent. Also the position-taking of the patient can be different, as in symptomatic psychoses like psycho-organic psychoses, where the patient is not passively overwhelmed by perplexity as in schizophrenia, but treats perplexity with some insight, or even dispassionately, as if she were a mere spectator.

A cognate phenomenon is the end-of-the-world experience. August Wetzel (1922), who was the first to describe this phenomenon (*Weltundergangserlebnis*), depicted it as a feeling of impending catastrophe, as if the world were about to end; an atmosphere of impending doom and sinister sense of dread, mixed up with feelings of happiness and redemption. Delusional mood and perplexity share a common ground with the

---

[3] We will develop this argument in a later section dedicated to schizophrenia as a disorder stemming from a crisis of embodiment and of the basic life-drive.

end-of-the-world experience, namely, 'the dissolution of the categorical structure [...] that is, of the category of symbolic contents of meaning. All experience departs from the normal meaning relationships with our world' (Callieri 1982, p. 47). But in the end-of-the-world experience a new meaning suddenly emerges. It is a 'new state of reality [...] in which all perceptions *acquire* a new abnormal content of meaning' (p. 73). The paradoxical mixture of feelings of doom and salvation 'tend to become rapidly attached to something concrete, in this case the end of the world, as a transition to something newer and grander' (Schmidt 1987, p. 109). Whereas delusional mood and perplexity are characterised by a latent meaning-awareness, or by an awareness of latent meanings, in the end-of-the-world experience a new meaning becomes *explicitly manifest*. Thus, the end-of-the-world experience is in itself a kind of delusion, whereas delusional mood and perplexity are pre-delusional states, since in these no fulfilment of meaning takes place.

The distinction between psychopathological states in which no precise intentional content is present (delusional mood and perplexity), and similar, yet distinct psychopathological states like the end-of-the-world experience, where a specific significance is attached to one's own experience, clearly overlaps with the classification of emotional experience into the two categories of moods and affects made in Part II of this book. Delusional mood and perplexity are mood states, whereas in the end-of-the-world experience the basic emotional experience takes the form of an affect and, as a consequence, the meanings that were latent in delusional mood and perplexity coagulate into an explicit and definite theme, namely, an eschatological one. The eschatological theme is typical for schizophrenia (Kepinski 1974) and consistent with the schizophrenic person's system of values and interests (Stanghellini and Ballerini 2007b). Wetzel, who believed that the precise content of the end-of-the-world experience was consistent with a preoccupation with cosmic events and grand relationships, was probably right to assume that it is exactly because schizophrenic persons are frequently attracted to philosophical questions and 'meaning connections' (*Bedeutungsbeziehungen*), involving mainly ontological, charismatic, and eschatological concerns, that the vague, fragmentary intimations that twinkle in delusional mood and perplexity can shape up into the full-blown delusional form that constitutes the end-of-the-world experience (Wetzel 1922, pp. 422–4).

The Unfathomed Flatness of Lived Space

In the following six sections, we will attempt to describe perplexity and delusional mood (hereafter we call these simply 'schizophrenic mood') in the light of the metamorphoses of the life-world that persons with schizophrenia live in, especially in early stages of this pathology.[4] Patients describe this situation as 'enigmatic', 'puzzling', 'weird',

---

[4] All sentences within single quotation marks, from this point onwards, if not otherwise specified, are taken from Giovanni Stanghellini's clinical conversations with patients with schizophrenia, especially acute schizophrenia in early stages of this disorder. We are also grateful to John Cutting who let us consult the files of his patients that he collected in many years of clinical work. Important additional sources of clinical material are his books and principally *Principles of Psychopathology* (1997), *Psychopathology and Modern Philosophy* (1999), *The Living, the Dead and the Never-Alive* (2002), and *A Critique of Psychopathology* (2011).

'confusing'. It is a 'conundrum', a 'cryptogram', a 'riddle', a 'chaos'. They use words like 'unreal', 'fake', 'strange' to describe the world, and 'meaningless' or 'inscrutable' to depict their lack of understanding. Some try to characterise their state of mind as 'stupefaction', 'disorientation', 'amazement', 'bewilderment', 'confusion', 'hesitancy', 'incertitude'; but also as 'alarm', 'trepidation', 'awe', 'dread'. They speak of 'suspense' and 'vacillation', 'tension' and 'oppression' to portray their bodily feelings, and of 'pressure' to describe the atmosphere surrounding them.

In our phenomenological characterisation of the life-world of persons who undergo the schizophrenic mood we will try to avoid all mentalistic, i.e. disembodied and disembedded, descriptions. Our aim is to secure the *sensorial dimension of the schizophrenic mood*, and to do so we will use six main descriptors, corresponding to the following six sections: lived space, temporality, embodiment, physiognomy of things and other persons, and understanding. Although the sixth existential may seem different from the first five, because of its cognitive nature, we will here treat understanding, or meaning-bestowing, as a special kind of embodied practice. Our point of departure in this section is Klaus Conrad's description (1958) of the initial stages of schizophrenia, and especially of the kind of mood he named *das Trema*. As Peter Berner writes:

> All hypotheses about delusional atmosphere presently discussed in German psychiatry refer in one way or another to Conrad's 'gestalt-psychological' analysis of *The Beginning Schizophrenia*. The state which we refer to as delusional atmosphere is, for Conrad, a modification of mood which, from its very beginning, is linked with the attribution of an abnormal—but as yet unidentified—significance of experiences.
>
> (Berner 1991, p. 88)

Conrad's theory is 'predominantly affective in nature' (Fuentenebro and Berrios 1995, p. 253). He assumes that an emotional state which he names 'trema' (a term that is usually translated as 'stage-fright') assumes the leading role in the development of schizophrenic delusions. In his staging of the schizophrenic metamorphosis of experience, Conrad accounts for trema as the initial stage of schizophrenia or its pre-psychotic state. The trema stage is followed by apophany in which the metamorphosis of the world and its objects bring about a revelation experience; apophany is followed by anastrophe (the stage in which the 'I' feels itself as the centre of the world), and finally the apocalyptic phase (where the 'cloud' of the essential properties that hide within all objects comes to a manifestation).

The constellation of feelings that characterises trema is a paradoxical blend of anguish, hope, despair, and suspicion. Conrad describes it as a highly complex mood: unbearable pressure, tension, inquietude and anguish, accompanied by inhibition and guilt feeling (as if one had committed a crime and castigation was impending) as well as suspicion, are all mixed up with euphoric and hopeful expectation. Some authors suggest that what is most characteristic of trema is:

> [A] fracturing and disintegration of previous meaning patterns, which is experienced by the patient as an uncanny sense of strangeness [. . .] a primary affect of mysterious significance [. . .] deeply perplexing and uncomfortable, promoting a powerful drive to understand what is being experienced.
>
> (Roberts 1992, p. 302)

This is only partly true. In fact, the disintegration of habitual meaning patterns of common sense understanding is just one aspect of trema, and probably not the most characteristic, at least not in Conrad's account. John Cutting suggests that what is essential to Conrad's description of the beginning schizophrenia is a dissolution of one's familiar way to experience space. In trema, there is a disruption fundamentally altering the patient's understanding of the world, and this deeply distorted understanding of the world 'could best be explained as a breakdown of Gestalt perception' (Cutting 1989, p. 430). Indeed, Conrad's descriptions of trema are an extraordinary resource to portray the transformation of space in the life-world of schizophrenic persons in the prodromal stages of this disorder.

In the trema stage, lived space undergoes a profound metamorphosis during which the neutrality of the background gets lost. In normal conditions, the things present in the surrounding space are distributed according to a hierarchical order: only a few of them are in the foreground, while all the others remain unperceived in the background. Lived space, which is organised around the vital necessities of the lived body, is first and foremost a structure of salience or relevance. Everything which remains in the background is neutral to perception. Trema, on the contrary, is characterised by:

> The failure to retain the space between perceived facts and what is behind them. The background loses its neutrality, and the patient becomes like an anxious child walking through a wood. Nothing is evident and natural anymore. The particularity of this suspicion is that the patient is not struck by what people do or say but what they don't do or say.
>
> (Berner 1991, p. 88)

Or as Conrad describes it himself:

> In the darkness, where one cannot see it, and behind the trees, 'it' lurks—one does not ask what it is that lurks there. It is something completely indeterminate, it is the lurking itself. The intermediate spaces [*Zwischenräume*] between the visible and what remains behind, all that is impalpable is no longer uncanny. The very background from which palpable things arise has lost its neutrality. What makes us tremble are not the trees and the bushes that we see, neither is it the whisper in the treetops nor the ululation of the owl that we hear, rather all that constitutes the background, all the surrounding space [*Umraum*] from which trees and bushes, whisper and ululation arise: they are precisely *the very obscurity and background*.
>
> (Conrad 1958, p. 41; our translation)

The fact that the background loses its neutrality does not merely imply that the background becomes threatening because of the obscurity that has become visible. Rather, as Conrad points out a paragraph later:

> All that remains out of the visual field of attention, all that is behind, all that is outside the theme of this moment, has become a barrier. It is not simply open, not a neutral possibility or something to which he can turn his attention at any moment. It has gained an aggressive character, has turned against him, has sealed itself from him or is lying in wait for him.
>
> (Conrad 1958, p. 42; our translation)

The experience of the background of lived space coming into the foreground also implies that lived space grows homogeneous, two-dimensional, losing its perspectival quality. It becomes—paradoxically—an *unfathomed flatness*. This uncanny experience of flatness is taken by the patient as an intimation and a warning: what appears is mere surface, facade, exteriority—a mask hiding a baffling profundity.

In Peter Handke's (1972) short novel *The Goalie's Anxiety at the Penalty Kick*, a story about the construction worker Joseph Bloch who one day for no apparent reason thinks that he is fired and then sets out on a bizarre and devastating journey, we find a detailed description of the increasing sense of unreality characterising the trema stage. In the space that Bloch moves through, everything looks staged. Most of the things that fill up this stage-like scenario look fake, as though they were 'carnival articles'; most of the events that take place look to him as 'reciprocal simulations'. Bloch's experience is similar to the feeling of a spectator walking through a movie in which he is the centre. The following describes how Bloch, towards the end of the novel, suddenly to his own surprise recovers his sense of 'reality':

> Everything had gone well for a while after that: the lip movements of the people he talked to coincided with what he heard them say; the houses were not just facades; heavy sacks of flour were being dragged from the loading ramp of the dairy into the storage room; when somebody shouted something far down the street, it sounded as though it actually came from down there. The people walking past on the sidewalk across the street did not appear to have been paid to walk past in the background; the man with the adhesive tape under his eye had a genuine scab; and the rain seemed to fall not just in the foreground of the picture but everywhere.
>
> (Handke 1972, p. 84 [81])

The 'miasma of unreality'—to use Louis Sass's eloquent expression—pervades Bloch's experience: disordered experience of time (lip movements are not synchronic with the sounds of the voice), of the materiality of things (houses looking like mere facades), of others (people looking like crowd artists), and of space (a two-dimensional rain falling) are all features of his world—a world depleted and fractured through the schizophrenic mood. Central to this pervasive feeling of fakeness and unreality is the breakdown of space *Gestalt*, as it is captured, for instance, in this uncannily beautiful episode in Bloch's odyssey:

> He sat down on the bed: just now that chair had been to his right, and now it was to his left. Was the picture reversed? He looked at it from left to right, then from right to left. He repeated the look from left to right; this look seemed to him like reading. He saw a 'wardrobe', 'then' 'a' 'wastebasket', 'then' 'a' 'drape'. (p. 124 [117])

The reader wonders what is going on here. The scene, so itemised in particulars disconnected from each other, has no unitary significance: it simply makes no sense. Handke's reconstruction of Bloch's subjective experience is full of these descriptions where a scene is fractured into snapshots apparently unrelated to each other. We may call this phenomenon the *itemisation of lived space*: the breakdown of space *Gestalt* reduces the ensemble of an episode to a list of itemised details or snapshots. Each snapshot hangs next to the other, as if they were a collection of photographs lacking a three-dimensional arrangement. Itemisation is part of what generates the feeling of unreality. The fragmentation of space *Gestalt* is furthermore accompanied by a feeling of disconnectedness from oneself. Last but not least, since meaningfulness requires the unification of details, the whole scene appears insignificant and motivationally flat.

Persons with schizophrenia usually lack words to illustrate this metamorphosis of lived space. Their descriptions span from a maximum of abstractness to more concrete characterisations of their lived experience. Many of them talk in a rather generic and abstract way of the surrounding world as 'fake' and 'unreal'. But when they are asked to explain why it looks so, only few of them are able to characterise these feelings of fakeness and unreality as related to *perceptual* changes: the world is like a 'stage', 'mere scenario', 'movie scenario', 'something like a theatre', 'as if everything was represented on a screen', 'people like cartoons', 'things like stage trappings', 'mere representations', 'buildings mere simulacra'. All these perceptual experiences refer to a flattening of perspective. Other persons report a different kind of strange and disturbing changes in perspective: 'distant things are moving towards me in a menacing way', 'flowers [in a picture in my office] are coming out of the picture'—alluding to an inversion of normal perspectivity. The 'world like a desert', 'like a lunar landscape', 'frozen like the Pole', 'no horizon', 'things out of reach' are also expressions of this mutation of spatiality in which the 'here' and the 'there' are not distinct. Finally, descriptions like 'a collection of photos', 'fragmented scene', 'things stand one next to the other', 'seeing things like reading one line after the other without grasping the whole meaning' also depict the itemisation of the life-world that takes place in the schizophrenic mood.

The experience of space that has lost its zones of neutrality, of appearance that has acquired the negative character of mere surface, also pervades the interpersonal space. Nothing anymore can be taken at face value, as in Case 54 described by Conrad:

> Be honest with me. Tell me what you want to tell me. I will do all you want, but at least tell me what is really going on, what is wanted from me. If you want money, you can have all my money. (1958, p. 43; our translation)

What matters, what is really important, is not what is actually said, rather what passes unsaid. Unfathomed flatness and suspicion are the two sides of the same coin.

To sum up: in trema, space-awareness instantly grows fuzzy, and lived space consequently undergoes a puzzling transformation. Worldly entities do not inhabit this perplexing space, rather they fill it. There is an itemisation of lived space which accompanies the flattening of perspectivity. As we will see in detail in the following sections, the transformation of lived space parallels profound changes in temporality and embodiment. Near and far, within reach and out of touch, are relative to one's bodily motility, including the body's capacities and limitations in its pursuit of its goals. As argued by Merleau-Ponty (1945, p. 116), the practical space is bodily space, oriented around the physical structure of the body and the projects undertaken to fulfil its needs. Dan Zahavi puts it eloquently:

> Our functioning body is present in such a fundamental and pervasive fashion that we only notice it explicitly when our smooth interaction with the world is disturbed, be it through voluntary reflections (philosophical or vain, e.g., when we gaze in a mirror), or in reflections forced upon us through limit-situations, such as sickness, pain, and fatigue. (1999, p. 101)

The appearance of space and worldly entities as three-dimensional is rooted in the integrity of kinaesthesia. Without the integrity of kinaesthesia and the practical reference to the body, space can grow unlimited, a 'boundless plain', the 'horizon infinite' (Sechehaye 1951, pp. 16–17 [22])—no more a lived space but a purely geometric space, an 'extension lacking magnitude and measurability' (Scheler 2008, p. 79 [73]).

The Objectualisation of Material Things

In this troubling flatness of lived space, things lose their incarnated givenness. There are two main features of this transformation of the physiognomy of worldly things: an objectualisation of things and their appearing as two-dimensional pictures or images. Things change into mere objects. An object is that which stands in front of oneself in its mere being-there, that is, without a practical relevance to one's bodily engagement with the world.[5] Whereas things inhabit the world and are part of it in virtue of their being related to an embodied self, and are thus experienced as 'something in order to', utensils relevant for one's bodily needs, objects are merely *within* the world, nearly like geometrical entities which fill up geometrical space. A person will see these objectified things as 'mere things' or 'a sum of real things' (Heidegger 2010, p. 68), and not as equipments for living. This quasi-ineffable and bewildering metamorphosis is sometimes encapsulated in sentences like 'in my room . . . [there are] mere objects', 'mere forms without meaning', 'like an abstract painting', 'just solid', 'just lines and angles', 'houses like cubes'. This alteration of the physiognomy of things (of their materiality) also involves the appearance of persons: 'trapezoid head', 'people truncated', '[people like] perpendicular lines'. Things and persons are 'stripped of their flesh', 'simply there', 'unrelated'. As with the transformation of lived space described above, there is a close relationship between the objectualisation of things and the metamorphosis of embodiment. To a disembodied self, the world becomes an indifferent collection of Cartesian extended objects equated with a 'constant presence-at-hand [*Vorhandenheit*], which mathematical knowledge is exceptionally well suited to grasp' (Heidegger 2010, p. 96; translation slightly modified). Devoid of their relation to one's own body, hence of their 'ready-to-hand' ('*zuhanden*'), one may perceive things as 'geometric cubes without meaning' (Sechehaye 1951, p. 24 [29]), 'cut off', 'detached from each other' (p. 34 [37]).

The other aspect of the metamorphosis of the materiality of things, the disconcerting ungraspable smoothness of things, is captured by Sechehaye's patient Renée: '[t]he trees and hedges were of *cardboard*, placed here and there, like stage accessories' (Sechehaye 1951, p. 17 [22]; emphasis added). It is difficult not to be disturbed by Renée's description of the uncanny world around her: '[o]bjects are *stage trappings* [*maquettes de décor*], placed here and there, geometric cubes without meaning' (p. 44

---

[5] In Latin '*ob-jectum*' literally means 'to be cast in the way of' or 'to oppose'. In German '*Gegenstand*' also means that which 'stands against' or 'opposes' (the senses). The Latin '*objectum*' as well as the German '*Gegenstand*' and the English 'object' all differ from a 'res', 'Ding', and 'thing' by being uncategorised, anonymous, and without any apparent relation to my practical engagement with the world. An object becomes a thing when it becomes part of this engagement.

[29]; emphasis added). Things lose their three-dimensional givenness and appear as two-dimensional images. Not only do things appear as geometric entities in a purely geometric space, we may also perceive the appearance of real things and persons as mere representations: 'flat', 'ungraspable', 'thin as plastic', 'immaterial', 'mere images on canvas', 'floating images', 'spooks', 'avatars', 'shells with nothing inside', 'no real houses but painted tents', 'as if they were painted on a window pane', 'stage trappings', 'a pasteboard house'.

As we have seen in Conrad's descriptions of trema, as lived space grows homogeneous and loses its perspectival quality, things may appear as mere surface, facade. As one's disembodied self cannot affect or grasp any object out there, the appearance of worldly entities is reduced to the realm of images—*Bildsphäre*, as Scheler calls it (2008, p. 82 [76]): 'I saw things, *smooth* as metal, so cut off, so detached from each other' (Sechehaye 1951, p. 34 [37]; emphasis added). Things appear unreal and fake because they are reduced to images, as 'advertisements for themselves'. Once again, Handke enters this feeling of disquieting unreality:

> On the square in front of the station he ran into a man he knew who told him he was going to the suburbs to referee a minor-league game. Bloch thought the idea was a joke and played along with it by saying that he might as well come too, as the linesman. When his friend opened the duffelbag and showed him the referee's uniform and a net bag full of lemons, Bloch saw even those things, in line with the initial idea, as some *kind of trick items* [*eine Art von Scherzartikel*].
>
> (Handke 1972, pp. 12–13 [16]; emphasis added)

Depending on the disappearance of the 'reality moment', the schizophrenic person experiences an ever more intuitively given fullness of free-floating qualities. The quality of a thing's colour becomes a quantified object in itself with no apparent relation to the original thing. In a similar manner, forms (roundness, triangularity, squareness) become independent objects. The schizophrenic mood enacts an essentialisation of the world, which transforms the world into an 'idea'. Spatial as well as temporal relations among bodies and objects, which are dynamically conditioned qualities intimately related to bodily movements, undergo a profound change. The world becomes perfectly adynamic.

The Disintegration of Temporality

In the trema stage, there is a profound metamorphosis of lived space and of the materiality of things that normally inhabit one's environment. The surrounding world loses its perspectival character, the perceptual distinction between foreground and background vanishes, things appear as smooth, ungraspable objects, or as mere geometric shapes. What about lived time? In the initial stages of schizophrenia, is there also a characteristic alteration of the experience of time? Are the metamorphoses of lived space and of lived time somehow related? What is the relation between these two and the schizophrenic mood, that is, the condition where the transformation is experienced in the perplexed person's lived body?

The following anecdote from Luciano Del Pistoia (2008, p. 155) will help us shed some light on the relationship between abnormal space perception and temporality:[6]

> The house of the Norman cousin is a white rustic cottage near the Seine. When we arrive, we can see its right side, part of the facade and of the roof. We say: 'Here it is!'. And we get off the car. Beyond the fence we see a lighthouse. It's new. Last summer it was not there. The Norman cousin explains that it's a scenario, a movie set. They just finished shooting a film, and tomorrow they will take everything away. Indeed, we only saw a part of the lighthouse, but we 'immediately *integrated it with memory and imagination*'. As a consequence, we took some wood frames for a three-dimensional lighthouse. Indeed, our perception works using hints that we immediately integrate with memory and imagination. Owing to this, the illusion of scenarios is possible. Also the cousin's cottage could have been a mere scenario: the side that it presented to us at our arrival did not guarantee all the rest. At the very moment we arrived, we just saw a part of it, a snapshot of the whole; nonetheless, we were sure that what we had in front of us was a real, three-dimensional building. As with the lighthouse scenario, we integrated our perspectival view of the cottage with memory and imagination. Here is another essential feature of perception: it is a form of understanding that implies *temporality*.

We always have partial views of things in the world. These partial views do not make things appear to us as mere two-dimensional figures or representations, because each snapshot of our perception is constantly integrated into a continuum which connects the present moment's 'adumbration' with *retention* (what we already know or have just perceived of that, or a similar, object) and *protention* (what we expect or imagine it to be). An intentional arc in consciousness bridges the retained past with the anticipated future, and thus makes possible our '*milieu humain*' (Merleau-Ponty 1945, p. 158). Consciousness at any moment stretches from the here-and-now backwards to the past and towards the future. This pre-reflective temporal structure of our experience was already noticed by Husserl in his lectures on the 'passive synthesis' of the various temporal modes. No experience and no coherence of consciousness is possible without the temporal constitution of 'primal presentational, retentional and protentional intentions [*urimpressionalen, retentionalen und protentionalen Intentionen*]' (Husserl 1966, p. 233). Dan Zahavi, however, in his careful analysis of this aspect of Husserl's thought, warns us that:

> Retention and protention should be distinguished from proper (thematic) *recollection* and *expectation* [. . .] Whereas the two latter performances are full-blown intentional experiences that presuppose the work of the retention and the protention, the protention and retention are dependent moments of any occurrent experience. They do not provide us with additional intentional objects, but with a consciousness of the temporal horizon of the present object.
>
> (Zahavi 2005, p. 58)

Hence, there are, at least, two levels in the temporal structure of our experience: both thematic articulations in the form of our active recollection and expectation, memory

---

[6] Our rendering of the anecdote borrowed from Del Pistoia is slightly modified to our purpose.

and imagination, and the implicit, pre-conceptual structuring in the form of the passive synthesis of retention and protention. The appropriate functioning of both these levels is necessary in order for us to perceive worldly things as three-dimensional (not as smooth and flat), and as meaningful entities as well.[7] We will return to the issue of meaningfulness later. For the moment, we will concentrate on the pre-conceptual relation between spatiality and temporality in perception.

A breakdown of the intentional arc that connects retention and protention with the present moment in perception results in a two-dimensional vision of the world. Obviously, when such a two-dimensional vision takes place, things appear as unreal, counterfeit, fake (the cousin's cottage is a mere theatrical scenario, and her face is just a mask). This is exactly what we observe in the course of the transformation of lived space and of the materiality of worldly entities as it takes place in the schizophrenic mood, and especially during the initial stages of schizophrenia.

Perceiving the world three-dimensionally presupposes an integration of perspectives across time. And this integration of perspectives presupposes the integrity of the lived body and motility. Perplexity, as a disorder of motility, entails the breakdown of this integration of perspectives. As a consequence, the world appears two-dimensional, flat, and worldly things smooth and ungraspable.

As we have seen in the section on lived space, what is most characteristic in the schizophrenic mood is a breakdown in space *Gestalt* resulting in an itemisation of the surrounding world: the whole scene loses its character of a meaningful ensemble, and we observe the appearance of fragmented details unrelated to each other and to ourselves. Parallel to this, there is a breakdown of time *Gestalt*. As with the itemisation of space, things will appear as mere objects (unrelated to one's body) and events merely as a collection of snapshots or representations (quasi-indiscernible from mental images). With the fracturing of the time-flow, we observe an itemisation of now-moments in consciousness.

Is there in the schizophrenic mood, besides the collapse of perspective in perception, making things appear flat and two-dimensional, a breakdown of the intentional unification of consciousness through time as well? Or put differently, a collapse of the implicit function that connects and integrates the present with retention and protention?

In a series of essays, the Japanese psychopathologist Bin Kimura (1992) attempts to define the kind of temporalisation that characterises persons with schizophrenia. The gist of his thesis is the following: the autonomisation of the anticipating moment, disconnected from its normal interrelation with the retentional one, is the essential character of schizophrenic temporality. He calls this existential mode typical for persons

---

[7] As discussed in Chapter 1, when we perceive an object we are always bound to a certain perspective. The object is always seen from a limited perspective, from the front, the side, or the back; we are never capable of seeing the object in its totality. However, we are immediately aware of our confined vision of the object as a result of our pre-reflective awareness of other possible perspectives on the object. This awareness somehow transcends our own perspective and reveals an understanding of the totality of perspectives on the object. This totality is the meaning of the perceived object. The capacity to form an idea of totality from a fragmentary perception is what Ricoeur calls our 'power to express a meaning' or 'intention to signify' (1987, p. 26 [44]).

with schizophrenia *ante festum* temporality. Although Kimura's analyses are not about the early stages of schizophrenia, his in-depth investigation of the changes of temporality in schizophrenic existence is nonetheless pertinent to the issue at hand. Quoting von Weizsaecker (1940), Kimura affirms that for persons with schizophrenia *to be a self* is not a safe, taken-for-granted possession, rather an 'endless achievement'. This statement comes very close to the ideas of the Italian philosopher and psychopathologist Ernesto De Martino (1997, pp. 96–105), who argued that in the schizophrenic world 'being present' or 'being there' is a reality to-be-built (*realtà condenda*). The achievement character of 'to be' for persons with schizophrenia makes them live in the temporal mode of the *gerundive* ('condenda' in Latin means 'due to be built'). Being-there is always in the making, it is an endless task. A schizophrenic person, like the sceptical or transcendental philosopher, is a perennial beginner. Like such traditional philosophers (and contrary to some of their pragmatic or science-inflated contemporary heirs), the schizophrenic lacks the ground for a stable and untroubled being, that is, a proportionate articulation between being rooted in the past and projected into the future. The ground for a secure being is for all of us our rootedness in our own past, our acquaintance with ourselves, and our familiarity with our own environment.

In Part I, we saw how Ricoeur, in his analysis of personal identity, addressed this part of our personal identity as 'sameness' (the *idem* and thing-like, involuntary, side of identity) as opposed to 'selfhood' (the *ipse* and personal, voluntary, side of identity). *Idem* identity is apparently absent, or at least heavily troubled, in persons with schizophrenia, and it is also voluntarily rejected by them. Kimura insists on the schizophrenic person's *choice to reject idem* identity as a menace to his or her own autonomy. Ricoeur, like many philosophers before and after him, warns us of the intriguing allure of habit (a well-known and weighty part of our *idem* identity). In fact, it is 'as if habit were a weak point offered to what is perhaps the most perfidious of passions, the passion to become a thing again [*la passion de redevenir chose*]' (Ricoeur 1966, p. 297 [280]). In the schizophrenic mood, this human tendency to fall into soothing habits is turned upside down. Where ossified habits threaten our identity as persons because they render us numb to the possibility of change, in ourselves as well in other people, a person with schizophrenia runs the risk of losing a sense of the sustaining (e.g. past achievements, persons with whom we have a common past) and binding (e.g. promises made, things said and done) factors involved in being a person. Kimura refers the case of a young schizophrenic who eloquently affirms:

> I cannot avoid feeling 'heteronomic'. Initially, I don't feel so forced, but little by little the feeling that I want to decide myself, autonomously, comes across me, and I want to do what I desire in an independent way.
>
> (Kimura 1992, p. 74; our translation)

Kimura explains further that when this person:

> [D]ecides to refuse being 'heteronomic' in order to become 'autonomous', he thinks he must leave behind, first and foremost, the 'present that has been' (*gewesene Gegenwart*) and search for his possibility of being in the future.
>
> (Kimura 1992, p. 75; our translation)

In persons with schizophrenia, we find a persistent refusal of the involuntary side of identity in terms of 'having' (been, said, or done) and the frantic affirming of the voluntary, autonomous aspect of identity in terms of 'being' (who we are or want to be). Schizophrenic existence is pervaded by the concern for being (or becoming who we want to be), whereas our own more prosaic, everyday existence is concerned with a more proportionate balance between having (been, said, or done) and being. In English, French, and German—Kimura remarks—the verbs that express possession, such as the verb 'to have', are also the auxiliary verbs for the past tense like 'have done'. Furthermore, they express a duty, like 'I have to do', 'I have promised', 'I have said'. 'To have' has thus three meanings: *possession*, *past*, and *duty*. In persons with schizophrenia these three dimensions of 'having' are firmly rejected for the sake of their strong heteronomic counterpart.

In non-schizophrenic forms of psychoses (e.g. melancholia), a crisis 'develops around the phenomenon of "having" in the three meanings of possession, past and duty; in schizophrenia it is a crisis concerning the question of "being"' (Kimura 1992, p. 78). One could say that persons with schizophrenia have ontological (questions about the nature and possibility of being) rather than ontical (questions about the factive and actual being) concerns: people are from another world, things are fake, everything looks unreal, the world is mere appearance. In other words, persons with schizophrenia are perplexed about the *status of reality* of those events which for us are 'facts' (Stanghellini 2008).

Kimura's analyses mainly highlight this pole of the schizophrenic person's mode of temporalisation: the schizophrenic mode of existence is *ante festum*. It is an existence that is disarticulated from all kinds of regimented identity (in terms of sameness and retention, that is, the sediment of one's past and the bonds of possession and duty); therefore it is disproportionately projected into identity as something that is not yet there but is about to happen: a revelation is on the verge to happen, the world is on the verge of ending, a new world is coming, one's own life is on the point of undergoing a radical change. The schizophrenic mood can be characterised as the dawn of a new reality, an eternally pregnant now in which what is most important is not present, what is really relevant is not already there, but is forever about to happen. Time in the schizophrenic mood is 'a state of suspense', 'pregnant now', 'being is hanging', 'something imminent', 'something . . . I didn't know what . . . was going to happen . . . between inspiration and expiration'. Thus, the schizophrenic mood is the dawn of a new reality. It is, however, also the 'dusk of reality' (Ey 1959), or, we could say, the *dawn of unreality*: 'A mineral, lunar country, cold as the wastes of the North Pole. In this stretching emptiness, all is unchangeable, immobile, congealed, crystallized' (Sechehaye 1951, p. 24 [29]).

Schizophrenic persons often describe their sense of temporal reality as: 'things to a standstill', 'immobility, but not calm', 'time going back to the same moment over and over', 'people like statues', 'frozen moment', 'out of time', 'marmoreal', 'unreal stillness'. We can thus see that time in the schizophrenic mood is fragmented, there is a breakdown in time *Gestalt*, and an itemisation of now-moments. The mere succession of conscious moments as such cannot establish the experience of continuity. The basic continuity of consciousness requires a pre-conceptual 'synthesis'. What we experience is, first and foremost, not a sequence of discrete snapshots, but rather a dynamic, integrated *Gestalt*.

If this temporal continuity collapses, each 'moment' in a person's stream of consciousness will be experienced as detached from the previous one and from the following, as well as extraneous to one's sense of selfhood. Each 'now' will be sensed as a free-floating fragment, going adrift. The continuity and temporal unity of conscious life—as explained by Fuchs (2010)—is thus connected or even synonymous with the *coherence of a basic sense of self*. If a breakdown in passive synthesis takes place, the 'nows' in consciousness will appear to the experiencing person as objects in an external space, rather than as parts of one's own stream of consciousness. This object-like appearance of now-moments in consciousness parallels the mineralisation of the life-world, which will be pervaded by unreal stillness and filled up by marmoreal objects.

In this dusk-dawn of reality (and of unreality), time is suspended. It is a paradoxical mixture of immobility and protention, a knot of stillness and frenzy, ecstatic astonishment, the zero hour between hesitancy and solution, calm and tension, emptiness and pressure, rest and unrest, stop and incipient movement. It is the time before the penalty kick, in which space and time *Gestalten* are in jeopardy

The Source of Vitality

As we have seen in the previous sections, the schizophrenic mood entails profound transformations of lived space and time and of the physiognomy of things. In this section we will describe the metamorphosis of embodiment. In the schizophrenic mood, the common sense framework in which body/world/action/meaning are usually set breaks down. The delusional world entailed by this breakdown instantiates a new enactment with its own specific (idiosyncratic) meanings.

It is important to note that what we are dealing with here is not simply a special type of 'bad mood', which, as we shall see in the next chapter, is the case in the borderline condition. Rather, it is a much more profound and drastic alteration of the possibility to be affected. Nevertheless, our analysis of bad moods in the previous chapter may help us to understand what is at stake in the schizophrenic mood. We arrived at the conclusion that bad moods are significant and possess an informative value for our understanding of human personhood, because they somehow inhibit and complicate our more intentional feelings, involved in affects such as anger, joy, pride, fear, desire, and jealousy. We argued that this complication of the emotional dimension of our intentional relation to the world, other people, and ourselves, reveals problems in the normative texture of our existence, and thus challenges our understanding of the person that we are. This inhibition or complication of our affective relation with the environment and ourselves is much more radical and dramatic in the schizophrenic mood. Here we have the almost literal switching off of a dispositive of our belonging to a world, our 'primordial *in esse*' (Ricoeur 1987, p. 103 [119]). This primordial *in esse* (in being), or basic sense of belonging to the world, is embodied in nature and experienced through feelings. Ricoeur's hermeneutical theory helps us understand the human person as an embodied biological self, provided with basic drives and an array of emotions. Our body is the *flesh* of our existence and the emotional anvil of our values. It is through the body that we first feel a motivation to do anything. Feelings of pleasure and pain are rooted in the very functioning of our body and account for a basic sense of positive and negative values, but the role of the body is not limited to such basic organic values:

> [B]odily existence reveals other values than those of pleasure and pain. These values are often hidden under the equivocal names of pleasure and pain which thereby lose their precise sense of organic satisfaction (related to an organic privation) and of physical pain (related to an aggression against the body). Pleasure and especially the act of pleasing oneself [*l'acte de se plaire*] become coextensive with value on the organic level and designate the entire field of affective valuation on this level. Further, emotion [*l'émotion*] gives to all valuation pertaining to other levels of value an organic echo [*un retentissement organique*], so that all sensibility can gradually adopt, by analogy or by resonance, the language of pleasure and pain [. . .] The agreeable and the disagreeable similarly cover an extremely ill-defined area of meaning [*signification*]: what suits me is, in a broad sense, that which awakens and touches positive affectivity [*l'affectivité positive*]. Thus to suit and to please becomes indiscernible, and pleasure in an organic sense is the lower stratum of the agreeable.
>
> (Ricoeur 1966, pp. 110–11 [106])

These bodily rooted values inform and orient our 'effort to exist' (1987, p. 137 [154]), our *originating affirmation*. The originating affirmation is the source of all vitality, the primitive and original will to live inherent in being an embodied self. In all its actions, the human self is characterised by this primitive will to exist which is 'the primitive act of consciousness' (Ricoeur 2007a, p. 218 [66]). The affirmation is primitive in the sense that it is an intrinsic part of embodied selfhood, and not a product of its activity. It is that which enables the self to act in the first place, and as such it has to be considered as an inescapable feature of human subjectivity. It is a dynamic force that drives the self to engage itself with the world and other people. The originating affirmation makes us strive to continue our existence with and through that which is not ourselves, i.e. otherness. It is the necessary precondition for *inter-esse* (being among that which is not ourselves).

As we saw in Chapter 7, Ricoeur's originating affirmation is somewhat akin to, and most probably inspired by, Spinoza's concept of *conatus*. It is, however, also rather similar to Scheler's *Lebensdrang* (life-drive): the basic drive through which factual reality is given and happens to us. Scheler's analysis of *Lebensdrang* is important because it enables us to see how our pre-reflective experience of reality and our ensuing reflective interpretation of this experience can be affected by a disturbance of the biological root of our engagement with the world. His analysis of the life-drive as the force that makes us vitally connected to the world complements Ricoeur's treatment of the originating affirmation, which we developed in Part I of this book. Also, Scheler's account of life-drive reduction, which he obtained during his quasi-mystical 'experiments' of suspension or neutralisation of the life-drive, resembles very closely the self-descriptions of the life-world that persons with schizophrenia live in (Stanghellini 2010),[8] and integrates the clinical-phenomenological descriptions of disconnectedness from reality provided (among others) by Minkowski and Blankenburg.

Scheler's analysis emphasises the role that this primordial emotional state plays in the embodied entanglement of self and world. Without this affective prerequisite no felt

---

[8] For the relevance of Scheler's account to psychopathology, see Cutting (2009a, 2009b).

readiness to act, no motivation to move is possible. The life-drive is what makes us feel vitally related to and practically engaged in the world, and thus enables us to see things in the world as affordances for our survival; for instance, a cave is a shelter, a stone is a weapon, a goat is food. Owing to the life-drive, a person experiences things in the world as provided with what we could call 'existentially-relative handles' by means of which we can manage them and put them to use. To say that things have handles means, first and foremost, that a person's vital-drive-based attention is directed to those features of the surrounding things that have a vital relevance to the living organism.

A person's body, animated by the life-drive, is the source of an appropriate and functional distance between the person and her world, which favours optimal perceptual distance, including figure-ground differentiation and the performance of relevant actions. The breakdown or serious impairment of the life-drive entails profound disorders of the self as an embodied self, of the self-world relation, and of the vital functions of conscious experience, in particular the implicit temporality, which—as we have seen above—is necessary for the basic continuity of consciousness and its directedness.

Most of the vital dimensions of human existence (pre-reflective self-awareness, object-awareness, meaning-bestowing, and attunement) undergo deep transformation if the life-drive becomes seriously impaired. These profound metamorphoses have their origin in the person's embodied emotional life. Scheler (2008, pp. 77–128 [72–117]) described in great detail the outcome of the *life-drive reduction*, i.e. the switching off of the 'urgency of life'—the root of all drives, needs, and vital attention—and new kinds of givenness are revealed in the life-drive reduction. The reduction of life-drive drastically affects the constitution of our life-world on several levels, the most important of which are our pre-reflective intuition (*Anschauung*) and the meaning (*Bedeutung*) that we reflectively derive from or bestow on this intuition. Scheler explains that these profound changes stem from the same vital root: '[t]he vital drive structure [*vitale Triebstruktur*] and its accompanying interest perspective is the selfsame, identical root of both the perspective inherent in intuition and meaning – and it is this [root] which is set out of function and out of course in the reduction' (2008, p. 85 [79]; translation modified). When the working of our vitality is impaired, our embodied relationship with the world and ourselves changes accordingly.

One of the results of this reduction of life-drive is a drastic transformation in how a person experiences her own body, which we also find in schizophrenic persons:

> The body [*Leib*] is switched off, and by a certain technique it then becomes increasingly objectified [*vergegenständlicht*], and accordingly so is all vitally animated being and becoming. This process is completely different from a merely logical setting aside of these matters. It has much more to do with excluding all influence of the body and of the vitally determined 'forms' of perception from the purely spiritual action (like the Indian technique of yoga). The end-point and ideal aim of this technique is the steady being and consciousness, so that 'I' am 'collected' and 'centralized' in the spiritual person [*in der geistigen Person*]. (2008, p. 112 [102]; translation modified)

In general, persons with schizophrenia experience throughout the course of their illness that the body loses what, in Chapter 3, we have described as its ambivalent status of being both an anonymous, physical object (a body as an object among other objects) and an integral part of our subjective experience (a personal body or lived body). The vital or 'animal' part of our embodiment becomes objectified: 'I am provided with an anal expeller', 'arms are just prostheses', 'hands disjointed from arms', '[I am] a bionic creature', 'a second body growing inside me', 'eyes are videocameras', 'instincts directed by electrodes'. As the body transforms into a deanimated object, the self loses its otherwise inescapable connection to the body, it becomes a purely spiritual person (*eine geistige Person*), that is, a person with only mental, intellectual dimensions who considers herself as *having* (not *being*) a body, possessing it, and accordingly having complete voluntary control over this animal part of her identity: 'like a cybernaut in my body', 'push button to activate brain', 'supervisor of my animal body', 'all these hairs . . . animal body', '[in my body] like an emperor in his pyramid', 'supernatural powers'. This Cartesian form of existence, in which embodied self-awareness is substituted by incorporeal *noetic* self-awareness (Stanghellini 2008), is a basic feature of schizophrenia throughout the course of this illness.

By means of a phenomenologically based qualitative method of inquiry, we (Stanghellini et al. 2012) have recognised two main properties of abnormal bodily experiences in early schizophrenia: dynamisation of bodily boundaries and construction, and morbid objectivisation/devitalisation.

The characterising feature of the first is a perplexing metamorphosis in one's corporeal borders and Gestalt. Patients complain about their body *being violated* by entities or forces coming from without their own bodily boundaries, e.g. about the intrusion or incorporation of extrapersonal things, forces, and events. Violation typically entails dynamism in the sense of experiencing something moving into oneself, not merely the static presence in oneself of something that should occupy a position external to the self. It also involves experiencing one's body as a thing-like entity, relating to the external world in a mechanical way. Persons with first-episode schizophrenia also experience a *dynamisation of bodily construction*. This is an experience of body disintegration which involves a shifting around of the usual spatial relationships between body parts, or a dynamic distortion of body Gestalt, i.e. of one's body as a unitary and integrated structure. Parts of the body are felt as moving away from their usual position. As in the experience of violation, one's body is felt as a spatialised thing-like entity functioning in a quasi-mechanical way. A third aspect of bodily dynamisation is the experience of *externalisation*, that is, feeling one's body or parts of it projected beyond one's ego boundaries into the outer space. As is the case with violation and distortion of body construction, externalisation is also not a static experience but it implies movement. Ego and corporeal boundaries, so to say, are violated from within by parts of the body that are felt as expelled into the outer space. In this type of experience as well, parts of one's body are experienced as thing-like entities in an outer space.

The characterising feature of the second category of anomalous bodily experiences is an uncanny *morbid objectivisation and devitalisation* of the body or its parts. In morbid objectivisation, parts of one's body that are usually silently and implicitly present and at work become explicitly experienced. Typically, morbid objectivisation goes together with the experience of devitalisation in the sense that parts of one's body are felt as devoid of life and/or substituted by some kind of mechanism. In general, the body or its parts are experienced as mere things, thing-like or corpse-like entities, rather than as living flesh. Parts of oneself are spatialised—experienced as if they were disintegrated from the living totality of one's body.

As remarked earlier, a striking image of perplexity is the gesture of the schizophrenic who looks again and again at his empty hands. The gesture signals the loss of the profound relationship between embodiment, manipulability, meaningfulness, and vital contact with the world. In perplexity states, schizophrenic persons experience the paralysis of their lived body in its capacity of being the pre-reflective medium through which one feels implicitly connected and attuned to the world. In acute phases of this illness, and especially in early stages, this immediate contact between a person's body and the world is lost. The fluid, reciprocal body/world interaction and interweaving is substituted by discontinuous, saccadic movements taking place in the no-body's land separating a deanimated body from a devitalised world: 'My body here, the world out there', 'body congealed standing in front of things out of touch', 'a kind of psychic paralysis'.

The intimate, pre-reflective awareness of my perceptions, actions, and thinking as my own is replaced by a second-order noetic awareness of something which perceives that I am perceiving, acting or thinking: 'The spectator of my body split from the world', 'One part of the brain talks to the other', 'the world is an illusion because it is seen *through* a brain'. Persons with schizophrenia often describe their condition as that of a *deanimated body* ('heart no more there', 'brain into ashes', 'nerves like strings pulling me up', 'people sucking blood from me'), or a *disembodied mind* ('like fog on quagmire', 'just ethereal, no body'). On the face of it, such self-descriptions may seem metaphorical, but—as Ricoeur noticed above—they contain a bodily 'organic echo' which reveals how these persons are actually feeling and experiencing. On the one hand, one's existence feels like that of a *cyborg* or a lifeless, purely mechanical body ('[I felt] like a puppet', 'No emotions, just impulses', '[the body] a mechanical engine', 'I didn't move it [the body] . . . it moved me'). On the other, one may feel like a *scanner* or disincarnated mind which lives as a mere spectator of one's own perceptions, actions, and thoughts ('[world] like a movie on the screen', 'mere representation of reality . . . [I am] not involved in it'). The self breaks down into an experiencing I-subject contemplating an experienced I-object while the latter is acting or perceiving ('[my] eyes watching TV', '[my] hand masturbating'). Acts of perception themselves are no more experienced from within, but *from without*, becoming objects of noetic awareness ('it was as if I could see my eyes watching the scene', 'I was like a receptor of stimuli'). The phenomenality of this experience is no longer implicitly embedded in itself, that is, characterised by a pre-reflective self-awareness. In other words, the act of experiencing turns out to be an explicitly intelligible object.

We have seen that there exists an intimate relationship between the transformation of lived space and temporality. Similarly, we can now ask if there is a relationship between anomalies in temporality and embodiment: how are temporality and embodiment related to each other in constituting a coherent sense of self? How can we connect the anomalies of embodiment with those of temporality analysed in the previous section?

To answer these questions, we make use of an example, borrowed from Fuchs (2010) in a slightly modified version:

> If we look at a child playing with his toys, lost in his game, we may assume that he does not experience the passing of time. He is completely immersed in his game and absorbed and directed towards his immediate goals. Time is inherent in his bodily commitment and engagement in this situation, with its valences and tasks. Lived time is the movement of life itself, implicit in the child's experience. Neither past nor future stands out as such from his pre-reflective existence. This implicit mode of temporality always remains the undercurrent of his experience. He is immersed entirely in his activity, as in flow experiences when the sense of time is lost in unimpeded, fluid performance. Time flows implicitly, his actions are silently grounded in his bodily awareness, in the sense that he is implicitly self-aware that his actions are his own.

As Fuchs goes on to explain, the implicit mode of temporality requires two key conditions on a transcendental level which can be designated *synthesis* and *conativity* of inner time consciousness: 'Together they form the intentional arc of attention, perception and action that bridges succeeding moments of consciousness by an intentional and affective directedness. At the same time, these are the prerequisites for a basic sense of a coherent self that is essentially temporal' (2010).

As we have seen in this and in the preceding sections, both synthesis and conativity are jeopardised in the schizophrenic mood. Synthesis, the prerequisite for the appearance of lived space and time as integrated and consequently meaningful *Gestalten*, is also the necessary condition for the continuity and temporal unity of conscious life, and as such it is synonymous with the *coherence of a basic sense of self*.

Conativity, the prerequisite for body-world relatedness or *inter-esse*, is also—as explicated throughout this section—the necessary condition for being and feeling an *embodied self*, for the existence of the body as an ambivalent part of our identity as persons, both as a physical object (the body as an object among other objects) and as an integral part of our subjective experience (a personal body capable of intentional position-taking).

Disattunement and Disincarnation

One characteristic feature of the feelings that persons with acute schizophrenia have of their social world is a paradoxical mixture of painful distance and fearful proximity to others.

The interpersonal space suffers a deep metamorphosis: the human world appears distant, there is a shutdown of the person's sense of cohesion with other human beings, and harrowing feelings of isolation: 'I feel disconnected', 'A wall of void isolated me from everybody', 'It is as if there were two worlds'. There is a lack of intuitive grip on social situations ('I simply cannot grasp what the others do') or *hypo-attunement* (Stanghellini and Ballerini 2011, p. 187), i.e. a feeling of detachment from other persons and social situations; an impaired ability to directly contact and intuitively decipher the behaviour of others and social situations. This feeling of being extraneous to the social world and of lacking an implicit, spontaneous, and emotional basis for sociality is sometimes accompanied by a numinous feeling of unity with others ('I felt the holy spirit of other persons'). Even though this phenomenon is rather uncommon, it nonetheless indicates that persons may not only suffer from feeling disconnected from other persons, but also (and quite paradoxically) for being unable to distance themselves from them. Others are not only experienced as 'belonging to another world', but also as oppressive ('people, folks oppress me'), their presence provoking distressful feelings ('being with people provokes in me an emotional crisis . . . an internal block, a block of feelings') and uncanny bodily sensations ('when I go out and meet other persons I am taken by obscurity. It is something in my head, not a pain, I feel suffocated, my mind is repressed, like a psychic pain'). *Invasiveness* in the sense of feeling oppressed and invaded by the others from without, as well as *coenesthopathic* or *emotional flooding* such as feeling oppressed and submerged from within by one's feelings and bodily sensations evoked by interpersonal contacts ('when people get too close to me I feel nervous') are common features of acute schizophrenia.

The sense that the other persons are living beings like oneself is also wrecked. The others (like oneself) may appear as deanimated bodies or mechanical entities: 'cold, implacable, inhuman, by dint of being without life' (Sechehaye 1951, p. 29 [33]), 'people's movements artificial', 'lifeless beings around', 'mechanic puppets', 'others moved by strings'. There is a cancellation of the meanings of other people's gestures in the sense that their movements often become purposeless and incomprehensible: 'Their movements were meaningless to me', 'I felt as one belonging to another race', 'I was unable to take part in things and situations as the others did'. We normally understand other people's actions as gestures, that is, as purposeful movements meant to handle things and put them to use, but to a disembodied self these gestures become movements without meaning. All this conveys the impression of an overall crisis of the embodied basis of sociality (Stanghellini and Ballerini 2011). These descriptions fit in the framework of embodied simulation theory. Here we find the claim that the source for our understanding of other people is to be found in our own embodied experience. We use our body to run simulations of the behaviours of others, and by so doing we are enabled to understand their mental state. This theory has recently received support from neuroscientists who claims to have identified the neural underpinning of our ability to simulate the behaviour of others, the so-called mirror neurons (Rizzolatti and Sinigaglia 2007). As one of the leading pioneers of this neuroscientific approach, Vittorio Gallese, writes:

> Anytime we meet someone, we are implicitly aware of his/her similarity to us, because we literally embody it. The very same neural substrate activated when actions are executed or emotions and sensations are subjectively experienced, is also activated when the same actions, emotions and sensations are executed or experienced by others. A common underlying functional mechanism—*embodied simulation*—mediates our capacity to share the meaning of actions, intentions, feelings, and emotions with others, thus grounding our identification with and connectedness to others.
>
> (Gallese 2010, p. 81)

Schizophrenic persons seem unable, so to say, to *use* their own bodies and their emotions to understand the emotions (thus the motivations to act in a given way) of the others. Abnormal bodily sensations, emotional flooding, and invasiveness may interfere with implicit body-to-body attunement.

Disorders of spatiality, embodiment, and otherness are parts of a unitary structure. A person's own self and the self of the other are experienced as devitalised and disincarnated, and they are thus disattuned from each other; lived space is a blend of detachment and closeness to other people. Usually, the strength of attunement as the force that *connects* the person with others is de-emphasised in the schizophrenic mood. Autism, a key-feature of the schizophrenic mood, is defined as a disturbance of attunement, i.e. of our pre-reflective ability to apprehend the existence of others and to see their mental structure as both overall similar to and yet different from our own; to make emotional contact and establish mutual relationships; to understand intuitively the manifestations of mental life of other persons; and to communicate with others using the shared meaning structures in a context-relevant manner. In the schizophrenic mood, not only our capacity to feel connected with the others is impaired, but also the possibility to *disconnect from* them. As we have argued in Part II, there is much more to emotional attunement than simply being connected. It implies what we may call the *dance* of corporeal identification/differentiation that allows both for understanding others and for the individuation of the borders between *self* and *other*. Connectedness *per se* is just one component of this *dance* joining with/disjoining from the others.

The metamorphoses of the experience of otherness and spatiality in schizophrenia reflect the fundamental fragility constitutive of the embodied nature of personhood that we have explored throughout the book. In schizophrenia this basic fragility is dramatically disturbed and develops into a full-blown fractured state which manifests itself in the fundamental feeling of incompleteness and, as a consequence, in problematic relations, meetings, and confrontations with the other persons. Detachment from the social world parallels the profound disturbance of the ontological setting of embodied selfhood (the fragile ambivalence of biological and personal factors), which is crucial for taking part in the self/other-than-self dialectic of social relations. The feelings of ambivalence constitutive of human personhood (selfhood and otherness) is stymied, and our feeling of being a person is thus somehow petrified and turns into a painful cognitive task, instead of being a seamless affective flow between self and others. In other words, the schizophrenic person loses the feeling of being a person, and compensates by thinking what is normally felt.

Disembodiment and Appearance of Things

We know, at least since Jaspers, that in the delusional experience of reality 'the environment offers *a world of new meanings*' (Jaspers 1997, p. 99 [83]). Being deluded is undergoing a radical transformation in the awareness of meaning. Experiences of 'primary' delusions are the seeing of new meanings. In the beginning of this chapter, we analysed the subtle changes that self and environment undergo before the eruption of delusions. The beginning of delusions implies a change in the awareness of reality:

> Everything gets a *new meaning* [*eine neue Bedeutsamkeit*]. The environment is somehow different—not to a gross degree—perception is unaltered in itself but there is some change which envelops everything with a subtle, pervasive and strangely uncertain light. A living-room which was formerly felt as neutral or friendly now becomes dominated by

some indefinable atmosphere [*Stimmung*]. Something seems to be in the air which the patient cannot account for, a distrustful, uncomfortable, uncanny tension [*Spannung*] fills him.

(Jaspers 1997, p. 98 [82]; translation slightly modified)

For the majority of psychopathologists, this change is a breakdown in meaning-bestowing, i.e. 'the dissolution of formal transcendental contents' of meaning. All experience departs from the normal-meaning relationships with our world (Callieri 1982, p. 30). Both the 'cognitive' and the 'dynamic' (or affective) theories of the delusional atmosphere hold that its central feature is a change in the normal attribution of meanings. Many authors embrace Jaspers's idea that in the delusional atmosphere (and in the delusional perceptions ensuing from it) perception is unaltered in itself: 'perception itself remains normal and unchanged' (Jaspers 1997, p. 100 [83]). Following Conrad's analyses of *trema*, we showed that this is not true. Perception changes radically in the course of incipient schizophrenia, and especially in the state we called 'schizophrenic mood'. In the schizophrenic mood there is a radical change in spatiality and temporality, hence a change of the experience of one's own self and external reality, and we suggested that these changes are primary with respect to changes in meaning-bestowing, and in particular with respect to the breakdown of the common sense understanding of self and world.

Meaningfulness requires an integration of spatial and temporal perspectives. Following Störring, we assumed that perplexity (as a basic component of the schizophrenic mood) should be interpreted as a disorder of motility. The power of organising experience is grounded in motility. A modification in the motility of a person's lived body implies a modification in the perception of the external world. As Husserl writes:

> The Body [*Leib*] then has, for its particular Ego, the unique distinction of bearing in itself the *zero point* of all these orientations. One of its spatial points, even if it is not an actually seen one, is always characterized in the mode of the ultimate central here: that is, a here which has no other here outside itself, in relation to which it would be a 'there'. It is thus that all things of the surrounding world possess an orientation to the Body, just as, accordingly, all expressions of orientation imply this relation.
>
> (Husserl 1989, p. 158)

By means of the integrity of kinaesthesia—the sense of the position and voluntary movement of muscles—my own body is the constant point of orientation in my perceptive field. The perceived object appears through the integration of a series of perspective appearances.

As we have seen above, a basic feature in the schizophrenic mood is a breakdown in space *Gestalt* implying an *itemisation* of the surrounding world: the situation in which the person finds herself loses its character of a meaningful ensemble; perception is shattered into a mere collection of fragmented details unrelated to each other and not in touch with the perceiving self. Such an itemised world appears as meaningless. Also, the integration of spatial perspectives is needed in order to perceive something as a concrete, three-dimensional 'utensil' (something to be used), not merely as a 'stage trapping' or a representation of a real thing. The disintegration of spatial perspectives makes things appear as unreal and without any relevance to the person, that is, without practical meaning (a house, for example, is there for people to inhabit, a mere scenario is not). Moreover, we described a disintegration of time *Gestalt*. As with the itemisation of space, where things appear as mere objects (unrelated to one's body) and events merely as a collection of snapshots or representations (quasi-indiscernible from mental images), the fracturing of the temporal stream of consciousness entails an itemisation of now-moments, each disconnected from the previous and the following ones, which results in them appearing as 'pieces' or 'quasi-objects' floating in consciousness unrelated to the experiencing person.

In a similar way, the understanding of a situation, be it a conversation or a football game, requires the integration of the present moment with retentions and protentions. If this is not the case, the outcome is, once again, the experience of something uncanny, unreal, and beyond understanding. Hence, meaningfulness requires the integrity of spatiality and temporality. In this section, we will explain how meaningfulness also requires the integrity of embodiment. We shall assume that what is meaningful for a human person is somehow inescapably connected with a rudimentary form of manipulability; or to put it differently, our reflective capacity to categorise and make sense of our experience of the world (meaning-bestowing) presupposes *corporeality*.

The lived body is not only the perspectival origin of my perceptions and the locus of their integration, it is also the means by which I own the world, insofar as it structures and organises the possibility of participating in the field of experience. The lived body perceives worldly objects as integral parts of a situation in which it is engaged, of a project to which it is committed, so that actions are responses to situations—rather than reactions to sporadic stimuli. The body seeks understanding from the things with which it interacts; the lived body is silently at work in whatever I do. I understand my environment as I inhabit it, and the meaningful organisation of the field of experience is possible because the active and receptive potentials of my own body are constantly projected into it (Sheets-Johnstone 1999). Cognition is enacted or action-specific because 'sensory and motor processes, perception and action, are fundamentally inseparable in lived cognition. Indeed, the two are not contingently linked in individuals; they have also evolved together' (Varela et al. 1991, p. 173; see also Thompson 2007, pp. 1–87). Similarly, perception is always entangled with specific possibilities of action, and thus 'should not (or, at least, should not always) be conceptualized independently of thinking about the class of *actions* which the creature needs to perform' (Clark 1997, p. 152). Perception is constantly geared up to tracing possibilities for action, or a set of affordances. Andy Clarke explains further:

> An affordance is an opportunity for use or interaction which some object or state of affairs presents to a certain kind of agent. For example, to a human a chair affords sitting, but to a woodpecker it may afford something quite different. (1997, p. 172)

Such affordances form the rudimentary constitution of what we called 'meaning', since the basic meaning of an object springs from how we put it to use. We owe this fundamental insight to Heidegger.[9] The basic kind of knowledge I have of the objects in the world is not a simple version of our more theoretical cognition of what is 'present-at-hand' (*vorhanden*), but reflects our concern with the world as expressed in our practical engagement with the things in the world. In Heidegger's words, 'the closest kind of association is not mere perceptual cognition [*Erkennen*], but, rather, a handling, using, and taking care of things [*das hantierende, gebrauchende Besorgen*] which has its own kind of "knowledge" ["*Erkenntnis*"]' (2010, p. 67). Objects appear to my embodied self as something 'in-order-to', as 'equipment', 'ready-to-hand' (*zuhanden*) for manipulating reality, i.e. for cutting, sewing, quenching my thirst, and so forth. In this way, I literally *grasp* the meaning of a thing or a situation, since this meaning is exactly the specific 'manipulability' (*Handlichkeit*) of a thing in the context of the larger web of our involvements (*Bewandtnisganzheit*) with the world (2010, p. 84).

The annihilation of practical meanings is one of the main features of the world disclosed by the schizophrenic mood as described in classical accounts—as in the case of the schizophrenic person watching his hands mentioned above. The following passage, once again from the *Autobiography of a Schizophrenic Girl*, can help to shed light on this phenomenon as the effect of the divorce of things from their ready-to-hand meanings:

> When, for example, I looked at a chair or a jug, I thought not of their use or function - a jug not as something to hold water and milk, a chair not as something to sit in—but as having lost their names, their functions and meanings [. . .] I attempted to escape their hold [*leur emprise*] by calling out their names. I said, 'chair, jug, table, it is a chair.' But the word echoed hollowly, deprived of all meaning; it had left the object, was divorced from it, so much that on one hand it was a living, mocking thing, on the other, a name, empty of sense [*vide de sens*], like an envelope emptied of content.
>
> (Sechehaye 1951, pp. 34–5 [37–8]; translation slightly modified)

Persons with schizophrenia describe this connection between disembodiment and the crisis of meaning-bestowing as 'I was here, things simply there, without meaning', 'things smooth, ungraspable', '[I and things] not rooted in the same environment', 'why should I call it a table, a table, a table? It means nothing to me!'.

The metamorphosis of meaning-bestowing is a consequence of this loss of practical grasp of the world. Scheler (2008, pp. 78–9 [73]) explains that the embodied life-drive blocks off all those potential significations which do not have a relevance for that living organism in a given situation. It infuses the world with a hierarchy of relevance, allowing the abridgement of competing perspectives, hence letting the figure emerge clearly from

---

[9] Clarke acknowledges this heritage, although he distances himself from Heidegger's metaphysical scruples about the human mind and maintains that his own version of affordances 'is significantly broader and includes all cases in which body and local environment appear as elements in extended problem-solving activity' (1997, p. 171). As we saw in Chapter 7, Ratcliffe makes even more significant (and more textually close) use of Heidegger's enactive or pragmatic conception of meaning. For more detail, see Ratcliffe 2007, pp. 62–74.

the background so that contextually relevant meanings may come into the foreground. From all the manifold meanings of things, the life-drive mobilises only that small fraction that is fitting to a person's situatedness, responding to that person's vital need, and appropriate in view of the cultural and historical environment. The suspension of the life-drive cancels all bodily-based projects, and thus allows for a new kind of enacted world to appear which is detached from our practical engagement and characterised by an unsettling focus on 'theoretical' aspects of experience (what makes reality appear as it appears? Why do people sit on that object? How am I to understand that colour?). This new metaphysical enactment of the world will be the topic of the last section, but first we will argue for the necessary step from a phenomenological to a hermeneutical approach in order to develop further our understanding of schizophrenic life-worlds.

A Hermeneutics of Schizophrenic Life-Worlds

In the preceding part of this chapter, we have provided a phenomenological characterisation of the schizophrenic mood as the experiential nucleus from which schizophrenic life-worlds originate. In this section, we will try to illustrate how a schizophrenic person takes up a position in front of this basic metamorphosis of experience in order to make sense of these dramatic transformations in his or her life-world. To do this, we will develop a hermeneutical account of the dialectic between the schizophrenic person and this experiential, emotion-centred nucleus. As explained in the first section, the task of clinical phenomenology is to characterise the personal level of experience, while the task of clinical hermeneutics is to articulate how the person *understands* her own experiences, that is, the meanings and values she attributes to them. The central idea of the dialectical model in psychopathology is that there exists an interplay between the person and the basic transformations of her field of experience. The dialectical model of mental disorders draws attention to the active role that the person, as a self-interpreting animal (Taylor 1985, pp. 45–76) engaged in a world shared with other persons, has in interacting with his or her basic disorder and in the shaping of psychopathological syndromes (Stanghellini 1997a, 1997b; Stanghellini and Rossi Monti 2009a).

The diversity of the manifestations of full-blown schizophrenic phenomena is a consequence of the way persons with schizophrenia make sense of the schizophrenic mood, and of the life-world that is enacted through a person's endeavour to bring about intelligibility. The different kinds of personal position-taking in front of the experience of this characteristic *Stimmung* engender the different forms of schizophrenic symptoms, syndromes, and courses. The principal theoretical references of the dialectical model in psychopathology are Bleuler, Wyrsch, and de Clérambault. The French alienist Philippe Pinel (1800) can be considered the founding father of the dialectical model of mental disorders. Pinel, physician and philanthropist, is perhaps most famous for having liberated the mad from the Parisian hospital of Bicêtre. Equally important, though, is his seminal work *Traité medico-philosophique sur l'aliénation mentale ou La manie* (Pinel 1800). In this book, Pinel lays down the cornerstones of a dynamic understanding of mental illness (Stanghellini 1997a). It will be helpful in what follows if we succinctly sum up the principal points of his theory of mental alienation.[10] First, there is the principle of the *partial nature* of alienation: no mad person is entirely so, but retains a part of selfhood that can be cognizant of his alienation, and thus enables the person to try to cope with it. Second, the principle of the *plasticity* of madness: each person stamps his identity onto the 'raw material' of the vulnerability from which alienation derives. Each case of pathology, each form of alienation, is the result of a dynamic relationship between the person and his vulnerability. Third, the principle of a *nosodromical* continuum of mental syndromes: the various psychopathological syndromes are not discrete entities, but steps along a continuum. The suffering person can, in different moments of his psychopathological course, be affected by different forms of alienation. Fourth, there is the potential for the *outcomes to be different* for different patients, depending on the character of the vulnerability and the resources that the person can muster to fight it. These principles have been reaffirmed in the later part of the twentieth century by Gladys Swain—a Pinel scholar and the author of *Le sujet de la folie*:[11]

> Mental alienation is never total: the alienated always preserves a distance from his alienation. Similarly the alienation is never partial as if it should only concern a part of the personality that one could completely and simply separate from the rest. It takes a hold on the entire subject without ever completely abolishing the subjective function. It happens in response to the flickering of the subject's capacity to support itself in such a state. When we understand this, recording and deciphering symptoms takes on a profoundly new meaning. There is a central source [*un foyer central*] by means of which we can organize them: they must be read as an expression of the subject's engagement in his madness, and of his relationship with his madness.
>
> (Swain 1997, pp. 71–2; our translation)

In a similar vein, Mario Rossi Monti sets out in full his 'genuinely dynamic' vision of mental illness:

> [B]y thinking of a subject who can in some way take up a position with regard to his own illness, an authentically dynamic understanding of mental illness is introduced. It involves seeing mental illness as the result of the interplay of forces and the consequence of the breakdown of equilibrium, in which life events and environment play an extremely important role.
>
> (Rossi Monti 2008, p. 124; our translation)

Fertile philosophical soil for a development of the dialectical model of mental pathology can be found in (our reformulation of) Ricoeur's hermeneutical phenomenology, with its focus on the fragile tension of selfhood and otherness, the voluntary and the involuntary, activity and passivity, in the constitution of our identity. We become the

---

[10] For a highly informative and critical account of Pinel's theory and its philosophical context, see Charland (2010); see also Weiner (2008a, 2008b) and Charland (2008) for the cultural and institutional setting in which Pinel's work was embedded.

[11] First published in 1977. We are here quoting from the re-edition from 1997. For a detailed review of Swain's (and her long-time collaborator Marcel Gauchet's) theory and the intellectual environment out of which it rose, see Moyn (2009).

person that we are through the confrontation, and sometimes the appropriation, of the otherness that is an inescapable part of our personhood, and yet this otherness is able to disturb the person that we want to be or consider ourselves to be. We saw how Ricoeur argued that a self does not simply coincide with itself. Selfhood, our pre-reflective awareness of being a self, is unstable, troubled, and often conflictual in nature. Selfhood is marked by the fragile tension inherent in our being both biological and personal; or in other words, by the interplay of our *bios* and our *ethos*. The dialectical model of mental pathology is grounded in this idea of a conflictual selfhood at the core of every person, healthy as well as disturbed. In the words of Samuel Moyn: 'Pinel's discovery opened the way for an era in which healthy selfhood, and not just deranged alienation, is understood as self-divided conflict' (2009, p. 329). For the self to be the person that it is depends on its ability to become that person through this 'self-divided conflict'. In Part II, we developed this idea of troubled selfhood into the full-blown notion of fragile personhood experienced, first and foremost, in our feelings of ambivalence. Emotions are part of both the *bios* and the *ethos* of a person, which we emphasised by adopting de Sousa's characterisation of emotions: 'of all the aspects of what we call the "mind", emotions are the most deeply embodied' (de Sousa 1987, p. 47). The fragile, often conflictual, and sometimes alienating nature of emotional experience stems from the fact that the array of a person's emotional experience envelops deeply heterogeneous feelings. In fact, our emotional life is so multifarious as to include feelings involved in warm-hearted parental love, blind rage, tenderness, jealousy, envy, compassion, as well as nauseating disgust. Our feelings play an important role in what we care about in our life. They are part of the constitution of the heterogeneous values that we live our life by, and because of their complexity (biological and personal) our feelings are thus one of the main reasons behind the fragile nature of personhood. In order to get a grip on the impalpable nature of many of the feelings involved in emotional experience, we made a phenomenological distinction between moods and affects, which allowed us to articulate aspects of emotional experience that are often neglected in philosophical theories of emotion. To make sense of these feelings, integrating the biological as well as the personal, we then developed this initial phenomenological analysis into a fully fledged hermeneutical approach. Combining the general lead from Ricoeur with Goldie's more particular emphasis on emotions, we proposed a narrative approach as one way to deal with the emotional ambivalence involved in being a person. Creating narratives provides a fecund means to cope with the often disturbing array of feelings involved in our emotional experience, and to interpret and speak about our feelings about the world, other people, and ourselves. This approach becomes obviously relevant in the dialectical model of mental pathology. The fragile, incipiently alienated, emotional core of personhood develops into a full-blown alienated manifestation in persons affected by mental pathology. The narratives that each person with schizophrenia makes about her emotional life and her awkward experiences are precisely such attempts to make sense of what is going on in her life, and establish who she is and who she wants to be.

Our emphasis on the active role that the schizophrenic person has in shaping her own psychotic pathways is also rooted in the empirical ground of clinical practice; for instance, in the findings concerning the extreme polymorphism of psychotic symptoms (Strauss 1969) and in the variability of schizophrenic courses (Strauss et al. 1985).

Both these findings support an argument against a linear pathogenetic process linking biological causes to a manifold and undulating symptomatology, and suggest instead the mediating role of the person.

We assume that Bleuler's (1911) distinction between primary and secondary symptoms can be considered as the theoretical foundation of this version of the dialectical model of schizophrenia. Kraepelin's (1899) and Bleuler's ideas on the aetio-pathogenesis of psychoses provide excellent examples of the antithesis between a naturalistic and a heuristic *Weltanschauung* that is still very much alive today. For Kraepelin, cases of illness originated by authentically similar causes should always show the same manifestations and the same anatomical findings, and apparent exceptions to this methodological rule only derive from the imperfections of our current state of knowledge about the sub-personal workings of the brain. Bleuler, on the contrary, held that:

> We can only understand a physically determined psychosis if we distinguish the symptoms stemming directly from the disease process [*Krankheitsprozeß*] itself from the secondary symptoms which only begin to operate when the sick psyche reacts to some internal or external processes [. . .] Therefore, the disease may remain symptomless for a long time. The primary symptoms are the necessary partial phenomena [*Teilerscheinungen*] of a disease; the secondary symptoms may be absent, at least potentially, or they may change without the disease process having to change at the same time [. . .] Which kind of symptoms develop—whether a particular chronic schizophrenic works peacefully today or wanders about or quarrels, whether he is neat or smears himself—depends mainly on past or present experiences, and not directly on the disease.
>
> (Bleuler 1911, p. 348 [284–5]; translation modified)

In fact, the nosology-imbibed Kraepelin considered Bleuler's psychopathological theory of primary and secondary symptoms as a purely artificial construct. In spite of Kraepelin's slighting treatment, Bleuler's distinction between primary and secondary symptoms remains a groundbreaking contribution to psychopathology. His theory has two main limitations, though: an insufficient assessment of basic phenomena and a blurred theory of the role of the person in the shaping of psychotic phenomena, courses, and outcomes. Nonetheless, it can be taken as the key to overcoming the apparent paradox with which we opened this chapter, namely, the idea of a common ground for the manifold manifestations of schizophrenia vs the idea that each patient has his own schizophrenia. These two apparently incompatible conceptions can be brought together if we assume that the persons affected by schizophrenia can take a position in front of the basic phenomena that belong to the common ground, namely, the transformations of the structure of their life-world brought about by the schizophrenic mood described in this chapter. In other words, then, the various forms of schizophrenia are a consequence of the multifarious ways in which persons with schizophrenia contribute to shaping their basic emotional disorder.

Gaëtan de Clérambault, who was one of the first to develop these ideas in modern psychopathology, noted that '[t]his conception helps us understand the variety of clinical forms' (1942, p. 541). A few years earlier, another pioneer Willy Mayer-Gross noticed the dialectical importance of position-taking (*Stellungnahme*) in the residing phase of psychosis. Mayer-Gross analysed the modes in which different patients elaborate their own experience of the acute psychosis in the post-acute phase. He identified five types of attitudes or secondary elaborations: despair, 'new life', forgetfulness, revelation, and integration. Common to these various attitudes is the way the person tries to take a position in front of the drastic destruction (*Zerstörung*) of our inmost 'values of existence' (*Existenzwerte*). For the person, this destruction of our most intimate values is in a painful tension with 'the drive for the intelligible unity of life-construction [*Der Drang zur verständlichen Einheitlichkeit der Lebensgestaltung*]' (Mayer-Gross 1920, p. 171). Mayer-Gross describes this painful tension in the following way:

> All that was 'sacred' to him, what gave him 'self-confidence', is destroyed because of his past vicissitudes [. . .] There is nothing at hand [*vorhanden*] whereby he can re-establish his broken self, the self is emptied; bewildered he finds no point of contact [*Anknüpfungspunkt*] from which he can continue his existence or re-establish it. Nevertheless, this search for an egress out of the despair remains as a task [*Aufgabe*], a demand [*Forderung*] of continuity.
>
> (Mayer-Gross 1920, p. 174; our translation)

Some thirty years later, the Swiss psychiatrist Jakob Wyrsch, who was concerned with the relationship between the person and the outburst of the psychosis during the acute phase of schizophrenia, distinguished four groups of patients (1949, pp. 95–112):[12] patients who try to objectify their own sufferings and conceive them as symptoms of a somatic illness; patients who are passive and unable of any reaction; patients who engage in a fight against their pathological experiences, displaying a stubborn and often desperate attempt to fit such experiences 'into the meaning context [*Sinnzusammenhang*] of their life-story' (p. 103); and a last group who is exalted by the novelty of the psychotic experience, which acquires for them a cosmic meaning: 'it is significant in the world order and not just for him' (p. 104). Wyrsch concludes the categorisation of his clinical observations by noting that these different reactions to the psychosis are 'only four of the many ways in which the person can deal [*sich auseinandersetzen*] with the illness that threatens his existence' (p. 105).

In a similar vein, Christoph Mundt's intentionality model (Mundt 1985, 1991) is a more recent contribution to the dialectical model of schizophrenia. Mundt pragmatically defines 'intentionality' as the act of conceptualising reality. The intentionality model in psychopathology emphasises the 'active, strategic character of constituting reality and building up inter-subjectivity'. It focuses on the role of the person in constituting basic psychopathological phenomena. Mundt (1991) points out three levels of intentionality performance: (a) a *sensory* level, i.e. the processing of sensory information to a *Gestalt*; (b) a level of *symbolic representation of reality* (based on language and cognitive performances), i.e. the effort of definition concerned both with expression and communication; (c) a level of *transcendental organisation* (concerned with the meanings and purposes of one's own existence), i.e. the effort to make the ideas of one's own self and its societal reality coincide. All three levels of performance are impaired in schizophrenia. We learn from Mundt that at stake are not only the modes in which the person faces acute psychosis *après-coup* (Mayer-Gross), but also the modes in which

---

[12] The quotes from Wyrsch are all our own translations.

the person shapes basic phenomena while they are breaking through (Wyrsch). On the one hand, basic phenomena are conceived by Mundt as the effects of the breakdown of intentionality; on the other, end-phenomena are thought of as the results of later attempts of intentionality to compensate for such a breakdown by means of the 'counter-reality' of delusion and neologism.

Of course, one should be very careful not to overestimate 'the importance of the constitutive element in the sense of the *active* constitution' of psychotic worlds by 'exaggerating the element of freedom and spontaneity involved in "projecting" these worlds' (Blankenburg 1980, p. 63). Indeed, especially chronic schizophrenic patients are forced back to levels of reduced intentional effort. However, the pivotal role of a 'repair' mechanism in the constitution of schizophrenic worlds is hardly disputable. The intentionality model draws attention to the capacity of symbolic representation of reality. In this perspective, the schizophrenic condition often shows the imbalance or disproportion between the complexity of experience and the personal capacity of representation, i.e. of adequate expression and understandable communication. The symbolic texture of our experience of reality accounts for the 'fundamental ambiguities of human existence [. . .] understanding them enables us to go beyond a purely descriptive phenomenology and enables us to develop a dynamic phenomenology, one that has a necessarily dialectical character' (Blankenburg 1982, p. 58).

This transition from a purely descriptive phenomenology to a dynamic phenomenology bears many similarities with Ricoeur's development of hermeneutical phenomenology against the backdrop of a more traditional phenomenology. The relation of a dialectical model of psychopathology to Ricoeur's theory of subjectivity will be treated in more detail in the concluding chapter of this book. For now, suffice it to say that the principal factor that binds the two together is the concern with the structural tension between selfhood and otherness in being a person.

Metaphysical Enactment

In the course of the schizophrenic metamorphosis of experience, an unusual perspective on the world is established. New concerns—the quest for what is real vs unreal, meaningful vs meaningless, true vs fake, subjective vs objective—emerge from this experience of self and world transformation. Things in the world and the behaviour of other people lose their incarnated givenness and their implicit meaningfulness: are things existing *per se* or are they the product of someone's mind, or perhaps the result of a cunning technological device? Are the meanings of things authentic or inauthentic and 'made up'? Are the others real persons in flesh and blood or mechanical puppets? Is their behaviour purposefully tricky and ambiguous?

Persons undergoing the schizophrenic mood can develop many different sorts of delusions—or not develop delusions at all. Delusions are *just one possible outcome* of the transformations in the structure of experiencing, and *typical schizophrenic* delusions are maybe not the most common delusional form in persons who are or have been affected by the schizophrenic mood.

Following a phase dominated by uncanny transformations in the life-world, by feelings of incoherence, incompleteness and fragility, and by profound existential doubts and uncertainties, typical schizophrenic delusions express 'philosophical' concerns (Jaspers 1997, pp. 283, 294–6 [238, 247–9]). 'Philosophical' delusions are probably the most characteristic form of schizophrenic delusion. But experienced clinicians know very well that persons with schizophrenia may develop much more *ontic* forms of delusions, like paranoid, hypochondriac or passivity delusions. De Clérambault (1942, pp. 534–5) gives the following example: three different persons are affected by a similar disorder of embodiment characterised by diffuse coenesthopathies. The first one, who is inclined to a continuous form of anxious introspection, will develop a hypochondriac form of delusion by which he explains his abnormal bodily sensations as the symptoms of a (usually severe) somatic illness. The second person, who has a more 'imaginative' character, will interpret analogous bodily disturbances as the outcome of some entity (e.g. a person, an animal, the devil) who is possessing her body and changing the place of her organs or doing other malicious deeds. The third, who has the tendency to give external or 'exogenous' explanations, will develop a persecutory delusion, believing, for example, that her somatic troubles derive from being poisoned by some conspirator. De Clérambault argues that the disparity in the content of delusions is more the effect of *different elaborations by the person* (on the sensible, affective, and reflective level) than of different basic transformations of bodily experience (p. 535).[13] Each person stamps his or her autograph onto the 'raw material' of abnormal bodily sensations. Each form of delusion is the result of a relationship between the person and her vulnerability—an attempt to establish an interpretation of the metamorphoses of self and world entailed by the schizophrenic mood. Thus, what is most characteristic and typically schizophrenic in these ontic delusions is *not* their ideational content—rather the existential metamorphosis that transpires through them and can be traced back to the radical transformation of the life-world described above. This is the underlying unitary modification, an expression of the basic vulnerability characteristic of the schizophrenic mode of existence.

Different personal attitudes such as individual cognitive characteristics, affective temperaments, and value-structures often lead to distinct clinical pictures. The person may have an *immunoplastic* role—moderating the pathogenetic impact of basic disorders and so protecting against psychotic breakdowns—or a *pathoplastic* role. In the latter category, the person may contribute to turning basic disorders into full-blown psychotic phenomena through a (pseudo-)explicative attitude. A patient affected, for instance, by cognitive concentration disturbances might interpret these disturbances delusionally and assert that his own thoughts are under the control of an alien force. Another patient, suffering from disorders of motricity, explains these as effects of other people's intention and consequently develops a delusion of alien control.

Persons who have an avoidant attitude, and those showing language impairments and alexithymic traits (the impairment of experiencing and expressing emotional

---

[13] De Clérambault writes: 'One observes these transitions in the sensitive order, the affective order, the reflective [*idéique*] order; in fact, the acceptance of one of these kinds of explanation, or a mixture of these, depends on: (1) the intrinsic modalities of the initial sensation, (2) the pre-established character of the subject, (3) the ideas of the subject and the surrounding ideas' (1925, p. 535; our translation).

states and bodily sensations, and the incapacity to distinguish between them) are less prone to have psychotic symptoms and more liable to develop non-delusional or sub-apophanic forms of schizophrenia (Stanghellini et al. 2001; Stanghellini and Ricca 1995). Typical schizophrenic delusions are missing in these forms of schizophrenia, as explained, among others, by Blankenburg and Minkowski. The essential disorder, or core-property, underlying schizophrenic phenomena manifests itself in the most explicit way, that is, without a delusional super-structure. Minkowski assumed that the basic feature of schizophrenic vulnerability is the loss of vital contact with reality. Vital contact with reality provides a latent awareness of reality 'making us adjust and modify our behavior in a contextually relevant manner but without distorting our overall goals, standards, and identity' (Urfer 2001, p. 282). Blankenburg characterised this phenomenon as a crisis of common sense. Persons with schizophrenia, he argued, lack an implicit understanding of the axioms or basic rules of everyday life, i.e. 'not only the knowledge of the naturally understood and matter-of-course things', but 'also the manner in which she understands things to be that way' (2001, p. 308). They do not share the background of tacit knowledge of their social group, through which its members conceptualise objects, situations, and the behaviour of other people. Also, they depart from the natural attitude that involves being attuned to the world as it appears in everyday experience. Instead of being absorbed by things as they spontaneously appear, they are focused on the condition of possibility of their appearance, on what makes them appear as they appear. One of us has called this the *noetic*, rather than noematic, attitude in persons with schizophrenia (Stanghellini 2008). The following statement by a patient affected by a sub-apophanic form of schizophrenia is a clear example of this:

> My attitude towards life can be summed up as follows: It is as if we were all in the theatre. But whereas all the others are focused on what happens on the stage, I cannot help thinking of what's going on backstage, what makes the scene possible.
>
> (Stanghellini and Ballerini 2007b, p. 136)

We see here a pragmatic impairment where the fundamental anomaly is understood to be in the person's intuitive grip on social situations, a kind of 'non-conceptual and non-reflective *indwelling* in the intersubjective world' (Parnas et al. 2002, p. 132). The overall attitude towards life held by persons with schizophrenia, as it becomes explicit in non-delusional forms, is dominated by morbid rationalism and the so-called 'antithetical attitude' (Minkowski 1997, p. 58). Morbid rationalism is an intellectualistic attitude that consists in trying to govern one's own life according to abstract principles and renouncing the non-rational feelings of consonance between oneself and the surrounding world. The antithetical attitude is the attempt to avoid all perturbations coming from without the person, feared as an attack on one's fragile sense of personhood.

In sub-apophanic forms of schizophrenia, a new, *metaphysical enactment* arises from the profound transformation of the life-world, where theoretical, rather than practical, concerns come into the foreground. This is also characteristic of delusional forms, especially in typical schizophrenic delusions. Here we observe a sort of *symbiosis* between the metamorphosis of lived experience and the kind of concerns and interpretations elicited by it—there exists an isomorphism between the feelings of unreality, strangeness, and uncanniness and the way the person who undergoes these feelings tries to make sense of them. The metamorphosis of reality takes place in a person who is, so to say, psychologically predisposed to develop an ontological, quasi-philosophical interpretation of this. Typical delusion in persons with schizophrenia are about the *being* of things, events, and persons, including themselves. They are not satisfied with what appears in immediate experience and are concerned with metaphysical questions. Many of these questions are ontological in nature. Ontology deals with the status of being, and considers the nature of the things that constitute reality, and especially their existence (vs non-existence) and their true meaning (vs ordinary, common sense meaning).

Next to an eerie preoccupation with ontology, we also find that eschatological, charismatic, and epistemological concerns dominate at the expense of worldly elements and the factuality of things (Bovet and Parnas 1993; Kepinski 1974; Parnas and Sass 2001; Stanghellini 2004; Stanghellini and Ballerini 2007a). We have already seen an example of eschatological delusion in the end-of-the-world experience. As explained earlier, in this form of eschatological delusions a new meaning suddenly emerges, the following pre-delusional states are characterised by an awareness of latent meanings—a new state of reality in which all phenomena acquire a new meaning. In eschatological delusions, the person feels involved in the transition to something newer and grander. Charismatic delusions often accompany eschatological ones, 'the world is about to end, my mission is saving it'. In epistemological delusions, the person feels that he has discovered the essence of reality whereas other people are ignorant and merely aware of the appearance of phenomena. Usually this new awareness comes in the form of a sudden revelation (Stanghellini and Ballerini 1992) that follows upon a phase of incertitude and tension.

These are the forms that the *metaphysical taint* of typical schizophrenic delusions may assume. This taint, better than all specific ideational contents, expresses the core of the schizophrenic life-world brought about by the schizophrenic mood. The schizophrenic mood—as we have seen—brings into the foreground essentially this kind of concerns: What does really exist, in contrast to what only seems to exist? What does exist independently and unconditionally, in contrast to what exists dependently and conditionally? And what does permanently exist, in contrast to what only temporarily exists? These concerns, which stem directly from the metamorphosis of experience, require adequate conceptual tools and linguistic competence to be expressed in some form of structured 'philosophical' delusion—be it dogmatic or mystical.

The metaphysical taint of schizophrenic delusions tells us that persons with schizophrenia have lost their 'ontic tie to the world and to the Other' (Bovet and Parnas 1993, p. 593). The 'ontic tie' that is missing is what throughout this chapter we have described as the 'original affirmation', 'conatus', or 'life-drive'. The schizophrenic mode of existence is the outcome of its cancellation—or its relegation out of the boundaries of the self—and the consequence of the disintegration of spatial perspectives, the loss of continuity and integration in temporality, the flattening of mundane things and the loss of the practical grasp on them, of the disembodiment of the self and the breakdown of the dance of intercorporeality that ensues from the schizophrenic mood.

Chapter 9

Borderland

People with borderline personality disorder are often described as affected by extreme emotional fluctuations and by the sudden emergence of incontrollable and disproportionate emotional reactions. Borderline persons often experience their own self as dim and fuzzy, and they feel deprived of a stable sense of identity and unable to be steadily involved in a given life project or social role. Often they complain of being insulted by the hypocrisy and insincerity of other people, or claim that they are mistreated because of their care for authenticity; in other words, they do not feel recognised and appreciated for their being the kind of person that they are. They may see others as caliginous, cloudy, and their faces as expressionless; and a moment later perceive them as dangerously ambivalent, suspect, tenebrous, with evil intent. The main purpose of this chapter is to provide a fine-grained and nuanced description of these rapid, abrupt, and dramatic emotional swings and of the changes of the life-world accompanying them. We will interpret these typical changes in the existence of borderline persons as fluctuations between a clearly normative emotion such as anger and the more diffuse and confusing background of a bad mood like dysphoria.

In the following sections, we will first provide a glossary for the varieties of emotions, and especially of bad moods, involved in the borderline condition, and in a concise manner illustrate their place in the spectrum of mood disorders. We will then pass to a discussion of the borderline condition as a disordered fabric of the person, that is, a disorder of the integration of selfhood and otherness in one narrative sense of personhood. Central to this discussion is the role of lived temporality. This will pave the way for the phenomenological description of the life-world borderline persons live in, with a special focus on the way they experience others and themselves, and more generally on their traumatic existence, i.e. on the way time, space, self, body, and things are constituted in a world characterised by daily traumas, and not only by early traumatic experiences. The concluding part will be about the difficulties which the borderline person encounters in working out an understanding of his own life-world in the sense of reconstructing a unitary and meaningful world out of the scattered fragments of his own existence; and finally about the help that a phenomenologically grounded clinical hermeneutics can provide to assist the borderline person in this complicated task.

Between Dysphoria and Anger

Our description of the life-world of borderline persons will focus on the emotions characterising it, arguing that emotions are the 'spatializing-temporalizing vortex' of the life-world. In Chapter 6, we argued that emotions can be conceived as kinetic, dynamic forces that drive us in our ongoing interactions with the environment. Emotions are functional states which motivate and may produce movements, and protentional states which project the person into the future providing a felt readiness for action. As such they organise the life-world, i.e. the lived space, time, self, otherness, and the physiognomy of things in the world that surrounds a person. Emotions are the core of the life-world. An emotion situates a person, allows him to perceive the things that surrounds him as disclosing certain (and not other) possibilities. There is a close resemblance between emotion as an impulse to move outwards and intentionality as an arrow directed at a target. Emotions, understood as embodied intentionality, provide our orientation in the life-world. They motivate us to turn our attention in a given direction, to be absorbed by a more or less defined object, to move in (or break away from) a given direction. Emotions also orient our receptivity. They contribute to our feeling of being involved in the world (engagement), to our grasping the meanings of worldly objects (enactment), and to our pre-reflective understanding of the behaviour of other people (attunement).

Dysphoria and anger engender very different kinds of existential orientation and enactment, thereby enacting very different configurations of the life-world. Dysphoria exerts a centrifugal force which fragments the borderline person's representations of herself and others, thus contributing to her painful experience of incoherence and inner emptiness, her threatening feeling of uncertainty and inauthenticity in interpersonal relationships, and her excruciating sense of insignificance, futility, and the inanity of life. But it also engenders a sense of vitality, although a disorganised, and an aimless and explosive one—a *desperate vitality* (*una disperata vitalità*), to use the words of the Italian novelist, poet, and filmmaker Pier Paolo Pasolini (1964). The centripetal force of anger restores the cohesion of the self, determines a clear-cut, unambiguous image of the other, and dissipates all doubts and sentiments of absurdity at the cost of acute, though transitory, persecutory delusions. Anger tends to preserve and maintain a precarious cohesion of the self (Pazzagli and Rossi Monti 2000, p. 223), in the same way that a small child might self-inflict physical pain in order to try to keep a sense of being alive and of cohesion.

As explained in Chapter 6, we use 'emotion' as an umbrella term covering the multifarious feelings involved in emotional experience. To try to get a grip on these feelings, we introduced a phenomenological distinction between affects and moods. Affects are focused and possess a specific directedness. They are felt as motivated, more determinate and articulated than moods. Affects normally do not open up a horizontal awareness, but occupy all my attentional space. In anger, for instance, I am completely absorbed by the phenomenon that agitates me. When I am angry, a relevant feature of the world (usually threatening my personal existence and the value I attach to it) captivates me, irrupts into my field of awareness without me having decided to turn my attention to it. I become fixated on the object of my anger, and all my attention is captured by it. I am moved by my affect in a specific direction, which in the case of anger may result in retaliation. Moods, on the contrary, are unfocused. They do not possess a specific directedness and aboutness. They are felt as unmotivated, and there are no 'felt causes' for them. They are more indefinite and indeterminate than affects. Moods do not direct us to anything specific in our relation to the environment, and we are not able to put our finger on what exactly causes our particular mood. This is precisely the case with dysphoria. Dysphoria manifests itself as a prolonged, unmotivated, indistinct, and quasi-ineffable constellation of feelings which convey a nebula of vague impulses, sensations, and perceptions that permeate a person's whole field of awareness. The normal distinction between self and other is blurred and hazy. Dysphoria has a horizontal absorption in the sense that it attends to the world as a whole, not focusing on any particular object or situation. No particular action is dictated by dysphoric mood. On the contrary, it complicates the relation between feeling and action because it introduces doubt, hesitation, and questions. This troubling aspect of dysphoric mood is eloquently captured by the English playwright Sarah Kane in her play *4.48 Psychosis*:

> Nowhere left to turn
> An ineffectual moral spasm
> The only alternative to murder
>
> (Kane 2001, p. 241)

The intentional structure that characterises much of human emotional experience is absent in dysphoria. If we imagine emotions as fluxes of intentionality that innervate the flesh and connect it to the world, moods are, so to say, pure intentionality devoid of the moderating power of language and representation. Moods are, to use Bin Kimura's terminology, pure noesis or noematically empty intentionality. By that we mean that if noematic representations function as a dispositive 'to control the noetic act so that it does not deviate from its relationship with life' (Kimura 2000, p. 88; our translation), then moods are noetic acts without any sort of representational, linguistic, or reflective control. This characterisation tallies perfectly with the experience that borderline persons have of their own dysphoric mood: an untamed source of vitality, a disturbing and an exuberant force, creative and destructive at the same time. A vigour that brings life as well as annihilation. A dramatic experience powerfully expressed by the Welsh poet Dylan Thomas in the opening lines of his poem *The Force That Through the Green Fuse Drives the Flower*:

> The force that through the green fuse drives the flower
> Drives my green age; that blasts the roots of trees
> Is my destroyer.
> And I am dumb to tell the crooked rose
> My youth is bent by the same wintry fever.
> The force that drives the water through the rocks
> Drives my red blood; that dries the mouthing streams
> Turns mine to wax.
> And I am dumb to mouth unto my veins
> How at the mountain spring the same mouth sucks.
>
> (Thomas 2003, p. 90)

This force brings life and death, and is experienced as ineffable and unrepresentable.[1] And perhaps most importantly, it is felt as an inseparable part of one's self.

---

[1] This view may complement the psychoanalytic concept of death drive (*Todestrieb*), i.e. the drive towards self-destruction or towards a return to the inorganic. In this vein, the death drive is not opposed to the life instinct, rather it is an ungovernable excess of vitality which—as Lacan would say—is not marked by the symbolic.

Anger and dysphoria may transform into one another. There is, we will see, a dialectic between anger and dysphoria in the existence of borderline persons. Anger, as an affect elicited by a given situation, may transform itself into a dysphoric mood that imposes itself on a person for days. Again, anger may transform itself into the corresponding mood, and finally become a permanent part of a person's character, the so-called irritable-dysphoric temperament. All this happens implicitly, that is, without explicit reflection and involuntarily. Inversely, dysphoric mood and temperament may passively and almost unconsciously determine angry affects, and thus provide a background which alters the way a person is affected by external events and by her own thoughts or memories. The transformation of dysphoric mood into anger may also take place in active reflection: a given mood may become an affect when in active reflection I am able to articulate it and find its motivations and 'felt causes'. In the course of a psychotherapy, for instance, a patient affected by a chronic state of dysphoria may become very angry at his parents when, reconstructing his life story, he recollects the way he felt mistreated by them in infancy.

In Part II, we argued that we are not simply passive with respect to our emotions. I can voluntarily relate myself to my emotions. My personhood is, in part, constituted by my active relation to my situatedness, including my emotions. Through narratives, emotions can also be incorporated actively, reflectively, and thematically into a person's identity. Moods are intimately connected to self-understanding. I understand who I am in the context of my practical engagement, as embedded in a certain world (private or social), and this engagement is primordially enveloped in a certain constellation of feelings. My questioning about myself is often elicited by my mood (and also by disturbing affects that disclose my mood) before my identity becomes an explicit problem. Moods may disclose to me what words and deeds do not. Feelings are no hindrance to more cognitive kinds of knowledge, but they are the *via regia* to understanding myself as embedded in a world shared with other persons. This is true in general, but not so for borderline persons who are overwhelmed by their emotions, and in particular by dysphoria and anger. Typical for these persons is an extreme difficulty to noematically represent dysphoria (it is 'dumb to tell', to use the words that Dylan Thomas repeats several times in his poem), to establish a connection between this emotion and the way they experience the world, as well as articulating their emotional experiences and actions in a coherent narrative pattern.

Varieties of Bad Moods and Mood Disorders

The basic emotions characterising the life-world of borderline persons are dysphoria and anger. In this section, we illustrate and discuss standard psychological and psychopathological definitions of these and other cognate emotions. Anger is an emotion normally conceived as involving a personal offence, or having been somehow wronged by another person, and as such it often motivates a desire for retaliation. In its Latin and Greek roots (*angor*, *anchō*), both referring to strangling, we can find a strong association with aggression. Anger is often considered less intense, but essentially similar to rage (from Latin *rabies* [rabies]) and fury (from Latin *furere* [getting mad]). The common feature shared by anger, rage, and fury is their connection with assaultive behaviour which summons anger as a sinister shadow. Anger and assaultive behaviours characterise the acute phases of the borderline person's existence. Despite its complex cognitive, personal, and social aspects (Solomon 2007, pp. 13–28), anger is, in most cases, a readily identified emotion because of its rather clear behavioural manifestations such as increase of muscle tension, scowling, grinding of teeth, glaring, clenching of fists, changes of arm position and body posture, flashing, paling (Tavris 1989). The psychological and psychopathological characterisation of dysphoria, on the other hand, requires more attention because of its more subdued manifestation and less direct connection to our behavioural patterns.

The word 'dysphoria' derives from the ancient Greek δύσφορος (*dysphoros*), formed as δυσ- (*dis-*), difficult, and φέρω (*phero*), to bear. It is an oppressive, burdensome, unbearable, heavy mood. Therefore, in its very etymological roots the word 'dysphoria' is quite polysemous, defining a condition in which a person is heavily oppressed, and she may, as a consequence, either react and vent her feelings, or passively suffer and submit to them (Stanghellini 2000). Phenomenal characterisations of dysphoria mainly focus on its being felt as a burden, but a burden one cannot get rid of because it is not external to one's own self. It is an obstacle to movement and, at the same time, it may generate impatience, discontent, restlessness, and an incoercible impulse to move away without a definite goal. It is also experienced as unpleasant or uncomfortable feelings characterised both by being painful and sorrowful, as well as discontented and indignant. This complexity again elicits opposite kinds of movement: inaction/action, resignation/resistance, suffering/retaliation, and more generally, flowing forwards and upwards/flowing backwards and inwards. Because of these *dissoi logoi* (double meanings) of dysphoria, its psychological and psychopathological definition has long been (and still is) quite controversial. Some use this term to simply qualify bad mood, or even as an equivalent for depressed mood. A more precise definition of dysphoria as a symptom is: 'a feeling state of unpleasant, nervous tenseness, a limitation of emotional resonance to hostile responses, and increased readiness to aggressive acting out' (Berner et al. 1987, p. 97). As a result of this semantic stipulation, dysphoria can be distinguished from cognate symptoms such as a depressed or euphoric mood.

A dysphoric person is sulky, unsatisfied, morose. Additionally, dysphoria is often accompanied by irritability which can be defined as oversensitivity or irascibility leading to explosive and aggressive reactions. Stimuli of low intensity, or better stimuli that are evaluated by others as having low intensity, are ill-tolerated by irritable persons. Irritability and dysphoria are often associated with internal agitation. Accordingly, dysphoric persons often complain of feelings of tension and uneasiness. Dysphoria, irritability, and internal agitation form together a symptom-complex that in borderline persons is also accompanied by emotional lability, i.e. a marked emotional instability characterised by short-lived emotional states and large emotional fluctuations, and by hyper-emotionality, i.e. the abrupt emergence of uncontrollable emotional reactions disproportionate to the intensity of the stimulus.

Similar constructs are emotional dysregulation (Putnam and Silk 2005) and affective instability (Koenigsberg et al. 2002). Borderline persons have very intense baseline emotions, a tendency to respond to life-events and environmental triggers with unusually strong emotions; they rapidly shift from one emotion to another, and have serious problems in regulating them. Emotional dysregulation and affective instability are considered a trait dimension, allegedly a feature of some kind of biological vulnerability underlying borderline personality disorder, present before the onset of symptoms. So far, though, no one has been able to identify this biological correlate (Paris 2000).

It has also been proposed that 'irritability' (Akiskal and Mallya 1987), or the irritable variant of cyclothymia (Akiskal 1994), is the typical temperamental variant in persons with borderline personality disorder. Central to persons with irritable temperament is being moody, irritable, and choleric, with a general tendency to angry outbursts; they infrequently enjoy periods of euthymia, have a tendency to brood, being hypercritical and complaining, with a characteristic penchant for ill-humoured jokes; they are obtrusive, dysphorically restless, and impulsive. The dysphoric-irritable temperament is supposed to be the red thread that runs through the borderline condition (Stone 1988), and at its biological core 'the morose temperamentality of the irritable cyclothymic provides the unstable base from which interpersonal tempests arise' (Akiskal 1994, p. 35).

The dysphoric emotional complex (dysphoria, irritability, internal agitation, and emotional lability) is the background *mood trait* characterising persons with borderline personality disorder. It is the long-lasting and profound emotional tonality or basic affective temperament in which the borderline person is enmeshed, and as such it influences both the voluntary (selfhood) and involuntary aspect (otherness) of that person. Anger is the affective state that intermittently punctuates the existence of the borderline person. Angry outbursts, emanating from the dysphoric background, may generate acute micro-psychotic episodes during which borderline persons may develop paranoid symptoms, including transitory delusion-like and hallucination-like phenomena. We will in a later section analyse in more detail the switch from dysphoria to anger, and the way it entails the metamorphosis of the life-world that borderline persons live in. For the moment, we confine our discussion to the importance of considering dysphoria and anger as varieties of emotions which do not overlap with other cognate phenomena indigenous to mood spectrum disorders. But before doing so, we illustrate four other emotions that may have a special importance in the experience of borderline persons, namely, despair, boredom, shame, and guilt.

Commonsense psychology usually defines despair as hopelessness and desperation. A more precise characterisation of this emotion is provided by Tellenbach who emphasises the intimate relation between the concept of 'despair' ('*Verzweiflung*') and the notion of 'doubt' ('*Zweifel*') as disintegration of something simple and definitive into something ambiguous:

> [T]he crucial emphasis, as also in the concept of *doubt* [*Zweifel*], shifts to the 'two', to the doubling. This doubling [*Zweiheitliche*] is also contained in *dubietas* and *dubium*. What we call despair [*Verzweiflung*] is remaining captured in doubt. From the doubling of despair results all *average* meanings of human states characterized by being shattered [*Zerrissenheit*]. To be precise, despair is *not* just hopelessness and desperation, not an ultimate or an arrival at an endpoint, but rather the movement backward and forward, an alternation, so that a definite decision [*endgültige Entscheidung*] is no longer possible. (Tellenbach 1980, p. 165 [149]; translation modified)

As a consequence of the ambiguity, the person experiences ambivalent feelings in the sense of being simultaneously moved towards two opposite directions. She is aware of this contradiction, but is not able to resolve it. The core of despair is therefore indecision, and its contrary mental state is not hope, but decision. This understanding of despair, rooted in movement, assimilates this emotion to dysphoria in the sense that despair shares with dysphoria the generation of opposite kinds of movement. In despair, this opposition comes to an extreme which results in a profound alteration of temporality: '[w]hat previously came about in the mode of *succession*, now appears only in the necessity of *simultaneity*' (Tellenbach 1980, p. 167 [151]). The same happens with lived space. Whereas we usually organise our actions in the mode of succession, in despair movements remain stuck in the indecisiveness of juxtaposition, that is, a kind of paralysis of action and thinking, but not a static one, rather a frenzied, restless, disconcerting paralysis.

Boredom is a mood characterised by a pervasive lack of interest in everything. The entire world is monotonous, and this monotonousness cannot be analysed by the person into further elements, but encloses the surroundings, things as well as persons, in a vague and unarticulated way: the world as a whole 'seeps towards me from the globe like a cosmic fog, deadening my mind, slackening my will, and depleting me of energy' (Smith 1986, p. 191). Boredom is central among the feelings involved in the dysphoric mood experienced by borderline persons. It shares with dysphoria the same temporal structure (monotonousness) and an analogous feeling of bluntness. In boredom as well as in dysphoria the world, other people, and oneself *just happen* and are void of significance. In other words, one's mind goes blank.

Whereas boredom is a mood that stymies my mind and dulls my attention, shame, on the other hand, is an affect that awakens and focuses my attention. When I feel ashamed, I am aware of being seen by another person whose gaze uncovers a part of who I am, usually a part that makes me feel embarrassed, inadequate, dishonoured, and humiliated. The effect of shame is that it reduces the complexity of the person that I am to one single aspect of it: when I feel ashamed, I know that for the other I am *nothing but* that specific feature of the complexities of who I am. In shame, I feel that *I* (i.e. my whole self) disappear, while that detail—the *stain*—of my self that made me feel ashamed is magnified, becomes over-conspicuous and gets the front-stage. Shame reveals to me my selfhood as an object for another; or shame is, as Sartre writes, 'shame of *self* [*honte de soi*]; it is the *recognition* of the fact that I *am* indeed that object which the Other is looking at and judging. I can be ashamed only as my freedom escapes me in order to become a *given* object' (Sartre 1956, p. 261 [319]). Lived space in shame is arranged like a circle that surrounds and towers above me. The other persons are piercing gazes that nail me to what awakened my feeling of shame, that is, something, like an act or an omission, or some failing or defect, which elicited contempt, derision, or avoidance from other people. Shame means to be utterly exposed to the present, to the painful presence of devaluating gazes, to annihilating disdain and contempt (Fuchs 2003, pp. 227–30). Lived time in shame is confined to the present moment, since no narrative articulation of what made me feel ashamed is possible. Narrative articulation would incorporate the partial feature of my self which made me feel derisory and mortified, into a meaningful story, or would at least help me to explain and justify myself in front of the others. But the affect of shame freezes my history in one single, isolated, de-narratised humiliating event. Shame lowers the person's self-respect, and may entail either the person's wish to hide or disappear or, more positively (and rarely), attempts to reconstruct one's narrative identity or improve oneself (Williams 1993, pp. 80–4). Shame as an affective state may accompany or (more exactly) *trigger* anger during acute psychotic exacerbations of borderline pathology. Anger and shame are typically accompanied by resentment, rancour, indignation, narcissistic rage associated with feelings of humiliation. The mixture of anger and shame may trigger persecutory delusions, and especially those sensitive delusions of reference first described by Ernst Kretschmer and then by many others (Ballerini and Rossi Monti 1990; Kohut 1978; Kretschmer 1966). Kretschmer was the first to describe—and to characterise in emotional terms—a type of personality that he called the 'sensitive character' that may represent the paranoid-prone feature of borderline personality. These are persons who are thin-skinned and suspicious, and at the same time proud, ambitious, and obstinate. They are characterised, as Kretschmer writes, by 'their *yielding susceptibility to influence,* their *reactive wavering,* their *fluctuating sense of reality* [*Realitätswert*], their *tendency to independent amendment,* and their *associative parallels to obsession*' (1966, p. 112; our translation). They are, furthermore, vulnerable to developing a kind of delusion in which they feel observed and spied on so that everyone may know their secret fault and insufficiency; they also fear pursuit by some religious or civil authority. They may oscillate between feelings of guilt and of indignation. These delusional ideas are the sequel of a key experience of humiliating insufficiency, in particular moral or sexual defeats. Psychotic episodes like these are acute and transient and usually accompanied by excitement and mania-like symptoms. These episodes are sometimes misdiagnosed as manic states with mood-incongruent delusions. Indeed, the type of delusions that arise in them is congruent to the prevailing emotion, namely, an explosive mixture of anger and shame.

All types of delusions or delusion-like ideas occurring in borderline persons have an *ontic*, rather than ontological, character. They are about the basic concerns that characterise our daily existence, including our fears of being abandoned and mistreated, and for the way we appear to others and their opinion about what kind of person we are. This brings the kind of delusions exhibited by borderline persons very close to those that are typical in other 'affective' psychoses, like melancholia (i.e. psychotic depression, where the main themes are moral guilt, impoverishment, and hypochondria) and mania (delusions of grandeur like genealogical and mystical ones). Borderline persons are deluded about reality, whereas schizophrenic persons are deluded about the reality of reality (Stanghellini 2008). As we saw in the previous chapter, ontological delusions are typical in schizophrenic psychoses.

Finally, guilt is a moral feeling which typically arises when we think that we have in some way wronged another person. As such, it is the fundamental theme in those forms of major depression affecting the melancholic type of personality.[2] Depressive

---

[2] The concept of *typus melancholicus* (TM) was formed with the help of phenomenological analyses in order to describe the personality of endogenous depressives (Tellenbach 1980). In continental European and Japanese psychopathology, it has been instrumental to the understanding of the major depressives' pre-morbid and inter-morbid lifestyle, social behaviours, values and beliefs, precipitating situations, and acute clinical pictures (Mundt et al. 1996;

episodes in borderline persons, though, are not characterised by guilt feeling. Another kind of delusional theme, similar to the one developed by the sensitive character, is sometimes called 'persecutory guilt' (Grinberg 1964). Grinberg explains that guilt is implicitly contained in all experience of loss. This theory is based on psychoanalytic observations and supported by the etymology of the English verb 'to lose', deriving from Old English *losian* which means 'to perish' as well as 'to destroy', and Italian and French verbs '*perdere*' and '*perdre*', deriving from Latin *perdo*. The proportion of guilt determines the persecutory or depressive taint in the experience of loss. Persecutory guilt is the delusional theme whereby the patient feels persecuted for a fault he believes to have really committed, and especially for the loss of his moral integrity. Persons who develop persecutory guilt exhibit a mixture of guilt and shame. They feel guilty for what they have done, for instance, if they believe they harmed another person, and ashamed, because they have fallen short of what they might have hoped of themselves.[3]

We have now identified an emotional complex manifested by borderline persons, the core of which is composed of dysphoric mood as an enduring and permanent trait, and angry affect as an intermittent state. Usually dysphoria is accompanied by irritability,

---

Stanghellini and Mundt 1997). It has, furthermore, been established by empirical studies that the melancholic type of personality is present in over 50% of unipolar depressives, ranging from 30 to 70 cross-sectional prevalence (Fukunishi et al. 1993; Mundt et al. 1997; Nakanishi et al. 1993; Sato et al. 1992, 1993; Sauer et al. 1989; Tölle, 1987; von Zerssen and Possl 1990; von Zerssen et al. 1994, 1997), supporting the hypothesis that TM is typical of a majority of depressed patients, plausibly constituting a specific vulnerability factor. An accurate assessment of the TM personality features in depressed patients represents a crucial step in identifying personality-related liability to major unipolar depression and thus clarifying the way in which personality influences the presentation of symptoms (Stanghellini et al. 2006). According to Tellenbach (1980) and Kraus (1977) the TM personality is characterised by the person's need for meticulous organisation of his or her own life-world and the fixation on harmony in interpersonal relationships (orderliness); the commitment to prevent guilt-attributions and guilt-feelings (conscientiousness); an exaggerated norm adaptation and external norm receptiveness (hyper/hetero-nomia); and by the emotional and cognitive incapacity to perceive opposite characteristics concerning the same object or person (intolerance of ambiguity). Such core-properties of TM have been operationalised in the 'Criteria for Typus Melancholicus' and empirically showed to underpin a coherent personality structure rather than a dimensional concept or a construct made up of separate dimensions (Stanghellini and Bertelli 2006).

[3] As Bernard Williams writes: 'We can feel both guilt and shame towards the same action. In a moment of cowardice, we let someone down; we feel guilty because we have let them down, ashamed because we have contemptibly fallen short of what we might have hoped of ourselves. As always, the action stands between the inner world of disposition, feeling, and decision and an outer world of harm and wrong' (1993, p. 92). Immediately after describing this interrelation between guilt and shame, Williams goes on to remark that what I have done points in one direction towards what has happened to others, in another direction to what I am; in other words, guilt looks primarily in the direction of others, while shame affects my understanding of the person that I am.

internal agitation, and hyper-emotionality, and sometimes by boredom. Anger may be accompanied by shame, and kindle acute crises of rage entailing transitory paranoid delusions.[4] The mixture of shame and guilt, on the other hand, may trigger acute episodes entailing persecutory guilt.

Usually, mood spectrum disorders are classified under two main categories: depression and mania. The dysphoria-anger complex must be kept distinct from euphoric and depressed moods. We will now briefly outline the basic features of euphoric and depressed moods with the sole purpose to establish clear-cut demarcations between them and similar, but not at all overlapping, emotions occurring in borderline persons. Euphoric mood consists of an excessive feeling of well-being, pleasure, gaiety, confidence, and vital drive. Euphoric mood is typical of acute manic episodes during which euphoria is usually accompanied by hyperactivity, disinhibition, flight of ideas, and grandiose thought contents or delusion-like ideas. These patients are ready to react aggressively if thwarted. Some authors describe a three-stage severity of manic states (Carlson and Goodwin 1973; Goodwin and Jamison 2007). Stage I is dominated by elation. Here euphoria predominates, and irritability may supervene if demands are not satisfied. Ideation is expansive, grandiose, and overconfident. Thinking remains coherent although tangential. Stage II, on the other hand, exhibits increasing hyperactivity and arousal. Feelings become more labile, characterised by a mixture of euphoria and irritability, which may turn into open hostility and explosive and assaultive behaviour. Cognition becomes increasingly disorganised and thought contents turn from grandiose to paranoid. Finally, stage III is a delirium-like state in which feelings turn into a terrified state, behaviour is completely disorganised and cognition becomes incoherent. The phenomenal features of all these stages of mania, although they may include anger and dysphoria, are radically different from those of the micro-psychotic episodes in borderline persons described above. One example of this radical difference is shame and its cohort of related feelings (resentment, rancour, indignation, etc.). These feelings play, as we have seen, a fundamental role in borderline experience, but are not typical in stages II and III of mania.

Depressed mood is a complex emotional state which includes, at least, four principal features: feeling of prostration (as in lack of vital drive), loss of pleasure and interest (anhedonia), helplessness, and moral pain. Its first component, lack of vital drive, is a feeling of diminished vitality, freshness, physical and psychical integrity, strength, vigour, vivacity. This lack, in turn, entails feelings of prostration, dejection, despondency, exhaustion, feebleness, fatigue, physical malaise.

Anhedonia (the incapacity to feel pleasure) is considered a feature of emotional anaesthesia, i.e. a painful feeling of the loss of the capacity of feeling. The person complains of his emotional void and his loss of emotional resonance: 'I have no feeling, everything is dead inside me', 'I am no more able to be happy or sad'. The type of anhedonia exhibited by borderline persons is different from the one affecting patients who undergo depressive episodes arising from the melancholic type of personality

---

[4] For a description of these short-lived delusions in borderline persons, typically involving significant others like the clinician herself (transfer psychosis), see Rossi Monti (2008). The clinician is ascribed the identity of a perpetrator, the patients being his victim.

(Tellenbach 1980). First of all, anhedonia is typically absent in the melancholic type of personality when not undergoing depressive episodes. The melancholic type usually exhibits hyperthymic temperamental traits (Stanghellini et al. 2006), including sociability, hyperactivity, and overinvolvement, but not anhedonia. Moreover, anhedonia may be an accompanying feature of dysphoria in borderline persons, but in that case it typically has a hyperbolic character (Zanarini and Frankenburg 1997), since it triggers an escalation of behaviours that are meant to contrast it, the most prevalent being alcohol and drug abuse, turbulent erotic life, and self-mutilations, which are not characteristic of the melancholic type of personality. And finally, when anhedonia appears in borderline persons, it is usually a feature of a depressive episode ('atypical depression') and typically consists in a kind of irritating emptiness which oscillates between desperate feelings of abandonment and angry self- and other-destructive acting-outs.

It is of the utmost importance to characterise the kind of depressive episodes occurring in borderline persons. Several attempts have of course been made. Gunderson and Philips (1991), for instance, contrasted 'empty' depressions, in borderline persons, with 'guilt' depressions. The latter normally occur in the melancholic type of personality. The main features of depression in the melancholic type of personality (henceforth, with Tellenbach (1980), simply 'melancholia' or 'melancholic depression') are guilty feelings, lack of vital drive, and exacerbated experience of loss of emotional grasp and resonance. Usually these patients show very low rates of anger and dysphoria. They complain about their lack of emotional resonance with the others and the environment, and, most importantly, they feel guilty for this lack of emotional involvement. On the contrary, the depressive experience of borderline patients is imbued with a tense, irritated mood, higher proneness to externalise anger, resentment towards the environment, relatively high reactivity to environmental solicitations, and usually low levels of guilt feelings (Stanghellini et al. 2006).

Another difference between melancholic and borderline depressions is found in their embodied features. Embodiment in melancholic persons is dominated by the structure of overidentification. They feel that they are *nothing but* their body which is experienced as abnormally materialised and reified, heavy and rigid, devoid of emotions, energies, drives, and all kinds of vitality and conation. This loss of bodily elasticity and resonance implies painful sensations of derealisation (feelings of detachment from other persons and external reality). In borderline depressions, we do not find this overidentification of oneself with one's own body. Rather, one's own body, as the source of vitality and conation, is felt as distant from oneself and out of voluntary control, lying somewhere between self and non-self—the land of otherness.[5]

An important feature that can help to disentangle borderline from melancholic depression is the kind of situation which generates each of them. Normally, the depressive decomposition of the melancholic type is triggered by experiences of *loss*, which she construes as *her own* wrong behaviour, whereas the borderline person is sensible to

---

[5] For the characterisation of the notion of otherness, see in particular Chapters 2, 3, and 6. The relevance of the notion of otherness, as developed in these chapters, to the life-world of the borderline person, will be a major theme in our interpretation of this psychopathological condition in the rest of this chapter.

experiences of *abandonment*, which he construes as wrong behaviour on the part of *the other person*.

To sum up, the dysphoria-anger emotional complex is radically different from the phenomena characterising manic-depressive spectrum disorders arising in non-borderline types of personality. This has important psychopathological as well as nosographical implications. Depressed moods, and especially the feelings of loss of feeling, imbued by guilt feelings, are the key features exhibited in melancholic depressions, while the kind of depression which usually develops out of borderline personality disorder is typically characterised by feelings of emptiness, irritation, and proneness to angry acting-outs. Acute episodes of excitement in borderline persons only superficially resemble 'pure' manic states. The latter are typically characterised by euphoric mood and mood-congruent grandiose delusions which are not present in the borderline's excitements. Moreover, although irritability is often present in stage I and anger in stage II of manic episodes, we hardly find here the mixture of anger, shame, resentment, rancour, indignation, humiliation, and the typical transitory paranoid phenomena characterising the borderline person's acute crisis.[6]

Lived Time, Other Persons, and Otherness

This and the following two sections will focus on a central feature of the clinical phenomenology of borderline persons, namely, the issue of lived time. Before we turn to unearthing the way the borderline person experiences himself, other people, material things, and the space in which they are immersed, we will start with an outline and discussion of three seminal contributions that help introduce the topic of the borderline life-world through a characterisation of the patients' lived temporality.

Once again, Bin Kimura (1992) provides, perhaps in greater detail than most, a description of lived time in persons affected by severe mental disorders. The clinical cases of mental disorders, he writes, show us that there are different ways of living time. Accurate phenomenological analyses show that different personality types exhibit specific anomalies of temporalisation. Patients may be unaware, or only partially aware, of such anomalies, since these need not be part of their conscious experience. Nonetheless, disorders of lived time become explicitly manifest in the ways people think, hope, live their present, remember their past, and project their future. His research, focusing mainly on severe disorders such as schizophrenia, manic-depressive psychoses, and borderline personality, is meant to establish that the way patients live time is of the outmost significance, both for anthropological (the existence of a person) and nosological

---

[6] Investigations into acute episodes of this kind have in some cases demonstrated high intra-episodic (persistence of the same symptom along the same episode) and inter-episodic (recurrence of the same symptom in subsequent episodes) occurrence of the anger-dysphoria complex (Gabriel 1987, Musalek et al. 1987). These findings are taken as indices of the nosographical distinction between depression, mania, and a third syndrome characterised by anger-dysphoria, as well as emblematic of the tripolarity (instead of bipolarity) of mood spectrum disorders (Berner et al. 1992).

purposes (the pathology of a person). Lived time is, so to say, the psychological and psychopathological fingerprint of these patients.

The borderline person, he writes, is absorbed in an unmediated instantaneity. By instantaneity he means a *pure* or *absolute now* devoid of past and future. Here he follows Husserl in defining 'retention' as the past as it is intentionally contained in the present, and 'protention' as the future as it is anticipated in the present, so that when both retention and protention are functioning, the present moment retains an implicit sense of both past and future. This is not the case for the borderline person, to whom *now*'s are pure presentification, lacking protention and retention. Presenting themselves independently from past and future, one cannot measure the 'length' of these nows, as it is possible with a present that develops out of the past and is directed towards the future. Each *now* thus becomes an infinity that in some sense 'communicates with eternity' (Kimura 1992, p. 150). This kind of absolute now has no temporal delimitation, no historical determination, and no linguistic-symbolic articulation. This isolated, ineffable, and absolute now is not able to carry any kind of relation to, or become an integrated part of, the narrative identity of a person. This type of temporality, which characterises the existence of borderline persons, is called by Bin Kimura *intra festum*. As in the atmosphere of a feast, here we find the irruption of spontaneity and ecstasy, oblivious of the past and the future. Blind spontaneity is the opposite of voluntary autonomy as the rapture of ecstasy is the opposite of engaged care. Moreover, borderline persons are unable to cope with the flux of immediateness, and this flux becomes paroxysmal, and immediateness chaotic. The borderline personality, immersed in the *intra festum*, is characterised by a short-circuit of selfhood in front of the paroxysm of chaotic immediateness. The absolute now is the night of the self and the disintegration of personhood, since continuity in time is fundamental for a self to be an integral part of the person that he or she is.

Kimura suggests that in borderline temporality there is no separation, no space in between the *now* and the person. On the contrary, the now-experience and the person are one:

> The general rule is that there is 'an absorption in immediateness'. The borderline patient absorbs himself in the immediate presence of the objects and does not try to establish, between himself and his objects, any relation, any *aïda* connecting independent entities. He does not try to go past this immediateness and to see beyond another person or another thing as the other side of difference (*aïda*), as something different from himself or, which is quite the same, to oppose himself to it as an independent subjective entity. This immediateness in which he finds himself is so to say an indifferent space, empty of all moments of negation; a negation which would be necessary for him in order to be able to transcend himself as a self [*Soi-même*] and individualise himself.
>
> (Kimura 1992, p. 109; our translation)

To understand this passage, and in general Kimura's ideas on the relationship between instantaneity (in time) and immediateness (of experience), it is necessary to clarify his conception of *aïda* (Kimura 2000), which could be translated as the 'in-between' (which is also the choice of the French translator, namely, *l'entre*), including not merely the space that stays in the middle, or the distance that separates two things. Rather, the *aïda* is a noetic (i.e. intentional) act which without mediation connects to other people and the source of life in oneself.

The *aïda* is the principle through which subjectivity is constituted. As the origin of subjectivity, Kimura poses what he calls the inter-subjective *aïda*, that is, the inter-subjective world as the ground and the first step of the development of the self. The discovery of a self in the other that defies my understanding is the prerequisite for my discovering in myself an-other, or an otherness, that remains unknown to me. The other-than-myself makes me discover the other-in-myself, or (which is the same) the inter-subjective *aïda* makes me discover the intra-subjective *aïda*.

In discovering otherness in myself, Kimura argues, I discover in myself an 'infinite interiority'. This is an 'amorphous' and untamed presence that I find in myself. It is a spontaneous vitality. Since this vitality is a *disordered* vitality, I feel it as a menace to my autonomy, i.e. to self-organisation. An infinite interiority is an 'impossibility' for the conscious self. It is felt as a threat by the self since it is unmanageable in its immediateness. But it is also, as the source of vitality, a vital force that we cannot renounce. To limit this danger, the self posits this infinite interiority as a finite interiority, or (which is the same) as *exteriority*. By becoming exteriority, this infinite interiority—this otherness or spontaneous vitality—can be managed and noematically represented.[7] Language can limit the power of infinite interiority, turning it into an object: 'Experience thus loses its immediacy through the mediation that it receives in language. Almost nothing in our everyday life remains of the immediate experience anterior to language' (1992, p. 130; our translation). Through the *mediating power of language* infinite interiority is confined to being an *object* of consciousness. Kimura goes on to explain how this limiting of our infinite interiority by language is what makes my selfhood unstable. My feeling of being me is disturbed by my feeling of the otherness that I am:

> Our everyday experience is already virtually determined through and through by the structure of the language. At the moment of reflective awareness the certainty of the sensible immediateness has already lost its immediacy and is mediated by the negation and thus opening the breach which contains the difference. Even *I* [*moi*], which apparently seems the most immediately given when it becomes conscious of itself as an 'I', is likewise constituted as an experience mediated by a negative differentiation. This differentiation is inserted between the 'I' in the process of becoming conscious and the 'I' of which one is conscious. That is, between the immediate experience of 'I' and the 'I' susceptible of explication in language, which to the immediate 'I' is nothing but the non-I [*n'est que le non-moi pour le moi immédiat*].
>
> (Kimura 1992, p. 132; our translation)

Kimura's analysis of the existence of borderline persons as the pathology of immediateness provides the coordinates to discuss a problem that is central in the clinical phenomenology of this disorder: the relationships between temporalisation, otherness (in the double sense of the other person and the otherness I discover in myself), and

---

[7] Kimura writes: 'the noematic images we have of the world are the traces of a pre-conscious noetic act'. And immediately after he specifies that, 'the noematic representations have as their function to recognize and control the [noetic] acts' (2000, pp. 86–7; our translation).

the fabric of the self, as this is observed in reflection and through the symbolic function of language and narrative. Kimura thus introduces us to these problems with which we will try to engage in the following sections.

Invalidation Trauma

In *Intimacy and Alienation* (2000), psychiatrist Russell Meares develops a theory of the pathogenesis of borderline personality disorder which includes an accurate description of the anomalies of self and temporalisation, connecting them with the issue of the *traumatic other* characterising these persons' existence. His principal claim is that the symptoms of borderline personality disorder can be best explained as the consequence of a splitting of the stream of consciousness deriving from a kind of traumatic experiences whose main feature is invalidation.

The fabric of the self as conceived by Meares is a delicate one. The development of a cohesive and continuous sense of self depends upon a special form of conversation. A non-linear, associative, and apparently purposeless form of dialogue, whose topic may at first glance seem banal. It is like a game, since it is apparently aimless. Or like an atmosphere, because it can be extremely difficult to answer questions about what is actually going on here or what we are really talking about. Intimacy is the basic emotion involved in this kind of conversation. Intimacy, Meares explains, is not to be equated to confession or incontinent revelation. Rather, it is the feelings in which this special kind of conversation is embedded, such as having a peculiar warmth or a form associated with a sense of well-being. Intimacy fundamentally depends upon the sharing of one's own inner experience with another. An intimate conversation is associated with a heightened feeling of being 'myself'. Thus, 'myself' develops extra-personally, in an early form of conversation in the sense of a particular form of relationship whose main characteristic is a special kind of emotion characterised as intimacy. In intimacy, I feel that the other person is attuned to my inner world; I feel that he recognises my inner life as valuable (Meares 2000, pp. 121–5).

The integrity of the self can be damaged by traumatic experience. The kind of trauma at issue here is not sexual abuse or some form of violent behaviour, but rather takes the form of an invalidating environment. An invalidating environment is one in which communication of private experiences is not met by appropriate responses. Instead of being validated, private experiences are trivialised, their expression is discouraged, and emotions (especially painful emotions) are disregarded. The kind of trauma that may jeopardise the development of a warm and intimate sense of self is the absence of *recognition*. One's sense of existence, then, goes on over a potential void:

> The threat of this void hangs over those whose development of self has been damaged by a traumatic environment. The mental activity underpinning the stream of consciousness seems barely developed. Self is stunted and fragile. At times it may vanish, leaving a static, painful, even frightening, vacancy, often described as a 'black hole'.
>
> (Meares 2000, p. 10)

The person is left with the experience of an internal void, of being no one—feeling the loss of his *own* value. Feelings of discontinuity over time, of inner emptiness, and a fragile sense of being 'myself' are indeed the principal symptoms of borderline personality disorder. Meares mainly focuses on the anomalies of temporalisation in these patients.[8]

These persons, he says, live in a restricted temporal horizon and are scarcely aware of a future or a past. There are three main aspects to this. First, borderline persons are frequently affected by rapid mood swings. They appear changeable, inconstant, voluble, 'moody', often prey to anger attacks (as we discussed in detail earlier in this chapter). Second, these persons are trapped in present stimuli so that their conversation is often a mere catalogue of recent events. Their awareness is captivated by the present moment, as if they were unable to ignore or switch off the stimuli that are coming from the environment or from their own body. These sensations may appear trivial, irrelevant or meaningless to an external observer, but for borderline patients themselves they are abnormally important and amplified. This phenomenon cannot be explained as abnormal arousal, as it is the case with anxious patients. The third feature of discontinuity of borderline personal existence analysed by Meares includes what he calls the 'traumatic system'. He explores the form and feeling of the self when it is disrupted in a traumatic way. From time to time, a system of traumatic memories intrudes into the stream of consciousness. These memories are not experienced as such, but as located in the present moment. The intrusion of this system of traumatic memory is alienating. It implies a disruption of the continuous movement of the stream of consciousness:

> These experiences are felt in the totality of self, which includes the body. In a state of alienation and disconnectedness, body feeling may change so that alterations occur in its rhythms, its 'smoothness', its density and shape. The individual may feel so insubstantial that he or she could be blown away by the wind.
>
> (Meares 2000, p. 57)

Usually, when a memory arises in the stream of consciousness, one is aware of the present moment and at the same time aware of a different domain of experience which belongs to the past. It is a blend of past and present, in which past and present can be distinguished. When the traumatic system irrupts into the mental life of borderline persons, this 'doubleness' is lost. The past experience is felt as entirely located in the present. Past experiences are stored in such a way that they cannot be acknowledged and processed as past feelings, thoughts, perceptions, etc. They intrude into consciousness as parts of the present, intermittently overthrowing the ongoing sense of personal being. According to Meares (pp. 90–2), perceptive distortions, for instance, hallucination-like phenomena that may occasionally occur in the course of borderline personality disorder, are a consequence of this.

We think that Meares's clinical study pinpoints an essential feature of the fabric of the human self that is missing in the life story of borderline persons. This is the issue of the other's recognition, which is missing in the circumstances that Meares calls the

---

[8] His descriptions of the metamorphosis of lived space is not convincing, since the case on which it is based, a self-description of the English protean writer Rebecca West, is probably better diagnosed as a delirious, psycho-organic psychosis (pp. 58–61).

invalidating trauma. My concern for the other originates in a lack in my own existence that generates a need for a dialogical coexistence with the other. We do not need the other merely as a means to satisfy our own desires. This need for others drastically affects the value I attach to myself. When the other person addresses me 'in the second person, I feel I am implicated in the first person' (Ricoeur 1992, p. 193 [225]); in Part I, we saw that selfhood is not constituted solely of mineness, since, as Ricoeur said, '[t]o say self is not to say myself' (1992, p. 180 [212]). The other person is fundamental to my own sense of being a self, to my self-esteem, and to my identity, because the world is a shared world whose meaning is, for a major part, constituted by the coexistence of different persons. *My identity as a person depends on the other's recognition of my being so.* The unity and coherence of my various actions with respect to the idea of myself as an individual person is deeply influenced by the reception of these actions by other persons—and this process is embedded in a special kind of intimate conversation during which I recognise the *other as a oneself* and the *oneself as an other* (Ricoeur 1992, p. 194 [226]). Meares's argument on this point is very close to the importance Kimura attributes to the interpersonal *aïda* in the constitution of the self, but compared to Kimura he adds a very important element. He sets the fabric of the self in an emotional atmosphere, since to him intimacy is a prerequisite for a mature self to develop, i.e. a self at ease in dialoguing with itself. Of course, this is also an extremely relevant point with respect to the issue of care. As we shall see in the next section, the presence of the other (and of intimacy) as a companion for my inner conversations is a prerequisite for the *temporal continuity* of my narrative identity.

Temporal Fragmentation and Narrative Identity

In this section, we shall discuss Thomas Fuchs's interpretation of the borderline person's temporal fragmentation (2007). As Meares did in his interpretation of the temporal splitting of the borderline person's self, Fuchs emphasises the centrality of interpersonal relationships in the pathogenesis of the borderline type of existence. He argues that the temporal fragmentation of the self is a way to avoid the necessity of tolerating the threatening ambiguity and uncertainty of interpersonal relationships. He also suggests that the increasing prevalence of the disorder may, at least in part, be attributed to the development of a mainly externally driven, fragmented character of post-modern society, whose main features, such as the acceleration of momentary events, the mobility of work life, the futility of communication, the fragility of relationships, the receding loyalty and commitment, overlap with the borderline type of existence.

As we have learnt from Kimura, borderline persons live unhistorically, bound to the stake of the present moment and not knowing about past or future. Their life is an unconnected series of fleeting events, instead of a continuous history. They are characterised by a peculiar atemporal mode of existing, switching from one present to the next, identifying totally with their momentary state of mind, torn by emerging wishes and impulses which flare up and vanish again. They suffer from a temporal splitting of the self which excludes past and future. They are unable to gain a distance from the present situation. Instead of projecting themselves into the future, they just *stumble* into it. They *are* only what they are experiencing at this moment, in an often intense, and yet excruciatingly empty and flat present. In spite of their constant struggle to create a 'world of feasts' or *intra festum*, borderline persons do not live in simple happiness. Rather, they often describe lasting feelings of dysphoria, emptiness, and boredom. The reason for this is that their transitory present has no depth. It lacks the fulfilment which only originates from the integration of past experience and anticipated future. Fuchs equates this atemporal mode of existence of the borderline persons to a *defence mechanism* in a psychodynamic sense: instead of repression, their means of defence consists in a temporal splitting of the self that excludes past and future as dimensions of object constancy, commitment, responsibility and identity. Thus, borderline individuals exhibit what may be called a '*fragmentation of the narrative self* (Fuchs 2007, p. 381).

In repression, one part of the self is discarded, and the only way it can express itself is by means of dreams, parapraxes (such as slips of the tongue and of the pen, mislaying, and misreading), and symptoms. In borderline persons, the ego is totally identified with *one* part or tendency for a period of time; the *other* part only lies dormant temporarily, not repressed, and may pop up at any time, now seemingly conforming to the ego just like the opposite part before. The temporal fragmentation of the self, Fuchs argues, avoids the necessity of tolerating the threatening ambiguity and uncertainty of interpersonal relationships. The price, however, consists in a chronic feeling of inner emptiness caused by the inability to integrate past and future into the present and, thus, to establish a coherent sense of identity.

Fuchs reads the borderline person's fragmentation of the narrative self in the light of the analyses of personal identity found in Frankfurt (1971) and Ricoeur (1992, pp. 113–39 [137–66]), the latter of which we discussed in detail in the first part of this book. Borderline persons are unable to form what Frankfurt calls 'second-order volitions', and are committed to 'first-order desires'. Only by forming overarching and enduring volitions, a person is able to endorse a particular set of first-order desires and voluntarily dismiss (or involuntarily repress) others. Being ruled only by their momentary impulses, i.e. first-order desires, borderline persons lack an essential feature of being a person, namely autonomy. Thus, apparently, the mode of existence of borderline persons is not just a defence in a strict sense, but a kind of necessity entailed by these persons' *lack of the strength* to establish a coherent personal identity through a labour of temporal integration.

Temporal integration and narrative identity, as we know, are closely intertwined. Narrative identity implies a meaningful coherence of the personal past, present, and future. This meaningful coherence is not already there. Rather, it is the product of an enduring labour striving to make one's life coherent and to fill it with meaningful behaviour. Narrative identity is different from mere constancy or sameness, since it is a temporal relation to oneself—in view of the continuing task of becoming the person that one is—by remaining faithful to one's commitments, promises, and responsibilities in front of other people (Ricoeur's 'keeping one's word' 1992, p. 118 [143]). It also requires the capacity of self-determination by forming durable second-order volitions, at the price, if necessary, of repression or neurosis. In the existence of borderline persons we find no consistent endeavour to do this. They lack the capacity to form enduring second-order volitions, in the light of which present impulses could be evaluated and selected.

An important point of Fuchs's discussion is that the capacity to establish a coherent narrative identity is 'essentially based on the presence of an implicit other who would understand our actions and projects, to whom we could tell our life story' (2007, p. 383). This implicit presence of the other presupposes early experiences of secure attachment to relevant others. In the case of the existence of a borderline person, as we have seen with Meares's ideas on invalidation trauma, an implicit other with whom one can share an 'intimate conversation', as well as a secure pattern of attachment, is radically lacking.

The hypothesis that the temporal splitting of the self in borderline persons is a defence against the ambiguity and uncertainty of personal relationships, as it is partly endorsed by Fuchs in his paper, is not entirely convincing to us. Also, it does not seem so convincing to Fuchs himself, since in another part of the paper he argues that the reason for this temporal splitting is that borderline persons 'lack the strength to establish a coherent self-concept' (2007, p. 381). This is quite another way of seeing it, consistent with Ricoeur's analysis of temporality. Remember that Ricoeur characterises human time as 'third-time' (1988, p. 245 [441]). This is time configured both by what affects the self involuntarily and by how the self acts voluntarily on it. These two aspects come together in narrative identity (1988, p. 246 [442]). On the one hand, we are affected by time through the involuntary events of our life, including our emotions, random thoughts, ideas, and impulses. On the other, we ourselves bring about time when we seek to understand our experiences and integrate them into our personal lifestory. Thus, the third-time, or human time, is time as it is narrated with reference to the identity of the person who speaks about and in time. Third-time is not merely implicit, passive, and involuntarily constituted. Rather, it is a reality *to-be-built* and thus requires some kind of strength or effort. Implicit, pre-reflective time is fragmented. It is time as it is passively constituted in the implicit dynamics linking the present moment with protention and retention. The narrative sense of time, the time of personhood, on the other hand, needs an effort to be actively, reflectively constituted through the constant dialectic of selfhood and otherness.

A prerequisite for this effort to be carried out, and to be effective, is the presence of an implicit other that helps to define and keep coherent one's own self over time: an *interlocutor,* in the sense of a person who engages in this intimate conversation. An additional reason for the borderline person's deficient narrative identity, as appropriately observed by Fuchs, may be seen in the absence of this companion in one's inner conversation as someone to whom we could tell our life story and with whom we could compare and possibly share memories and experiences. The failure to sustain intimate social relationships will thus lead to a precarious sense of identity (Wilkinson-Ryan and Westen 2000).[9]

---

[9] Clearly, this theory reverses the standard view which sees problems in interpersonal relationships as consequences of emotional dysregulation. In the present theory, problems in regulating emotions are interpreted as the consequence of difficulties in contextualising one's emotions and in organising them into a coherent narrative pattern, and these difficulties are seen as consequences of the failure to establish an intimate dialogue with another person.

The presence of a traumatic system involves some kind of interpersonal as well as temporal fragmentation, as we shall see in detail in the next sections. In the present section and the two preceding ones, we have tried to show how the inter-subjective and intra-subjective lives are deeply intertwined, that is, how the development of stable and reliable ways of being-with-others are relevant to establishing effective modes of being-with-oneself which the 'third-time' of narrative identity can deploy. We suggest that the disproportion between the fragmentation of implicit time entailed by the traumatic system, and the strength of will needed to restore an explicit temporal continuity through an actively constituted narrative identity, is the key for understanding the borderline person's split temporality.

Otherness Lost and Found

The existence of borderline persons exhibits prolonged states dominated by dysphoric mood. This is a noetically full and noematically empty emotional state, characterised by brimming constellations of feelings, a state of tension which may lead to 'impulsive' outbursts as well as to standstill and stagnation; an enduring, though precarious, condition of desperate vitality which contains the seeds of creativity as well as destruction. Intermittently, borderline persons enter acute episodes of excitement in which anger may prevail. Ontic persecutory delusions may develop out of these episodes, in which the persecutor is typically a significant other (the patient's partner, relative, or therapist). Alternatively, they may collapse into acute episodes during which dysphoric mood exacerbates, culminating in a painful paralysis of action characterised by feelings of emptiness, boredom, dissatisfaction; a mixture of, or a rapid oscillation between, dysphoric mood and more focused affects like disgust, fear, and anger (concerning oneself or others). This may entail tormenting ideas of meaninglessness, persecutory guilt, and, in the most severe cases, suicidal ideation.

The purpose of this and the following sections is to provide a description of the life-world inhabited by borderline persons, and to document the shift between the kind of lived worlds enacted alternatively by dysphoria and anger. To guide us through the fragmented world of the borderline person, we have chosen Sarah Kane's last play *4.48 Psychosis* (Kane 2001, pp. 203–45). It is a drama about suicide that tries to represent intense human despair, written by a dramatist who took her own life shortly after completing it (Saunders 2002, pp. 109–10). The lines from this play may serve as an unsettling red thread running through the troubled world of the borderline person. In particular, they can be read as a compassionate and disturbing description of the state of dysphoric depression:

> I am sad
> I feel that the future is hopeless and that things cannot improve
> I am bored and dissatisfied with everything
> I am a complete failure as a person
> I am guilty, I am being punished
> I would like to kill myself
> I used to be able to cry but now I am beyond tears
> I have lost interest in other people

I can't make decisions
I can't eat
I can't sleep
I can't think
I cannot overcome my loneliness, my fear, my disgust
I am fat
I cannot write
I cannot love
My brother is dying, my lover is dying, I am killing them both
I am charging towards my death
I am terrified of medication
I cannot make love
I cannot fuck
I cannot be alone
I cannot be with others
My hips are too big
I dislike my genitals
At 4.48
when desperation visits
I shall hang myself
to the sound of my lover's breathing

(Kane 2001, pp. 206–7)

These lines are part of 'a report from a region of the mind that most of us hope never to visit but from which many people cannot escape' (Grieg 2001, p. xvii), telling about 'the fragility of love' and 'the search for selfhood' (Saunders 2002, p. 113). What is it like to inhabit this region of the mind? How does it feel to be a person living in it? How does a person who dwells in it live her own body? Are the others friendly or hostile? What is the physiognomy of the surrounding things? How are others and things located in space? And events distributed in time?

At the heart of Kane's drama, as in the existence of borderline persons, resides the excruciating experience of the other. The main concern of the borderline person is 'to receive attention/to be seen and heard/to excite, amaze, fascinate, shock, intrigue, amuse, entertain or entice others' (Kane 2001, p. 234).[10] Also, to avoid pain and shame, repress fear, maintain self-respect; all this is needed to overcome past traumatic experiences, 'to obliterate past humiliation by resumed action' (p. 234). The other is indispensable for living: 'I go out at six in the morning and start my search for you' (p. 214). It is needed as a *source of recognition*: 'Validate me/Witness me/See me/Love me' (p. 243). The absence of the other makes the presence of the self impossible. The other is absent when she is not totally present. Her absence, or incomplete presence, is often the reason of feelings of non-recognition and desperate loss of selfhood: 'I'm dying for one who doesn't care/I'm dying for one who doesn't know' (p. 243). Here, the absent other is nothing but an abandoning other. The other who does not donate her entire self is an inauthentic other: 'And while I was believing that you were different and that you

---

[10] If not otherwise specified, the quotations are from Kane (2001). To distinguish Kane's quotations from phrases taken from patients the latter are written in italics.

maybe even felt the distress that sometimes flickered across your face and threatened to erupt, you were covering your arse too. Like every other stupid mortal cunt./To my mind that's betrayal' (p. 210). The other is also the source of aching shame, since her gaze is permanently on the razor's edge between recognition (*If he sees me, then I exist, at least for him*) and humiliation (*He watches me because he despises me*): 'Watching me, judging me [. . .] I gape in horror at the world and wonder why everyone is smiling and looking at me with secret knowledge of my aching shame/Shame shame shame./Drown in your fucking shame' (p. 209).

The values that are at play in the interpersonal world of borderline persons are directed to achieve apparently standard (but in fact unattainable) goals like 'to belong/ to be accepted/to draw close and enjoyably reciprocate with another/to converse in a friendly manner, to tell stories, exchange sentiments, ideas, secrets/to communicate, to converse/to laugh and make jokes' (pp. 234–5). These goals are felt by borderline persons as standard, basic aspirations of what, with Meares, we may call intimacy ('*If you think this is asking too much, doctor, then you are like all the others!*')—but these aspirations are often unrealistic and almost unattainable. More intimate, personal values are also entailed in the borderline person's ideal of being with the others:

> to win affection of desired Other
> to adhere and remain loyal to Other
> to enjoy sensuous experiences with cathected Other
> to feed, help, protect, comfort, console, support, nurse or heal
> to be fed, helped, protected, comforted, consoled, supported, nursed or healed
> to form mutually enjoyable, enduring, cooperating and reciprocating relationship with Other, with an equal
> to be forgiven
> to be loved
> to be free
>
> (Kane 2001, p. 235)

As if this interminable list of expectations was not enough, the bonds of loyalty and the promise of reciprocal care must be accompanied by its antonym, namely, spontaneity, that is, being free from social conventions and acting according to the vital impulses of the present moment: 'to be free from social restrictions/to resist coercion and constriction/to be independent and act according to desire/to defy convention' (p. 234).

Feelings of admiration and irritation mix together while reading these lines, exactly as it happens while listening to borderline persons. One can be fascinated by their absolute, uncontaminated vitality, and disturbed by their stubborn, ruinous *naïveté*. An unarmed, individualistic kind of rebellion that will surely lead to self-destruction: 'Every man worthy of this name/has in his heart a yellow serpent/Installed as if upon a throne,/Who if he says "I will" answers "No!"' (Baudelaire 1951, p. 240; our translation).[11] With these lines,

---

[11] 'Tout homme digne de ce nom/A dans le cœur un Serpent jaune,/Installé comme sur un trône,/Qui, s'il dit: «Je veux,» répond: «Non!»' (Baudelaire 1951, p. 240).

from *L'Avertisseur*, Baudelaire attests the rebellion of the poets as an epiphany of humanity, and thus inaugurates the fragmented condition of the modern person. Modern identity is held in check between two fires: on one side, an identity ever more swallowed up by the disorder of the interior world of affections and drives, on the other, a social role charmed by the conventions and decorum of urban life. The troubled person, embedded in a society which demands individualism but discourages being coherent with one's own personal identity, may try to find cohesion in indignation, if not liberation in rebellion (Stanghellini 2000). As Sarah Kane herself admitted:

> In order to function, you have to cut out at least one part of your mind. Otherwise you'd be chronically sane in a society which is chronically insane [. . .] Go mad and die, or function but be insane.
>
> (Saunders 2002, p. 114)

Cutting out a part of one's mind so as not to go mad and die. This is a compromise which borderline persons can hardly make in their life. The part of one's mind one should cut out, Kane explains, is a special kind of sensibility, 'of ability to feel and perceive' (Saunders 2002, p. 114). The other in borderline existence, first and foremost, appears as dim and fuzzy (as we will shortly demonstrate through the words of our patients), and yet the very same other remains a prerequisite for being a self and establishing a narrative identity (as we explained in the preceding sections, and as it is evident through Sarah Kane's words). Remember that a necessary condition for being a self is *becoming a person* in and through the presence of another person that enables one to feel oneself and stay coherent with one's sense of self over time. Hence, the failure of an intimate relationship leads to breakdown of one's sense of identity. The reason for the impossibility of this compromise can be articulated as a practical syllogism: a reliable other, someone to trust, is needed for me to exist as a person, to survive; to establish if he is reliable I can only trust my feelings; if I renounce my sensibility, I renounce life itself.

Another reason for the borderline person's incapacity to renounce her sensibility is that she cannot perceive the other as a social role, that is, as an external representative of identity. To give a very simple example, if a patient focuses on my social role then for him I am a doctor. If, on the other hand, he focuses on my identity as a person, I am a person with my own life story, values, emotions, and so on. Social roles are mainly established and consolidated through the symbolic use of language, and we have seen that in borderline existence there is an excess of noetic intentionality or 'pure' feelings with respect to noematic representation. Moreover, borderline persons feel overt distrust towards social norms and conventions, and social roles are part of these. Consequently, they cannot establish if someone is reliable or not according to the way (appropriate or inappropriate) he performs his social role. The only way that remains to ascertain the other's dependability is via one's emotional sensibility. Here surfaces another, tremendous problem, since the way the other appears in the course of the borderline person's existence is constantly changing due to the influence of his emotions.

We have seen that the other in the life-world of borderline persons oscillates between opposite polarities: a hoped-for source of selfhood through recognition, but also of humiliation and thus of disunion and despair; a partner from whom both loyalty and spontaneity are expected. Another essential feature of the antinomies of otherness in borderline existence is the double appearance of the other as a dim and fuzzy person or as a tenebrous and suspect one. As Sarah Kane powerfully portrays it, the others are at one moment 'expressionless faces staring blankly at my pain'; and immediately after, a tenebrous individual 'so devoid of meaning there must be evil intent' (p. 209). This instability in the appearance of the other is in synchrony with the drastic fluctuation of feelings, and more specifically with the swing between dysphoric mood and angry affect. In the penumbra of dysphoria, the other may appear as the a mere shadow. To use the words spoken by the patients themselves, the other is experienced as indefinite, indeterminate, indistinct, ill-defined ('*Most of the times they are out of focus*'; '*I can't grasp their physiognomy and what they mean to me*'). All these qualities that the borderline person perceives unmediated in the other persons express in semi-sensorial terms the unintelligibility of the other. The indefiniteness of the other is the norm in borderline existence, and it worsens in acute dysphoric-depressive episodes during which the other may become lightless and opaque: fuzzy, blurred, caliginous, cloudy, foggy, gray, hazy ('*When I feel bad the others become misty, shadowy*'; '*They are in a dim light*'). When the dysphoric mood turns into anger, the other changes from being opaque to being tenebrous: he is ambivalent, evasive, obscure, puzzling, unexplicit, and suspect ('*You are ambiguous, doctor! I don't trust you anymore!*'; '*You don't have the spunk to tell me the truth!*'). This paves the way to persecutory delusions ('*Why don't you say explicitly you want to harm me!*').

Indignation, Resignation, and Retaliation

A similar shift happens in the way borderline persons perceive their own self. Identity disturbance is one of the criteria for the diagnosis of borderline personality disorder in DSM-IV. The major theoretical and clinical descriptions of identity confusion in borderline personality disorder come from the psychoanalytic literature.[12] According to Kernberg (1984), identity diffusion in borderline patients reflects their inability to integrate positive and negative representations of the self and the other. The result is a shifting view of the self, with sharp discontinuities, rapidly shifting roles (e.g. victim and victimiser, dominant and submissive), and a sense of inner emptiness. Wilkinson-Ryan and Westen (2000) empirically demonstrated that identity disturbance in borderline personality disorder is characterised by a painful sense of incoherence, objective inconsistencies in beliefs and behaviours, overidentification with groups or roles, and, to a lesser extent, difficulties with commitment to jobs, values, and goals.

Our concern, here, is to show how this shifting view of the self is related to variations of other components of the life-world, namely otherness, lived time, body, and in general the physiognomic appearance of the outside world; and, moreover, how all these variations are related to intense oscillations in feelings: 'I will drown in dysphoria/in the

---

[12] For example, Erikson (1968) defined 'identity confusion' as a subjective sense of incoherence, difficulty committing to roles and occupational choices, along with a tendency to confuse one's own attributes, feelings, and desires with those of another person in intimate relationships, hence, to fear a loss of personal identity when a relationship dissolves.

cold black pond of my self/the pit of my immaterial mind/How can I return to form/ now my formal thought has gone?' (Kane 2001, p. 213). Dysphoric mood brings about a formless and immaterial sense of one's own self; a cold, black pond into which the self is drawn. As we have seen, the existence of borderline persons exhibits prolonged states in which dysphoric mood prevails, a noetically full and noematically empty emotional state. The problem is how to come back from this painful state. Anger is one possible way. Another and, to our view, more effective solution is to articulate the dysphoric mood into a coherent and responsible narrative account of one's own actions and experiences. But before discussing this narrative option, we shall first shed some light on an often neglected feature of dysphoria.

What some clinicians and researchers fail to appreciate is that, first and foremost, this emotional state is characterised by brimming waves of feelings—and not by feelings of void and inner emptiness. Before feeling empty, borderline persons feel too full of emotions. Kimura captures this brimming emotional state in his description of the *intra festum*:

> [T]he feast constitutes the most privileged occasion for the realization of ecstasy as excess or chaotic immediateness. Here one witnesses, among other things, the manifestation of vital exaltation, inebriation, rapture, sexual debauchery, play, violence, crime and death; we could say the destruction of everyday routine in general by means of a passion for the sacred or, conversely, for the sacrilege. In short, it is a triumph of *Chaos* over *Nomos* and *Cosmos* which characterizes the region of the feast. Here, the principles of life and death are in no way antagonists and they do not exclude one another. On the contrary, the correlation between them is such that an increase in one elicits that of the other.
>
> (Kimura 1992, p. 148; our translation)

They feel full of spontaneity, of a disordered vitality, which is also felt as a menace to autonomy, i.e. self-organisation. Prior to their feeling of 'void in my heart' that 'nothing can fill' (Kane 2001, p. 219), which many clinicians and researchers have noted, there is a state of wild emotional tension—a paradoxical spams of moral engagement, self-harming untamed liveliness, and nefarious skinless sensibility not modulated by reasonableness and unmediated by rationality—conveying a sense of authenticity as well as of suffering which Pasolini (1964) in one of his most famous poems represented as a *desperate vitality*.

Focusing on the vital character of dysphoria implies being able to see in the precarious sense of selfhood and identity of borderline persons a positive aspect, a less deadly feature than mere identity confusion and the manifestation of death instinct. Borderline persons feel that they have the right to receive a compensation for the traumas they have suffered; they have the right to rebel against the hypocrisy of social conventions, and thus to change the world (Correale 2007). This is the tragic horizon in which the bad mood of borderline persons is inscribed (Stanghellini 2000). One of the aims in our discussion of bad moods was to *urbanise* them, that is, to reconstruct the philosophical as well as psychopathological question of bad moods. Dysphoria stays on the delicate edge between the formation of personhood and its bloody catastrophe. In the borderline person's dysphoric mood a spark of revolt, a life impulse, burns desperately attempting to dismantle the rules and conventions of sociality.

This approach draws attention to the ambivalence at work in the emotional life of the borderline person. Dysphoria is the characterising mood trait accompanying borderline persons in the unfolding of their existence. As we have seen, it generates opposite kinds of movement: inaction/action, resignation/resistance, suffering/retaliation, and more generally, flowing forwards and upwards (indignation)/flowing backwards and inwards (resignation). It is an obstacle to movement and at the same time it may generate impatience, discontent, restlessness, and an incoercible impulse to move away without a definite goal. Thus, dysphoric mood as a desperate, untamed, and inane source of vitality is the emotional root of the well-known borderline stable instability. The dysphoria complex is precariously suspended between indignation, resignation, and retaliation, and thereby marks off a region of the mind within which the combat for personal identity is fought.

As *indignation*, it defends the limits of that which is tolerable, the border upon which to keep watch, the trench from which to fight. Indignation finds its origin in the borderline person's care for spontaneity in interpersonal relationships which he himself would sometimes call 'authenticity'; and especially in his ecstatic and tragic sense of love: '*If I renounce to love I cannot be myself*'; '*Don't ask me, doctor, to stop with him. I know it harms me, but I need to love in order to feel myself*'. Or as Kane describes it: 'Cut out my tongue/tear out my hair/cut off my limbs/but leave me my love/I would rather have lost my legs/pulled out my teeth/gouged out my eyes/than lost my love' (p. 230), where 'love' means the source of the borderline person's vitality, the 'vital need for which I would die' (p. 242). It is the flux of spontaneity that chaotically irrupts into the borderline person's life, the vital force that innervates her sense of being alive, the very principle through which her selfhood is constituted.

As *resignation*, it paves the way to the sense of void that characterises borderline depressions, or the micro-depressive episodes which may punctuate the borderline person's daily existence. These are the episodes, often described in the literature, during which deep feelings of depersonalisation add up to the permanent lack of a stable, integral identity. The latter is characterised by the experience of one's life, and especially one's past, as a collection of disarticulated events (as we have seen in the preceding sections). The former is the here-and-now vanishing of the flux of spontaneity, entailing feelings of auto-, somato-, and allo-psychic depersonalisation, i.e. sensations of emptiness, numbness, fragmentation, vanishing of one's own self ('*My head empty, my self empty*'; '*Nothing inside, just like a big hole, as if they'd cut a piece of me*'); experiences of separation from one's own body as the source of one's disordered vitality ('*My mind here, my body there*'; '*Arms and legs drained*'; '*As if [I were] all frozen*'); and feelings of abandonment and aloneness—all immersed in an atmosphere of 'corrosive doubt/futile despair/horror in repose' that engenders a devastating sense of resignation: 'I can fill my space/fill my time/but nothing can fill this void in my heart'(p. 219).

As *retaliation*, in the *hybris* of the blind and insensitively stubborn affirmation of one's own existence, it restores a coherent sense of one's own self and of identity. At the same time, though, it incarnates the wreckage and the bloody fall of one's human frailty, and the sense of tenderness and admiration that it can inspire in us. Anger, as we have seen, is to a certain extent a self-defining emotion ('*Now I feel better: I know you are a cunt!*'; '*I know what I must do: I will humiliate him [her lover] in front of his family and *friends!*). A numb and empty body becomes a body filled with anger. A self filled with anger[13] is a self that can finally feel itself, a strong and hard embodied self that repays the suffered insults—but at the cost of losing its humanity, and thus wrecking the fragile dialectic of selfhood and otherness constitutive of personhood. It is a self that is insensitive to the voice and the face of the other person, a self without innocence, a self that has lost the humanity endemic to personhood. Tragic is the existence which, in pursuing a plan, acts in such a way that it brings the same plan inexorably to destruction. This is the case for the borderline person's anger, which seems to be situated at the point where an intention swings into its opposite: fragile doubts about oneself and the other into incorrigible convictions, moral indignation into the shame of aggression, the fire of love into the stake of intolerance.

Give Us Our Daily Trauma

It is customary that therapeutic conversations with borderline persons are about some stressful event that has just happened during the days or hours before the therapy session. It is also common that, if the therapist asks about that specific event during the following therapy session, the patient will hardly remember the event itself and the circumstances under which it took place.

Borderline persons, as we have seen, are mainly focused on the present moment. They live in an *intra festum* temporality. There are two main features of this: the present moment is neither articulated with the retention of past moments nor integrated by the protention into the future; '[t]heir transitory present has no depth. It lacks the fulfilment which only originates from the integration of past experience and anticipated future' (Fuchs 2007, p. 381). The present moment, lived as an absolute now, lacks depth, value, and existential meaning. It is a flat present, reminiscent of death: 'Everything passes/Everything perishes/Everything palls/my thought walks away with a killing smile/leaving discordant anxiety/which roars in my soul/No hope No hope No hope No hope No hope No hope No hope' (Kane 2001, p. 218). In these moments, an acute feeling of despair, i.e. discordant directions of intentionality leading to a paralysis of thinking and action, accompanies dysphoria.

---

[13] In many cultures, as we have already seen in the last chapter, anger is conceptualised through the *hot fluid in a container* metaphor. This metaphor captures a great number of aspects and properties of anger. It allows us to conceptualise intensity (*filled with*), control (*contain*), loss of control (*could not keep inside*), dangerousness (*brim with*), expression (*express/show*), and so on. In fact, it appears that no other conceptual metaphor associated with anger can provide us with an understanding of all these facets of anger. It is also the metaphor that appears to be the most popular both as a folk theory and as a scientific theory of emotion. The hot fluid in a container metaphor has the following structure: the container with the fluid is the person who is angry, the fluid in the container is the anger, the pressure of the fluid in the container is the force of the anger on the angry person, the cause of the pressure is the cause of the anger force, trying to keep the fluid inside the container is trying to control the anger, the fluid going out of the container is the expression of the anger, the physical dysfunctionality of the container is the social dysfunctionality of the angry person (Kövecses 2000a, 2000b).

The present moment is to the borderline person *momentary* in the sense that it is lived as evanescent, fast, flying, fugaceous, ephemeral, fleeting, impermanent: '*Sometimes it's like in a flash*', '*I live in a meteoric time*', '*Everything important is short-lived, instantaneous – all the rest is boredom*'. Lived time in the existence of a borderline person is '*islands of feast*' in a stagnant '*ocean of spleen*'. It is being 'dead for a long time' (p. 214) interrupted by transient, vanishing, volatile moments of intensity. The prevailing mood is obviously dysphoria, typically accompanied by feelings of boredom, punctuated with moments of excitement, thrill, during which one's blind vitality finds its fulfilment.

Next to this volatile and empty character of temporality, sometimes the events that happen to the borderline person are not just momentary, but also *momentous*, that is, overwhelmingly significant to him. The present moment can be spasmodic, urgent, clamant: '*When my telephone rings, it's him; it's imperative to me, I cannot escape from it*', '*Time is pressing me, I must seize the moment*', '*Time is clamant, opportunities come rarely and call me with a loud voice*', '*Doc, I need to see you now!*'. At their extreme, during these moments, events—including the appearing of a person in the room, someone's way of moving, the tone of his voice—may acquire an offensive, thing-like physiognomy, and become intruding, perforating. Obliviously absorbed in immediateness, for the borderline person there is no space in between the *now* and himself.

The now-experience and the person are one. The space of security that usually separates us from significant events, allowing us to see them from a certain distance, abruptly breaks down. In short, there is a sudden change in the structure of lived space that accompanies the metamorphosis of lived time. A patient may report that she dreamt of my office as an impersonal medical facility, with walls painted in white, and anonymously furnished. Time passes during the dreamt session and nothing happens. The same patient may report about another dream during which other persons enter my office during our session, the door is wide open, anyone can listen and watch inside. In this second dream the session finishes immediately after having started.

Dysphoric space is usually experienced as indifferent extension, a space devoid of salience that offers no directions and no way out.[14] When dysphoria turns into spleen, the surrounding world is '*moribund, reminds me of Death in Venice*'. One's life appears as meaningless, without scope. It is like 'still black water/as deep as forever/as cold as the sky/as still as my heart when your voice is gone/I shall freeze in hell' (p. 239). In despair, space undergoes an even deeper metamorphosis. As we have seen, movements remain stuck in the indecisiveness of juxtaposition. Despair in the borderline life-world is a kind of frenetic palsy. Dysphoric mood, ignited by shame, may turn into anger; then, space offers no protection. Events are described as 'wounding', 'biting', 'stinging'. Someone's remark may be felt as 'caustic', 'corrosive', 'dissecting'; her behaviour, 'pointed', 'raw', 'sharp'—and these, of course, are not *just* metaphors. Changes in

---

[14] We find an apparently similar phenomenon describing lived space in persons with schizophrenia. The basic difference between these two is that whereas in the schizophrenic mood lived space conveys a feeling of unreality, in borderline persons it conveys a feeling of meaninglessness.

lived space make it possible to experience someone's comportment as piercing; the piercing metaphors arise from alterations of lived space. As Kane explains, 'the defining feature of a metaphor is that it's real' (p. 211). In general, the physiognomy of things in the life-world of borderline persons reflects the fluctuation in lived time between evanescence and urgency: things show themselves on the edge between melting and blasting. They are dissolving, liquefying as well as ardent, combusting, conflagrating: 'In a moment things around me are glowing, and a moment later reduced to ashes', 'My life is as if I were walking on burning coals', 'Feverish moments, during which something makes me feel fervent'.

An essential feature of the borderline persons' life-world is that typically these persons are not able to distance themselves from present events. As space offers little or no protection from piercing objects, neither does time protect from wounding memories. This is the key to understanding the traumatic existence of borderline persons. The present moment—be it an event taking place in the external world or a bit of memory intruding into the field of consciousness—irrupts *without mediation* into the existence of borderline persons. Borderline persons are not able to liberate themselves from what they are thinking, experiencing, or suffering right now. The incapacity to distance oneself from an event, to take a stance in front of it, to integrate it into a narrative sequence and by doing so to give a personal meaning to it, are defining characteristics of trauma.

Our existence is moved forward by what happens in our life. Events happen to us as a part of involuntary otherness involved in a human life, and we appropriate these events, or we define ourselves in opposition to these events; but no matter how we relate ourselves to the events of a life, our sheer relation, our position-taking, instils personal meaning in them, and by this activity we affirm our selfhood. This dialectic of otherness and selfhood is at the heart of the construction of our narrative identity. If an event loses this capacity to 'move', the dialectic of identity shatters because the person is not able to integrate this event into the historicity of his existence. The event becomes a *traumatic* event, it becomes pathogenic. An event is traumatic when it does not kindle the dialectic of narrative identity—rather, it arrests the historicity of existence (Stanghellini and Rossi Monti 2009a). As Deleuze once wrote paraphrasing Foucault: 'Thought thinks its own history (the past), but does so in order to free itself from what it thinks (the present) and, finally, to be able "to think otherwise" (the future)' (Deleuze 1986, p. 127; our translation).[15]

Borderline persons live out a traumatic existence because they are not able to *think otherwise*. They cannot articulate the present with their past—they cannot view their present experience as the product of past ones. Also, they are incapable to distance themselves from the present experience and by doing so to take a different stance

---

[15] Foucault emphasised that his extensive inquiry into the history of human culture, science, and self-understanding was not that of a historian, but 'it was a philosophical exercise. What was at stake was to learn to what extent the labour of thinking one's own past can liberate thought from what it thinks silently and thus allow it to think otherwise' (Foucault 1984, p. 15; our translation).

towards it, that is, to view their present from a different angle. As argued by Meares (2000, pp. 59–61), when a memory arises in consciousness we are usually able to distinguish between this memory, as a fragment coming from the past, and a present experience like a perception of something going on here and now in the outside world. When the traumatic system irrupts into the psychic life of borderline persons, this capacity is lost. The past experience is felt as entirely located in the present. Past experiences intrude into the field of consciousness and are experienced as aspects of the present.

In human existence, the meaning of an experience is set within a temporal dynamic that is highly *non-linear*. Not only do past experiences have influence on the future, but also what is expected affects the meaning of past experiences. Borderline persons lack the future-orientated attitude integral to protection, which is a necessary prerequisite for attributing new meanings to one's own past and to its re-enactment in present traumatic experiences, and thus for overcoming one's past and moving away from the present. The orientation towards the future bestows new meaning(s) upon the past and makes it possible to 'think otherwise' about one's present. As the process of recovery is based on restoring meaningfulness, or attributing new meanings to one's experiences, the integrity of protection can be seen as a prerequisite for recovery (Schrank et al. 2008).

A Hermeneutics of Traumatic Existence

Usually, the relationship between trauma and borderline existence is conceived in terms of cause-effect: a trauma located in the past may cause the present suffering. This is certainly plausible, as epidemiological studies suggest. The majority of patients with borderline personality disorder report some form of child abuse, including physical and sexual abuse, or neglect (Zanarini 2000). The frequency is significantly higher than in other personality disorders or in depression. However, borderline personality disorder can develop without any trauma history (Paris 1994), and trauma is a risk factor for many other mental disorders (Paris 2000). Moreover, around 80% of people exposed to early trauma do not develop mental disorders (Fergusson and Mullen 1999). The idea that borderline personality disorder is rooted in early trauma is probably overrated and may lead to wrong interpretations. Clinicians should not automatically assume that present traumatic experiences are re-enactments of early traumatic experiences. Correale (2007) advises clinicians to transfer the focus of attention during therapy sessions from the search of early psychological adversities to the daily traumas suffered by these patients. This is not to deny the importance of child abuse or neglect in the pathogenesis of this condition. Rather, it is a way to meet the patients' need to recount their traumatic existence (and share its burden with a significant other) and to enhance the patients' capacity to describe their experiences and reflect upon them by placing them in time and history. This, of course, will also improve the clinician's understanding of what is actually going on in the patient's life-world. He suggests focusing on what he calls *traumatic sequence*, performing with the patient a kind of slow-motion recollection of one of the daily traumatic events that constellate the borderline person's existence.[16] An example of this could be the following:[17] the patient recounts that her new boyfriend arrived thirty minutes late for their appointment and that they had a horrible quarrel. That is the fact, and it leads her to conclude that she has been mistreated as usual, and that it was a dreadful mistake to have an affair with him. The clinician then asks her to explicate this, to give further details about the traumatic sequence and the emotions involved in it.[18] The traumatic sequence typically includes four steps:

1. The traumatic experience which usually originates in the context of a traumatic relationship. The relationships of borderline persons are often traumatic. The reasons for this, as we tried to explain, are of two primary kinds. First, there is a difficulty in establishing an image or representation of one's partner coherent over time, since the dysphoria-anger complex entails an oscillation between an *opaque* (fuzzy, blurred, hazy) image of the other, and an image of the other as *tenebrous* (ambivalent, evasive, obscure, puzzling, suspect). Second, the values at play in the interpersonal world of borderline persons are not only difficult to attain, but in conflict with one another. The borderline person requires the other to be present and loyal, and capable of recognition, that is, a source of validation. In addition, presence, loyalty, and recognition must be accompanied by the other's spontaneity, being free from social conventions and acting according to the vital impulses of the present moment. Furthermore, as we have seen, the borderline person is not capable of autonomy in the sense of establishing a coherent enough representation of herself and remaining faithful to it, and thus takes to an extreme the value of spontaneity. She conceives of partnerships as the encounter between two *spontaneities*, not regulated by any sort of internal or external *nomos*.

2. A phase of emotional dissonance and cognitive indecision. The traumatic sequence typically starts with an unexpected event of disappointment and disillusion. The other does something (or omits to do something) and thereby hurts the borderline person's sensibility. The patient notices that while waiting for her boyfriend she was overwhelmed by a quasi-ineffable variety of bad moods, including dysphoria, anxiety, and despair, characterised on the cognitive level by a state of dissonance

---

[16] Slow-motion (*moviola*) is also the method devised by the Italian psychotherapist Vittorio Guidano (1991). A similar approach was then developed in a series of articles by one of us with the name of 'explication' (Stanghellini 2007a; Stanghellini 2010; Stanghellini and Rossi Monti 2009b).

[17] This clinical vignette is taken from a seminar held by Antonello Correale at University of Urbino, during the course 'Phenomenology and Psychotherapy' in June 2009. It has been slightly modified to fit our purpose.

[18] 'Explication' here means bringing out the raw feelings of the patient's experiences and the personal meanings that the patient attributes to them. It is an accurate unfolding of subjective experiences and the organisation of these experiences according to a meaningful pattern immanent to the experiences themselves; the interpretation or the explanation of these experiences according to a model that is not immanent in the clinical material itself may come as a later step (Stanghellini and Rossi Monti 2009b).

and indecision. She could not construct any consistent and stable explanation of her boyfriend's behaviour: 'What's going on?', 'Is he stuck in traffic?', 'Did he have a car accident?', 'Did he forget about our appointment?', 'Was he distracted by something or someone else?', 'Another woman?', 'Is that an ambiguous way of letting me down?', and so on. This is an initial manifestation of what is sometimes called the borderline patient's deficit of reflective function (Fonagy and Target 1997, pp. 693–6). We prefer to talk of her difficulty to *situate* her emotions. To situate one's emotions means to recognise and relate them to the present situation, to understand them as one's own personal way of being attuned to that given situation; and eventually to grasp the connection between one's emotions, the present situation in which they are elicited, and one's life-history as the background from which they arise. Borderline persons fail to see in their emotional reactions the involuntary *manifestation of otherness*, that is, the re-enactment of one's past and the manifestation of one's character. Thus, they fail to engage in a proper 'hermeneutics of the *I am*'.

3   Emotional dissonance is prodromal to a phase of despair, in the sense posited above: a kind of frenzied paralysis of action and thinking. The person notices that while she was waiting for her boyfriend, her thinking completely collapsed. She could make no decision at all. She was entirely passive, in a kind of psychic paralysis. She felt that she was getting mad and that she simply could not cope with it. Only during the recollection of the traumatic sequence, she realises that what was profoundly disturbing to her was the idea that events are random, reality uncontrollable, the behaviour of other persons unintelligible, and the whole world nonsensical. The outside world, as well as her own actions and reactions, were lived as if they were entirely out of control. The situation she found herself in appeared in the mode of the unpredictable. Despair may be the ingress into dissociation, which is often considered a desperate defence or adaptation to traumatic experiences. In the state of dissociation there is a collapse of the capacity of mentalisation. Dissociation may imply amnesia, and therefore this phase may be absent in the patient's spontaneous recollection of the traumatic sequence.

4   The last step of the traumatic sequence is a mechanical, routine interpretation of the traumatic event. We will develop it in the next section, which also concludes this chapter.

A Miscarried Hermeneutics of the *I Am*

The traumatic sequence typically concludes its trajectory in a miscarried self-interpretation. It characteristically implies a traumatic identification, i.e. the assumption of a traumatic identity. During the recollection of the episode, the patient may, for instance, tell that after the terrible quarrel with her boyfriend she finally came to an overall interpretation of the situation: she realised that her destiny is having relationships with bad persons, and that in order to defend herself from this destiny she needs to over-react and become bad herself.

Borderline persons typically place themselves in the narrative they construct of the sequence in which they are involved in one of three stereotyped roles which we, once again with Sarah Kane, can call: 'Victim. Perpetrator. Bystander.' (Kane 2001, p. 231). This is the rigid interpretative framework for their *miscarried hermeneutics of the I am*. As we anticipated in the introduction to this chapter, we conceive of the borderline condition as a disordered fabric of personhood—a disorder of the integration of selfhood and otherness (the other person as well as the otherness intrinsic to personhood itself, which is here manifested in time, body, and character) in one's sense of being a person. The capacity to develop an implicitly functioning sense of one's own self and to establish a coherent narrative of being a person is essentially based on the presence of an implicit other that is modelled on the basis of the internalisation of secure figures of attachment or, more accurately, of secure schemes of self-other relationships. This secure basis is lacking in the life story of borderline persons. Thus, the constitution of the implicit other with whom one can share an 'intimate conversation', and to whom one would also feel responsible, is missing too. This has two principal consequences: first, borderline persons have great difficulties in developing a sense of their own self and in establishing a coherent narrative of personal identity based on the internal dialogue with an implicit other. Second, the flesh-and-blood other is constituted according to stereotyped schemes of self-other interaction, seemingly reminiscent of early distressing experiences.

In the preceding sections, we have also discussed the puzzling manifestation of otherness, in terms of an involuntary source of one's actions, in the existence of borderline persons. In discovering otherness in themselves, borderline persons discover in themselves an amorphous and untamed presence.[19] This presence is felt as a spring of disordered vitality that is a menace to autonomy in the sense of self-organisation. Otherness is an impossibility for borderline persons. It is both a threat to the self and the source of vitality, the vital force that they cannot renounce. Thus, it is impossible both to appropriate one's otherness and to distance oneself from it.

With this in mind, let us try to explicate the basic types of interpretations that borderline persons may develop of the manifestation of otherness in the traumatic situations in which they are repeatedly involved. At the centre of the mindscape borderline persons live in, there is a moral question: 'Whose fault is it?', 'Who is to be held responsible for my own and the other's sufferings?'. Shame and guilt, the voluntary and the involuntary, fate and necessity are the protagonists in the play in which the borderline person is involved.

In the traumatic situation, one may identify with the role of the victim, and in this case feel passively involved and totally without responsibility for what happens. If *I* am the victim, then the other is the perpetrator: 'He is bad, I am the victim'.

---

[19] It could be of some help at this point to remember our analysis of a-rationality in Chapter 1, and especially the third scenario of the story with the broken eggs. I was suddenly overtaken by a feeling of despair, and the meaning of my life was shattered in an instant. I took the eggs out of the pack and dropped them. I explain that 'it simply happened, as if a piece of my brain caused me to do so'. An anonymous event, simultaneously something external and internal, made me behave like this. It felt like a kind of otherness in myself, impersonal and personal at the same time, with no clear-cut distinction between my self and otherness, something that belonged to me but was not under my control.

Feelings of abandonment, or lack of attention, acceptance, help, protection, reciprocity, support—or in short, lack of recognition—are typical in the borderline traumatic existence. The borderline person looks primarily in the direction of the other. It is the other who is guilty, since he or she acted out of voluntary intention. These feelings may kindle acute emotional states characterised by anger, resentment, and indignation. The self-other relationship may take the form of a transitory persecutory delusion. Usually, the persecutor is a *significant* other. This makes the persecutory delusions of borderline persons radically different from paranoid delusions in persons with schizophrenia, which typically involve *anonymous* others. Borderline persons who are more vulnerable to develop feelings of shame are probably more prone to assume the role of the victim rather than other types of traumatic identities, thus to exhibit persecutory delusions. We may then suppose a pathoplastic role of personality[20] in assuming the role of the victim rather than another type of traumatic identity. This is especially pertinent to the subtype of borderline personality that we named 'sensitive character' according to Kretschmer. The mixture of anger and shame that characterises the Kretschmerian personality traits may trigger persecutory delusions in borderline persons, and especially delusions of reference, which typically arise in the type of borderline persons who are particularly vulnerable to narcissistic rage associated with feelings of humiliation.

Other persons may identify with the role of the perpetrator. In our example, the patient admits she misbehaved. Her reaction to the wrong suffered, she says, was extreme, exaggerated—nonetheless, she thinks she cannot be held entirely responsible. It was for her a sort of reflex, an automatic response she simply could not control: 'I am bad, but I am not guilty because it's not my fault'. Indeed, borderline persons seldom develop feelings of guilt or guilt delusions as melancholic persons do (with the exception of paranoid guilt as we have seen, but that involves shame as in the previous reaction-type). Guilt presupposes responsibility. Borderline persons do not hold themselves responsible for their actions, since they basically experience these as *re-actions*. If asked about the source of the harm they did, they would respond that it was a kind of fit, or seizure—like an epileptic seizure, kindled by the wrong they previously suffered. They experience their action as an *expression of the involuntary*. Rather than feeling guilty, they may feel under the spell of some malignant power coming from within them. They do not develop, as persons with schizophrenia typically do, delusions of alien control (they do not feel under the influence of an agency coming from without their self). Responsibility is placed neither on a flesh-and-blood other (one's partner, the therapist, or a friend, as is the case with borderline persons who identify with the role of the victim) nor on an anonymous, generalised other, or a mechanism (as is the case with schizophrenic paranoid delusions of alien control). Rather, they experience the influx in their life of an uncontrollable destructive force that comes from within. A sub-personal force that cannot be separated from their own self is responsible for their deeds. Borderline persons are the witnesses of an

---

[20] We refer to the final part of the previous chapter on schizophrenic mood, where we use Ricoeur's theory of the dialectic of narrative identity as a framework for discussing the concept of the pathoplastic role of the person in shaping full-blown psychopathological pictures.

ultimate truth: they feel the alienating power of the involuntary, of the otherness that is constitutive of our personhood.

Finally, other borderline persons may identify with the role of the bystander, a merely passive spectator of the ineluctable and unpredictable events. They feel they cannot decide, control, or change the course of their life: 'It always goes like this. This happened again. I can do nothing to avoid it'. These persons are prone to develop feelings of impotence and helplessness, and to conceive of life as nonsensical. They are oppressed with tedium, their mind becomes a mirror that reflects the ineluctability of the world and one's own powerlessness, the futility of existence. The world and life itself simply *is*, it just happens. Tedium may be interrupted by cynical, sarcastic, or auto-sarcastic remarks. In this case, neither is the other construed as a perpetrator nor is the self felt as dominated by otherness. The responsibility is *on life itself*, on its inescapable as well as unpredictable nature. This variant of borderline persons may conceive of their existence as a *tragic* existence. One of the characterising features of the tragic is that one feels near to one's own destiny, so much that one can see it, touch it, nearly manipulate it, and maybe avoid it. Nonetheless, one can merely watch oneself thrown into this without any brakes. The nightmare is the most common paradigm of the tragic. In every nightmare there is always a moment in which powerlessly I see myself being hurled into the jaws of the destructive power from which I was trying to escape. Borderline persons construe themselves as *just* the bystanders of their tragic destiny.

In the next and final chapter, we return to the relation between philosophy and psychopathology that we introduced in Chapter 1. We argue that the hermeneutical theory of emotions and personhood developed throughout the first two parts of book illustrates how both philosophy and psychopathology can benefit from a mutual exchange. The question of naturalism is pertinent to the current state of both disciplines and thus provides a common ground for such an exchange. Whereas philosophy can provide a theoretical framework for an exploration of this ambivalence, psychopathology helps us understand that vulnerability to mental pathology is not a question of malfunctioning, but a rather dramatic expression of the fragility inherent in being a human person. We use the analysis, carried out in this and the previous chapter, of the difficulties schizophrenic and borderline persons encounter in working out an understanding of their own life-world to argue that the 'end-products' (like ontologic delusions in persons with schizophrenia and ontic ones in borderline persons) are the results of a miscarried hermeneutics of their own self. By way of conclusion, we will argue that a phenomenologically grounded clinical hermeneutics, a therapy of care, can accompany and help these persons in their complicated task to understand and communicate their experience and make sense of it.

Chapter 10

Emotions, Vulnerability, and a Therapy of Care

The entanglement of emotions and rationality is at the heart of human fragility and, consequently, a major factor in our vulnerability to mental illness. Human beings are personal animals. We are neither purely rational beings nor merely emotional ones. Rather, human rationality is an emotional rationality—and as such a vulnerable rationality. In this final chapter, we shall try to make explicit what this vulnerable entanglement of emotions and rationality means for the therapeutic approach to mental illness.

The aim of this chapter is twofold: to recapitulate the principal points of our theory of emotions and personhood, and to show the therapeutic implications of this theory. We begin with revisiting the question of naturalism. Chapter 1 advanced the claim that the ambiguity of subjectivity and biology is at the heart of contemporary psychopathology, and that our best way to understand the 'wounded' thinking involved in mental illness is to confront and examine the experience of emotional fragility, the ambivalent dialectic of selfhood and otherness, brought about by this ambiguity. Hence, a major part of the following explorations was dedicated to the many ways a person experiences and deals with this emotional fragility. At the end of Part II, we ventured the claim that a better understanding of the fragility of human personhood can help to make sense of our peculiar vulnerability to mental illness. In the present chapter, we develop this conception of vulnerability. We argue that the uncanny metamorphoses in the life-worlds of schizophrenic and borderline persons, described in Chapters 8 and 9, are brought about by an extreme disproportion of emotions and rationality, and that the end-products of mental illnesses are a result of the person's miscarried hermeneutics of intrinsic emotional experiences. With the fixation in a pathological life-world, the dialectic of selfhood and otherness constitutive of human personhood collapses. This understanding of the vulnerability to mental illness contains a rudimentary framework for engaging with this fragility by means of hermeneutical therapy. A phenomenologically grounded clinical hermeneutics can accompany and help persons affected by mental illnesses in their complicated task of understanding and communicating their experiences and making sense of them. The aim of such a therapy is to re-establish the dialectic of selfhood and otherness that will help the suffering person to become who she or he is.

The Fragile Dialectic of Selfhood and Otherness

The scope and limits of naturalistic explanations of mental illness remain an open question for psychopathology. How we integrate the subjective experience of mental illness with the (neuro)biological underpinning of that illness is vital for our understanding of mental disorders, and whatever model we choose has a significant bearing on how we approach the therapeutic aspect of mental suffering. We began the book with the claim that the question of naturalism is particularly urgent for psychopathology. On the one hand, neuroscience has helped us to understand that our mental illness is inescapably connected with the way the neurological functioning of our brain gums up our thinking and feeling. On the other hand, although neuroscience has proved an indispensable resource for psychopathology, investigations of subjectivity still remain necessary if we want to understand the suffering involved in mental illness. The fact that we are persons with a subjective sense of autonomy (a sense of agency and ownership) *and* biological organisms restricted by and exposed to the same natural conditions as other biological organisms is undeniably at the heart of our endeavours to understand and live with our peculiarly human vulnerability.

Throughout this book, we have argued for the view that this ambiguity of subjectivity and biology is responsible for the fragile sense of ambivalence constitutive of human personhood. To be a person is to be both an individual self and an anonymous biological organism. Most of us acknowledge that the peculiarity of our personal identity is, to a large extent, determined by our biological constitution. Aspects of our physical constitution and features of our character traits are inscribed in our genetic material, and have developed throughout our personal history in terms of an obscure blend of chance and necessity without explicit interference from our voluntary decisions. Nevertheless, an equally decisive—and perhaps even more significant—part of who we are is the result of exactly such voluntary choices, or more precisely, of *how we relate ourselves* to what and who we are, to other people, and to our environment. The personal character of our existence relies on the dialectic of selfhood and otherness, i.e. our involuntary, embodied, situated *dispositions* and the voluntary, reflective, normative *position* we take in front of them. This fragile dialectic of passivity and activity is the defining feature of being a person.

We have not attempted to solve the hackneyed question of nature vs nurture, or to answer the intricate mind-body problem that is at the core of that question. Naturalistic explanations of the mind entail a plethora of vital, but also frustrating questions that lie at the heart of our attempts to understand mental illness. Some twenty years ago, Colin McGinn elegantly described this situation:

> How is it possible for conscious states to depend upon brain states? How can technicolour phenomenology arise from soggy grey matter? What makes the bodily organ we call the brain so radically different from other bodily organs, say the kidneys—the body parts without a trace of consciousness? How could the aggregation of millions of individually insentient neurons generate subjective awareness? We know that brains are the *de facto* causal basis of consciousness, but we have, it seems, no understanding whatever of how this is so. It strikes us as miraculous, eerie, even faintly comic. Somehow, we feel, the water of the physical brain is turned into the wine of consciousness, but we draw a total blank on the nature of this conversion.
>
> (McGinn 1989, p. 349)

Despite the philosophical importance of dealing with such general issues, they are beyond both our ability and the interest of this book. Moreover, we suspect that McGinn was right when he concluded that a definitive solution to the mind-body problem is impossible due to the 'cognitive closure' of our human mind. Against the background of the previous explorations of our emotional mind, we would say that it seems a misguided belief in cognitive transparency to insist that the human mind is capable of fully understanding the reality of itself or of the nature of which it is a part; in other words, '[i]t is deplorably anthropocentric to insist that reality be constrained by what the human mind can conceive' (p. 366). We therefore agree with McGinn that '[a] deep fact about our own nature as a form of embodied consciousness is thus necessarily hidden from us' (p. 366). Nevertheless, we believe that one of the fundamental issues in the contemporary discussions about naturalism, namely, how to explain the presence of both rational and a-rational factors in human thinking, feeling, and behaviour, is—or at least should be—central to our endeavours of understanding mental illness.

Thus, instead of struggling with what seems to be a theoretical deadlock, we chose to focus on how the ambiguity of subjectivity and biology surfaces in the experience of fragility that characterises the existence of human persons. And we have argued that the root of this fragility is emotional and that it stems from the basic feelings of ambivalence of selfhood and otherness constitutive of human personhood. We are personal animals whose experience is characterised by ambivalent, often troubling and conflictual, feelings of selfhood (agency and ownership) and otherness (body, world, and other people). To understand our fragile sense of personhood, we have explored this ambivalent character of human experience by investigating the interplay of personal and anonymous factors involved in our emotional life.

We have used Ricoeur's theory of subjectivity as the theoretical framework for our account of personhood because it provides a solid foundation for investigating the ontological (What am I?), phenomenological (How do I feel?), and normative (What shall I do?) aspects of human subjectivity. It is precisely the interplay of these three dimensions of human subjectivity that makes Ricoeur's theory valuable. In our reformulation of his theory, we have emphasised the troubled nature of human selfhood, namely, the conflictual sense of being a self in terms of the tension between otherness (the involuntary) and selfhood (the voluntary), and we have examined how this tension plays out in the ontological, phenomenological, and normative aspects of human selfhood. We reformulated Ricoeur's theory as, on the one hand, a phenomenological diagnosis of the troubled character of human selfhood, and, on the other, a more hermeneutical, therapeutic effort to deal with this troubled selfhood in terms of an ontology of care.

Ricoeur approaches the troubled awareness of being a self in terms of personhood. To be a human self is to be a person. But to be a person is not simply to be a self. There is more to personhood than a sense of being a self. Selfhood is troubled by the constant interference of otherness as it is manifested by our body, the world, and other people. We can never quite be the self that we want to be. Our affirmation of selfhood is inevitably disturbed by the otherness that is an integral part of who we are as embodied persons in a world shared with other people. I care about being a person, and this care binds me to the otherness (my body, the world, and other people) that makes me the person that I am.

A person's values and concerns are constituted by voluntary and involuntary factors. I do not always choose what I care about. Many of my values and concerns are involuntary, and as such they reveal the otherness that interferes with who I think I am or who I want to be, and yet the same values also inevitably constitute the person that I am. Love and hate are not under the sway of my will, and neither are hunger and sexual arousal. My desires can be both vital and spiritual. They stem from the anonymous biological constitution of my body as well as from my personal engagement with the world and other people over time. This ambivalence is expressed, for instance, in the fact that my desire for another person can be a sexual desire, a desire for power, for love, or for recognition—in fact, most of the time, our desires are undecipherable mixtures of all these, and innumerable other, cares and concerns. The ambivalence of what we care about is thus often cognitively impenetrable, and frequently the heterogeneous values that are revealed and engendered by our care are in conflict with one another. This complexity and lack of transparency makes many of our feelings hard to understand and difficult to cope with. In short, our sense of personhood is ambivalent and fragile because of these deeply heterogeneous values that make up what a person cares about.

Our body bears witness to the ambivalence of our care. We are complex organisms evolved over millions of years that have left vestigial traces in our emotional behaviour. The 'tinkering' of evolutionary development (Jacob 1977) helps to explain the disparity, and often conflictual nature, of these vestigial traces in our emotional life. There are obvious biological sources of disharmony, as de Sousa observes, at work in the affective churn of our emotional life:

> Our emotions have been cobbled together at different times in response to different selective pressures. As a result, our most basic emotional capacities are very likely to be relatively independent modules, often driven by unrelated biological needs. There is no reason to think that they will work harmoniously together, any more than we can hope that the need to flee an enemy will never interfere with peaceful digestion.
>
> (de Sousa 2011, p. 22)

Not surprisingly, Panksepp argues for the same organisational complexity involved in the development of the affective brain:

> In envisioning the affective brain, we need to explicitly recognize that the brain, unlike any other organ of the body, is an evolutionarily layered tissue where we can see the imprints of evolutionary progressions within its anatomical organization.
>
> (Panksepp 2011, p. 557)

We cannot expect a natural hierarchy or any sovereign arbiter that organises and controls our emotional life. We have argued against attempts to establish such organisational structures of our emotional life, be that in terms of rationality (the cognitive theories, e.g. Robert Solomon), core evolutionary themes (the feeling theories, e.g. Jesse Prinz) or pragmatic possibilities (Ratcliffe's phenomenological alternative). On the contrary, as a consequence of our explorations of emotional fragility, we find more plausible de Sousa's suggestion that '[e]ach of us may comprise a radical *heterarchy*, in which many partial systems work in parallel, of which any one can take over control according to need' (1987, p. 74). What makes us human is our peculiar rational capacity to take responsibility for our own emotional fragility, to recognise ourselves through our emotions, to articulate them, to make sense(s) of them, to appropriate them by integrating them into our narrative identity, to *hierarchise* them, to reflect upon our thoughts about them, and thus to (try to) behave according to rational patterns. However, these rational capacities are only one aspect of what and who we are. Our heterarchic nature is experienced as a diffuse ambivalence of rational and a-rational feelings in our emotional life, and becomes *conceptually articulated* as ambiguities, contradictions, self-deceptions, and paradoxes, when we reflectively try to make sense of our existence by means of our rational resources.

The ambivalence of our emotional life makes the rational appropriation of the norms by which we live our life a major part of the fragility constitutive of our personhood. We constantly evaluate the norms by which we live our life. Over time we learn to abide by some norms and reject others. The dialectic of selfhood and otherness is central to our experience of the norms that govern our rationality. The objectivity constitutive of norms can alienate and exclude, as well as liberate and include, the subjectivity of the person whose thoughts, feelings, and behaviour are informed and orientated by these norms. Without norms my existence as a person would shatter. I communicate and interact with other people through moral, rational, conventional, social, and pragmatic norms. Norms create an interpersonal space for thought and behaviour that would disintegrate without the constant safeguarding of rational thought and behaviour according to such norms. Nevertheless, the objective demands involved in norms can also be experienced as an oppressive or alienating otherness. I can feel that who I am, my personal values and my most intimate desires, are quenched by the objective demands imposed by the norms that structure my existence. This is not only the case with explicitly moral norms. Already the norms constitutive of the language by means of which we communicate can become alienating. We may feel that the words we use or the sentences we construct are inadequate for capturing how we feel or how we feel about the way we feel. This is probably what Sartre wants to bring out with the famous words from the short story *Érostrate*, where the tormented narrator Paul Hibert—in his 102 letters to 102 famous French authors—writes that 'I wanted *my own* words [*de mots à moi*]. But the ones I use have dragged through I don't know how many consciences; they arrange themselves in my head by virtue of the habits I have picked up from others [*chez les autres*]' (1975, p. 49 [89]).

My rationality binds me to the otherness of the norms that orient and inform the dialectic of selfhood and otherness involved in becoming the person that I am. The norms that discipline my rational thinking are, however, often at odds with my most intimate desires, values, and concerns. The intimate feelings that qualify my subjectivity are not always 'rational', 'appropriate', 'sane' or 'considerate' in the sense that what I feel and care about does not always tally well with my own reflective norms, the norms of other people, or simply the norms of the society in which I live. Faulkner's *As I Lay Dying* can be read as a painful testimony as to how our sense of selfhood is constantly struggling with the norms of rational thinking and behaviour. Particularly penetrating are Cash Bundren's reflections upon the madness of his brother Darl who, in spite of his profound 'natural affection' for other human beings, continues to defy the norms that govern the normal patterns of how to think and behave in the Deep South in the first decades of the twentieth century:

> Sometimes I think it aint none of us pure crazy and aint none of us pure sane until the balance of us talks him that-a-way. It's like it aint so much what a fellow does, but it's the way the majority of folks is looking at him when he does it [...] I aint so sho that ere a man has the right to say what is crazy and what aint. It's like there was a fellow in every man that's done a-past the sanity or the insanity, that watches the sane and the insane doings of that man with the same horror and the same astonishment.
>
> (Faulkner 1930, pp. 226, 232)

With the last sentence, Faulkner brings out the complexity of otherness of the norms that have the power to guide, liberate, trouble, and at times destroy our sense of selfhood. What oppresses or destroys us is not simply an otherness expressed in the norms of the 'majority'; it is an otherness that we feel in ourselves and which can become a source of reflective discomposure 'a-past the sanity or the insanity'.[1] The norms by which I live my life as a person challenge my sense of selfhood. I cannot divert the encroaching challenges of otherness ingrained in these norms by simply clinging to the intimacy of my heterogeneous feelings of selfhood. I am not simply a self. My inarticulate sense of self is too heterogeneous, and my sense of being a self would be lost in such an attempt to be myself in spite of otherness. I am a self who is a person. I can only become myself through the norms that guide my existence as a person in a world shared with other people.

We placed emotions at the heart of the appropriation of otherness that drives human existence. Emotions, we argued, are felt as embodied motivations for actions. We are moved by them, they provide us with an existential orientation which has its roots in both our anonymous biology and our personal history. Emotions, understood as embodied intentionality, motivate us to turn our attention to (or away from) a given object, to move in (or break away from) a given direction. They contribute to our feeling of being involved in the world (engagement), to our grasping the meanings of worldly things and situations (enactment), and to our pre-reflective understanding of other people (attunement).

Emotions arise involuntarily in ourselves and as such they are part of the otherness we experience in ourselves. There are many (or few) things we can choose in our lives, but emotions are not one of them. We cannot choose our emotions. They just happen to us. And yet, we feel that the emotion that we are feeling is *ours*. It is not a pure accident, or something external, which intrudes into our self. It can be a disturbing emotion, a perplexing or even a disrupting one, a momentary affect or a long-lasting mood; an emotion is felt as personal not merely in the sense that we feel it as intimately our own, but also in the sense that it *concerns* us. All that we feel, in some way or other, matters to us, and thus has some kind of significance for the kind of person that we are.

---

[1] Remember Ricoeur's suggestion that 'feeling interiorizes reason and shows me that reason is my reason, for through it I appropriate reason for myself', that is, feeling 'personalizes reason' (1987, p. 102 [118]).

Although emotions belong to the *pathic* dimension of our life, in that they affect us involuntarily, we are not merely passive with respect to our emotions. My emotions constantly challenge the person that I consider myself to be and make my self-understanding an infinite reappropriation of my sense of self. Our cares and concerns can express themselves as feelings over which we have little or no control, but as they come into our consciousness we can *appropriate* them as part of our personal identity. Appropriation involves responsibility. We are responsible for the way we live with our emotions, for the otherness they reveal in ourselves, and for the way in which we integrate this in our personal history. In order to appropriate our emotions, we need rationality and language. To appropriate an emotion is to make a *logos* out of the *pathos*. Paraphrasing with a slight twist Kant's famous dictum, we could say that emotions without rationality are blind, and rationality without emotions is powerless.

Narratives are a way to appropriate our emotions, to articulate, interpret, and communicate our feelings about the world, other people, and ourselves. Narratives provide us with a language for our emotions, a language through which we can appropriate our feelings through an articulation of what we care about. The narratives that we make of our emotional life are attempts to make sense of who we are, who we were, and who we want to be. Once appropriated, our emotions become part of who we think ourselves to be, and thus become integrated, in part at least, into our voluntary decisions and actions.

Disintegration of *Logos* and *Pathos*

Our exploration of this fragile sense of personhood concluded with the claim that this emotional fragility is at the heart of our particular human vulnerability to mental illness. Mental illness is a disorder of rationality, of how we rationally cope with our emotional experience—and this rational endeavour is embedded in the emotional dialectic of selfhood and otherness. To pinpoint our ideas concerning human vulnerability to mental illness, it can be of help to recapitulate our analyses of the schizophrenic and borderline types of existence as extreme instances of the disintegration of emotions and rationality.

To make sense of human emotional experience requires acknowledging that we are personal animals whose emotions include rational as well as a-rational factors. To be a person is neither to be a disembodied, rational spirit nor an a-rational body. On the contrary, we are embodied spirits in the sense that our rational capacities are enmeshed in and motivated by the a-rational mechanisms of our body. Human rationality does not spin in a reflective void, but is saturated with pre-reflective, a-rational feelings that inform and shape our rational attempt to come to terms with the person that we are. If exercised in an emotional void, human rationality may take the form of a disembodied existence disconnected from the basic source of vitality, unrelated to one's own self and to other people, and disengaged from the world—as it happens with the schizophrenic type of existence. In schizophrenia, we find the switching off of the dispositive that makes us feel that we belong to the world, our 'primordial *in esse*'—as Ricoeur calls it. If this basic sense of belonging to the world, this very possibility to be bodily affected, through feelings, is switched off, then a hyper-rational form of existence may arise, characterised—as described in Chapter 8—by morbid rationalism and hyper-reflexivity. Self, body, others, and world are experienced as devitalised and objectified, and the source of one's volitions, movements, and actions may be experienced as an anonymous mechanism, external to one's self.

At the opposite extreme of this disintegration of emotions and rationality, we described the borderline type of existence. Here, emotions are experienced as disordered fluxes, an untamed source of vitality, a disturbing, exuberant force, creative and destructive at the same time. A vigour that engenders life as well as annihilation. Dysphoric mood in borderline persons speaks—in the words of Deleuze—of a 'profound and almost unlivable Power [*Puissance*]' erupting through the body with a transformative effect that makes the normally lived body (*le corps vécu*) 'a paltry thing in comparison' (Deleuze 2003, p. 44 [47]). Commenting on the works of painter Francis Bacon, Deleuze shows that this power is 'conveyed through the nervous wave or vital emotion', and that it can be discovered only by going 'beyond the organism', in a 'chaos where forms are contingent or accessory', since the 'organism is not life, it is what imprisons life' (p. 45 [48]). When this overwhelming power ripples through this body without organs, mere 'flesh and nerve', it produces a violent '"affective athleticism", a scream-breath [*cri-souffle*]' (p. 45 [48])—making conceptual representation impossible.[2] It is, as we argued in Chapter 9, pure intentionality devoid of the moderating power of language and representation, or (to use Bin Kimura's words), pure noesis or noematically empty intentionality. If the noematic representation does not function as a dispositive to control the noetic act, the noetic act will deviate from its relationship with life.

Feeling vulnerable, or the experiential dimension of mental pathology, can be experienced as feeling faintly anchored in oneself—as it is the case with persons with schizophrenia—or feeling overwhelmed by an emotional turmoil without being able to articulate, appropriate, and cope with these troubling emotions—as it is the case with borderline persons. Our emotional life is palpitating with multifarious normative stirrings that involve both biological and personal values, and being a person depends on our constant endeavour to interpret, understand, and cope with these heterogeneous values in the light of the norms (e.g. cultural, societal, ethical, aesthetic) that sustain and orient our existence in a world shared with other people. Central to this interpretive endeavour are our rational capacities to make sense of our emotional experiences and to deal with the values disclosed by our emotions and feelings. Our rational capacities draw upon the reflective resources we find in the norms that are an intrinsic part of our personhood. Persons affected by mental pathologies are at odds with rationality, both their own rational capacities and the rationality of the norms that govern human coexistence. Their rationality is more easily 'wounded' than our own, probably because there exists a troubling *disproportion* between the pervasive quality of their abnormal emotional experiences and the norms that allow them to make sense of their feelings and appropriate them as part of their identity.

---

[2] Deleuze writes that Bacon's paintings evoke hysteria. This is, we think, a diagnostic mistake.

Although our investigation in this book has mainly been about (some of) the ways emotions inform, sustain, and complicate personhood, it goes without saying that rationality remains central to understanding mental illness. We did, however, criticise cognitive theories of emotions for their ambition to find a basic rational fabric ingrained in our emotional life, or some kind of underlying intentional structure that shapes and directs our emotions. Our emotions, we argued, are steeped in the biological functioning of our body to the extent that many of our feelings cannot be brought under the sway of our rational strategies or acquire immediate intelligibility through the intentional structures of our experience. The fact that our emotions are prone to spiral out of rational or reason-responsive control is not a mere unimportant flaw in our rational engagement with the world. On the contrary, the emotional disturbance of our rational dispositions is constitutive of what it means to be a person, and carries informative value about who and what we are. We are rational creatures, and rationality is indeed the hallmark of our humanity, but we cannot hope to explain nor understand rationality in isolation from the innumerable biological features that we share with other higher mammals. Due to this intimate kinship with our evolutionary cousins, our peculiar rational capacities are highly exposed to a-rational disturbances. Our experience and behaviour are characterised by rational dispositions, but, as most of us know too well, these dispositions are intrinsically prone to frustration and very easily disturbed. And as Dominic Murphy cogently puts it:

> We are animals with an evolutionary past, and understanding our normal psychology likely will involve seeing how that past has shaped it. Hence, understanding breakdowns in that psychology will be, at least in part, based on our understanding of how evolved minds are organized. (2006, p. 305)

In a sense, our explorations in this book have been an attempt to clarify and articulate this vulnerable character of rationality as we find it expressed in the fragile character of our emotional life. As explained towards the end of Chapter 1, the conception of rationality, against the background of which we went on to develop our account of emotions and personhood, is inspired by Ronald de Sousa's distinction of *categorical* and *normative* rationality. Categorical rationality accounts for the basic difference between the 'a-rationality' and 'rationality', where 'a-rationality' refers to the anonymous causal functioning which governs most of what goes on in physical nature, and 'rationality' refers to the rational patterns particular to human nature. Normative rationality, on the other hand, explores the unstable character of this particularly human rationality, accounting for our frustrated attempts to distinguish between 'irrational' and 'rational' thoughts, feelings, and behaviour. We argued that we cannot account for human rationality merely in terms of the thin, skeletal kind of rationality responsible for the strict norms that govern logical or mathematical reasoning. Human rationality is a thicker, fleshier, kind of rationality that besides the strict norms of logic involves a more complex web of normative concerns (heterogeneous values, conventions, and norms) that do not possess the stability of the other, more peeled rationality. Human thoughts, feelings, and behaviour are never simply 'rational' or 'irrational', 'right' or 'wrong', 'true' or 'false', 'correct' or 'incorrect', but can also be 'appropriate' or 'inappropriate', 'shallow' or 'deep', 'functional' or 'dysfunctional', 'sensible' or 'insensible', 'adaptive' or 'non-adaptive', 'sentimental' or 'sober'.

This unstable normative texture of human rationality entails that 'reason is'—as Simon Blackburn puts it—'every bit as pliable as sentiment' (2010, p. 25).[3] And it is exactly in this pliable character of our rational capacities that we find a major factor of our vulnerability to mental illness. The rational certainty involved in mathematical or logical reasoning provides a solid foundation for understanding many features of the world in which we human creatures live. This rational certainty turns brittle and problematic, though, the moment we attempt to understand the unstable character of our rationality when it comes to our personal thinking, feeling, and behaviour.

To understand how this rationality becomes disordered or 'wounded' in mental illness, we suggested an exploration of the emotional fragility at the core of our vulnerability to mental suffering. In this exploration, we have attempted to maintain a reflective equilibrium that adopts a naturalistic perspective while focusing on the subjectivity of human experience. As we suggested at the beginning of Chapter 1, this approach can be viewed as a version of what Tim Thornton, following McDowell, has called 'relaxed naturalism'. Although we are basically sympathetic towards this methodological approach, we also expressed some concern that a relaxed version of naturalism runs the risk of transforming too readily the a-rational, causal workings of our biophysical nature into problems of rationality that can be solved by a cognitive approach. The main problem, at least to our view, of a 'relaxed naturalism' is that it tends to downplay the significance of a-rational, causal factors for the functioning of the human mind. Conceiving disorders of rationality as a matter merely of cognitive malfunctioning does not take seriously the cognitively impenetrable aspects of the human mind, particularly evident in our emotional life, and thereby forecloses the possibility that the instability of human rationality, and the problems entailed by this instability, may originate precisely from the basic ambivalence of a-rational and rational factors involved in human experience and thinking.

Our alternative to a cognitive approach, i.e. our model involving the ambivalence of subjectivity and biology in our emotional life, allowed us to examine the irreducible

---

[3] In other words, a major reason for our vulnerability to mental illness lies in the brittle character of our rational attempts to cope with our emotional fluctuations. In the paragraph leading up to this statement, Blackburn explains why it is so important to be aware of this unstable character of rationality: 'If we throw away attention to the particular nature of peoples' flaws, preferring a blanket diagnosis of "unreasonable" or "irrational" whenever their minds move in ways we think inferior, we not only lose important textures and distinctions, but we also lose most chances of engagement and improvement. For "unreasonable" and still more "irrational" not only function as general terms for denigrating the movement of peoples' minds. They usually have further, sinister connotations that the defect is irredeemable, that it is not sensitive to discursive pressures, that it licenses us to treat the subject as a patient or in other ways that are beyond the human pale, or out of the game' (Blackburn 2010, p. 25).

heterogeneity of the rational and a-rational factors at work in mental suffering—and thus to follow George Graham's recent advice for an approach to mental suffering:

> Seek for explanations of a mental disorder that combine references to brute, a-rational neural mechanisms and to the rationality of persons. Examination of the immediate forces behind a mental disorder reveals that they carry two distinct inscriptions. 'Made by unreason' and 'Made by reason'.
>
> (Graham 2010, p. 7)

A Dialectical Conception of Mental Illness

Drawing upon our development of Ricoeur's theory, we employed the dialectical model of selfhood and otherness in the constitution of personal identity to describe, assess, and make sense of the life-world of persons with schizophrenia and borderline personality disorder. Our theory of emotions and personhood provides philosophical support to, and thus strengthens, the dialectical model of mental illness as it has been employed and developed in psychopathology since Pinel first introduced this model in 1800. In fact, Pinel's insistence on the importance of personhood in mental alienation can be seen as an early attempt to bring out the conflictual sense of selfhood involved in mental suffering. Gladys Swain points out this conflictual core in Pinel's understanding of mental alienation:

> [O]ne could say that it is a *reflective dimension* which Pinel introduces into madness: not a complete coincidence of the alienated with himself within the alienation, but a relation between self and self [*un rapport de soi à soi*] maintained in spite of the menace of his effacement present as the horizon of alienation [. . .] thus in essence, two things are both made thinkable: the internal conflict at play in alienation, and the alienation itself as the manifestation of a conflict. (1997, p. 123; our translation)

The reflective dimension that Pinel insists on in mental suffering is exactly what we have explored in the preceding chapters in terms of personhood and emotions. The ambivalence involved in our sense of being a person stems from the emotional complications of being an embodied self. The minimal, pre-reflective sense of selfhood is inherently troubled. That is, the subjective experience of being a self, characterised by a pre-reflective minimal sense of agency and ownership, is awash with emotions, feelings, and moods. Emotions root the self in itself, in its biological constitution. The source of our basic sense of being a self, i.e. of being a vital and self-identical subject of experience, is affective in nature. Also, emotions bind the self to, make it feel attuned to and engaged with, the world, other people, and itself. At the same time, though, the affective dimension of pre-reflective subjective experience discloses the dialectical interplay of the voluntary (selfhood) and the involuntary (otherness) that is at the heart of human vulnerability. To be a *self* is to feel rooted in one's emotional life. The feelings of selfhood are complicated by troubling, and often conflictual and alienating, feelings of otherness that make the self lose itself and thus reveal the need to reflectively reappropriate oneself as a self by *becoming a person* through that otherness. This dialectic of selfhood and otherness brings out the particular vulnerability involved in being a person that is both a biological organism and a conscious self.

Being the self-interpreting animals that we are, we continuously strive to make a *logos* of our *pathos*. This dynamic relation of *logos* and *pathos* is the engine which drives the dialectic of selfhood and otherness at the core of personal identity. A collapse of this dialectic, due to an excess of one or the other, reduces our identity to an identity of immutable sameness.

Psychopathology, that is, all psychopathology and not merely that of psychotic experiences, bears testimony to the many ways in which a collapse of this dialectic entails a loss of our sense of self, a descent into boundless suffering, a removal from human fellowship, a detachment from a shared reality entailing ossified, stereotyped, or simply uncannily unusable experiences of the world. Without going into the details of the dramatic effect of this collapse, which we have already done in the two previous chapters, the excess of *logos* yields a world—paraphrasing Minkowski—in which the dead prevail over the living, the stagnant over the flowing, being over becoming, lived space over lived time. In this kind of world, the dialectic of *logos* and *pathos* is crystallised in a hyper-logic or hypo-pathic configuration, where that prevails which is definable, measurable, abstract, and rationalisable. The person who lives in this world is one who prefers to conceive herself not in relation to the passing train, but in relation to the solid bulk of the roadbed that was there before and after the train has passed. The schizophrenic life-world is a deadened world which corresponds to a paralysed identity, that is, a self that simply *is*—and not a self that is becoming the person through the restless movement of otherness intrinsic to our emotional life.

The life-world of borderline persons appears completely different. However, the identity collapse at the heart of borderline personality disorder is also the result of an identity fossilised in an immutable sameness. Here, too, the paralysed identity is the product of a frustrated disproportion of *logos* and *pathos*, but in this case it stems from an inability to integrate the *pathos* by means of the *logos*. In the previous chapter, we have interpreted the stable instability of the borderline personality disorder as the effect of an untamed vitality—contrary to those who interpret this disorder principally as a mood heedlessly oscillating, punctuated and mixed with a paradoxical apathy. We understand the emotional dimension of the borderline person as the most pregnant epiphany of human vitality. It is a desperate vitality, though, because the borderline person cannot—or will not—let his bouts of energy be restricted by or conformed to the needs of the other person, ethical norms, or societal conventions. He considers such normative restrictions of his vital self-affirmation as inauthentic and therefore as expressions of an unwarranted submission of his truly natural being, of his candour, of his spontaneity. The absence, and the intense contempt, of the *logos* capable of organising his emotions and feelings condemns the borderline person to a series of traumatic experiences of relational failures, romantic bankruptcies, sexual frustrations, and eventually a series of amorous solitudes constantly repeating themselves; in other words, another example of the collapse of personal identity.

These two examples illustrate not only diverse types of the frustrated disproportion between reason and sensibility in human existence, but also different phases of this disproportion along a psychopathological and pathogenic trajectory.[4]

The fixation achieved in the schizophrenic condition, exemplified by preferring the solid bulk of the roadbed upon which the train passes to the passing train itself, is the consequence of a profound transformation of the life-world at the centre of which is a constellation of feelings that we have called the schizophrenic mood. This transformation disrupts the experience of a common world, dodging the logical and linguistic means by which we normally try to organise and understand our experience of the world. The sense of losing reality, the uncanny perplexity, the feelings of alienation from humanity are so radical in the initial phases of schizophrenia that these feelings are to a disturbing extent ineffable, adamant to 'normal' rational explanations, and unable to be articulated in intelligible narratives.[5]

It is in front of this loss of discursive common sense and rational explication that the incipient transformation of the world and one's sense of selfhood generates models of explicative and narrative comprehension, which privilege—in the emblematic case translated by Minkowski—a search for sense mediated exclusively by logical categories at the expense of the comprehension provided by intuitive and emotional dispositions. These logical categories concentrate principally on that which is stable and thus measurable, instead of that which is dynamic and therefore elusive. The life-world engendered by the schizophrenic mood is a reality in which temporal and spatial organisations are typically highly disarticulated: the paradoxical unity of, on the one hand, feelings which fixate on and exalt the detail, the fraction, the particular, the instant, the twinkling of an eye at the cost of totality and continuity, and, on the other hand, a rationality petrifying the perturbing experiences into a world view and a conception of selfhood,

---

[4] In the previous two chapters, our examination of the life-worlds of schizophrenic and borderline persons showed how the dramatic emotional problems involved in these disorders cannot be understood in isolation from the normative challenges particular to the dramatic transformation of the patients' life-worlds. Their experience of body, time, space, and other people are disturbed in the sense that the dialectic of selfhood and otherness is severely disrupted, and so they lose their sense of being a self. We suggested understanding this loss of self as a problem of feeling. Their interpretation of who and what they are is seriously troubled by the drastic changes of their emotional life. In other words, their miscarried hermeneutics of their own self (e.g. ontological delusions in persons with schizophrenia and ontic ones in borderline persons) is inescapably connected with how they feel about their body, the world, and other people.

[5] As Thomas Fuchs observes: 'The languageless character [*Sprachlosigkeit*] of mental suffering and in particular of traumatic experiences points at the limits of language in general. Not all experiences can find their expression in words. Like every medium, language [*Sprache*] both discloses and conceals reality. It never allows us to discern the issues except in a pre-structured way. In language the world is always "premeditated" ["*vorgedacht*"], and that so fundamentally that language can appear as the absolutely all-encompassing [*das schlecthin Umgreifende*] which shapes all human feeling [*Empfinden*], perception [*Wahrnehmen*], and thinking [*Denken*]. Hence, the inherent limits of language are not easy to recognize and to name. That such limits exist, is confirmed by the suffering from lack of language itself: mentally ill persons often complain that they are not able to conceive their experience in words' (Fuchs 2008, p. 134; our translation).

which privileges sameness over change and alienation in selfhood over alienation in otherness. As such, it is a world which lends itself to be understood through separately parcelled categories. A hyper-logical and hypo-pathic world made of solid and immovable bulks of roadbed, and not trains, may therefore be considered an effect and not the original cause of the existential transformation which we call schizophrenic.[6]

The fixation that we find in borderline persons illustrates another kind of extreme disproportion of *logos* and *pathos*. Here, as we have seen, the initial cause is the presence of a vital drive that does not accommodate to the conditions of common sense; in fact, the borderline person refuses such conditions and wilfully enters into brash collision with the hypocrisy and the inauthenticity of the pallid emotions by which other people live. In a sense it is a kind of *absolute pathos* that we are allowed to experience in the borderline existence: the uncompromising and defying energy with which the borderline person afflicts, irritates, terrorises the other person while also being flattering, exciting, and inflaming. It is an emotional energy that throws itself at the other with overwhelming intensity. Often, this impulse takes on a sexual form which the borderline person defines as 'love'. And the borderline person is not able to detach himself from the object (and we are, in fact, dealing with an object and *not* a person). The 'loved' one is part of him. He cannot live without it. He is not able to separate himself from it any more than he is able to separate himself from his arm or leg. He cannot forget about it. It would be like forgetting about his own life or the meaning of his being alive. The object of his love, so claims the borderline person, is the very source of his vitality.

The loved object is the form that the desperate vitality takes for the borderline person, that is, it is the collector of the flux of pathic intentionality, noetically dense but otherwise noematically depleted. One could say that the loved object is the manageable form of the *pathos* of the borderline person, and as such it represents a relief for the torment involved in feeling pervaded by an aimless vitality. This is the principal reason why it is impossible for the borderline person to separate himself from the loved object in spite of the pain that this inflicts because of the lack of recognition or the encroaching abandonment, the ambiguities, suspicions, frustrations, humiliations, failures, and so on. The borderline person thus achieves a miscarried hermeneutics of his own *pathos*, using the category 'love' to denominate this disturbed bond. With this name, he ennobles his feelings, assigns them to the most prestigious position according to his scheme of values, and thereby finds a strong and definitive collocation for his fragile sense of identity.

What we find expressed in these psychopathological conditions is a collapse of the fragile dialectic of selfhood and otherness constitutive of human personhood. We are vulnerable because we care about being the persons that we are. And we can only become who we are through the otherness that we are. Due to this inescapable presence of otherness in the heart of our selfhood, our identity is not a fact but a task, which we have to accomplish through a constant interaction with the otherness that we are not. In this sense, we are fragile beings characterised by the constitutive ambivalence

---

[6] In fact, at the beginning of this transformation, one may suppose that persons with schizophrenia are probably dealing with an opposite disproportion of *pathos* and *logos*, in which prevails an overpowering *pathos* unmanageable for the logical structures of reason and common sense. Thus, ultimately, what is achieved is a troubling welding of an abnormal and disproportionate emotional experience and the search for a *logos* able to dominate the emotional intensity.

of selfhood and otherness. It is an inescapable ambivalence that can produce a healthy dialectic of opposites: being and wanting to be, being and appearing to be, the voluntary and involuntary, emotions and rationality, sensibility and understanding, and all the innumerable expressions of our becoming the person that we are.

In this perspective, pathology is not the contrast of irreducible oppositions, but exactly the collapse of the contrast. That is, pathology is the collapse of the non-coincidence, the conflictual tension, of the dialectic nourished by the contrast—and in particular the inability of the person to achieve the constant mediation of his or her own conflictual non-coincidence. The pathology therefore consists in the inability (due to the enhanced existential fragility), on part of the person, to exercise a moderation and an integration by means of his or her own reflective capacities. In other word, health is not something given, a *datum*, but a practice, an *ethics*, established through a reappropriation of the non-coincidence, the conflictual and vulnerable character, constitutive of the person that every one of us is. Health, and the fragile freedom which characterises health, 'is, in each of its moments, activity and receptivity. It constitutes itself in receiving what it does not create: values, capacities, and sheer nature' (Ricoeur 1966, p. 384 [454]).

Towards a Therapy of Care

Appreciating the fragile character of personhood may lead to a therapeutic sensibility to the vulnerability underlying psychopathological trajectories. This, in turn, enables us to understand that the psychopathological configurations which human existence takes on in the clinic, are the outcome of a miscarried hermeneutics of one's feelings and of the transformations of the life-world that those feelings bring about. The development of a pathogenetic trajectory might be the following: (1) a disentanglement of emotions and rationality from each other, bringing about an uncanny metamorphosis of the life-world, (2) a person's miscarried hermeneutics of the transformed life-world, (3) the fixation in a pathological life-world in which the dialectic of selfhood and otherness collapses. This understanding of our vulnerability to mental illness contains a rudimentary framework for engaging with such a fragility by means of hermeneutical therapy. The aim of such a therapy is to re-establish the dialectic of selfhood and otherness that will allow the suffering person to become who she or he is. It goes without saying, though, that these concluding pages are nothing but a suggestive proposal. To work out properly a therapeutic approach to mental illness in terms of care would be an enterprise far beyond the scope of the present book.

Against the background of the previous explorations, our proposal can be boiled down to the claim that our best way to deal with a person's mental illness is to use the *fragility of personhood* as a point of departure for understanding and coping with mental suffering.[7]

---

[7] Also Thomas Fuchs has singled out the vulnerability of human personhood as a crucial aspect of mental illness, and, accordingly, the notion of personhood as indispensable to psychiatry: 'Persons are endangered beings. In fact, one could say that a human being becomes mentally ill because he is a person, that is, he stands in a relation to himself and therefore carries within him the possibility for self-disruption [*Selbstentzweiung*] up to self-loss [*Selbstverlust*]. In order to find himself again, he is in need of others who understand what it means to be a person. Psychiatry cannot renounce the notion of personhood' (Fuchs 2002, p. 159; our translation).

To help a suffering mind we must start by acknowledging that mental suffering is not merely a matter of thinking nor can its causes be limited to the activation or inhibition of the neurological webs of our brain. Our mental torments are embodied and *personal*. To find the origin and cause of pain is a bewildering challenge even when it comes to suffering caused by a fairly obvious physical event. When I stub my toe against the table leg or hit my thumb with a hammer, I experience a radiance of pain that seems to originate in either my toe or my thumb but soon ripples through my entire body; it can make me dizzy, nauseous, euphoric, angry, sad, leave me indifferent, make me cry, or even make me laugh. I might know or be told that the pain which I am feeling does indeed originate in the damaged nerve tissue of my thumb and that my feeling of pain is caused by noxious stimulation that activates certain parts of my brain (e.g. Vogt 2005). But even though we are convinced by this physical location and tracking of pain, most of us are aware of the experiential complexity of these physical facts. Truls Wyller articulates this awareness eloquently:

> It is certainly true that as living beings we feel pain in particular limbs and not 'in' the 'person'. But, equally true, without a person feeling the pain there would be no pain. That the pain is in my thumb is a natural thing to say. But so is my saying that I feel the pain, and I would not say my thumb feels it. That is why we comfort persons and not their thumbs—except, perhaps, when we care for small children: 'Oh poor thumb, are you hurting so much? Let me give you a kiss'.
>
> (Wyller 2005, pp. 385–6)

Attempts to locate and individuate the causes for mental pain are, obviously, even more precarious. What Wyller observes about clearly circumscribed physical pain, namely, that when we are in pain '[s]omehow the *whole* person experiences the pain as painful' (2005, p. 336), is more readily obvious when it comes to mental pain. While we may be able to comfort small children—and perhaps also adults—by paying careful attention to a broken arm or a sore bruise, it seems an awkward, even absurd, endeavour trying to help a troubled mind by paying exclusive attention to 'the broken brain' (Andreasen 2001). One of the principal features which makes our mental pain more bewildering than their physical counterpart is that the origins and causes of our mental suffering seem to involve the person more radically. Our identity is what is at stake in mental illness. We may lose ourselves in our mental pain more easily than we can by hitting our thumb with a hammer. This may be an obvious, but not in any way a trivial difference. While in most cases the question 'how do you feel?' is ridiculous when asked of a person who has just hit her thumb with a hammer, it remains a crucial question every time we want to understand and help a person suffering from mental pain. The subjectivity of pain surfaces as an increasingly concrete explanatory problem as our means of objectively individuating the cause of pain (e.g. the hammer blow) diminishes; in other words, the person involved in the experience of mental pain is a more significant factor in explaining the painful experience than when we are dealing with physical pain where potential causes are more readily identified. Mental pain is personal to an extent that physical pain is not. We care about our mental suffering because the pain we feel in mental illness is a pain which is an intimate and inescapable part of the person that we are. It is the entire person who suffers from a pain that rarely finds an explicit cause or origin. The unexplainable character of mental suffering becomes an additional cause that often only enhances suffering.

To reach the person who is engulfed or paralysed by the suffering of mental illness, we should pay attention to the expressions of *care* that still remain as distorted echoes of the person whom suffering has rendered unrecognisable. We suggest a hermeneutical therapy which is worked out on the basis of the account of the intimate and intimidating relationship of emotions and personhood developed in this book. It is an approach to mental suffering that approaches the 'end-products' of mental illness in terms of the normative vulnerability that characterises the fragility of human personhood, that is, a dynamic approach that understands those 'end-products' as the suffering person's miscarried hermeneutics of their own selves, and which proposes a therapy of these painful interpretative endeavours in terms of the notion of care.

In our view, such a therapeutic approach has the advantage of taking seriously the complex fragility at the core of human vulnerability while still being able to propose concrete therapeutic means to deal with this vulnerability. To use the fragility of personhood to make sense of vulnerability has the further advantage of respecting the suffering person's sense of being an autonomous self without neglecting the a-personal factors involved in mental alienation. In fact, it should not come as a surprise that at the heart of our therapeutic outline is exactly the interplay of self and otherness that we have spent so much time on.

A therapy of care is founded on an ontology of care: we propose an understanding of what it is to be a human being through the complexity of what a person cares about. The ontology of care sketched by Ricoeur and further developed by us in this book insists on the affective generation of our heterogeneous values and concerns, i.e. the ambivalence of rational and a-rational factors at the heart of our emotional life, and traces the experiential tension and conflict that this ambivalence effectuates in our troubled awareness of selfhood. Our originating affirmation of selfhood is constantly troubled by the otherness revealed by our ambivalent feelings. Our feelings are *intimate* in the sense that they make our experiences matter to us and thereby make them our experiences, and yet our feelings are also *intimidating* because of the otherness they reveal in ourselves. My feelings make me aware that I am who I am because of the otherness of my body, the world, and other people. I care about otherness because my care reveals that I am that which I am not. In short, an ontology of care understands what it is to be a human person in terms of the dialectic of selfhood and otherness disclosed by the importance of what a person cares about.

Against this ontological background, a therapy of care involves two fundamental attitudes to mental illness. It is a therapeutic approach that acknowledges the fragility constitutive of human personhood. It also insists, however, on our responsibility for being the person that we are. To become the person that we are, we must become aware of what we care about, because being a person is to take upon oneself the responsibility involved in what one cares about. Thus, a therapy of care is a therapeutic approach that respects the constitutional fragility of who and what we are, and thus conceives of mental illness as the result of a normative vulnerability intrinsic to being a human person, while insisting that to help a suffering person is to help that person accept and live with the responsibility involved in that which she or he cares about.

Our emotions represent a fundamental aspect of the otherness that is part of who and what we are, or in other words, the involuntary factors of our identity that trouble our sense of selfhood and are at the core of the dialectic constitutive of personhood. The role played by our emotions in this dialectic is somewhat paradoxical.

On the one hand, our emotions are stable dispositions, behavioural patterns which are repeated over time, involuntary procedures profoundly rooted in the biological body as well as the personal story characterising a certain individual. They are thus a constant, an element of the 'sameness' of my character in the dialectic of identity. In this sense, my emotions characterise who I am. A person can be recognised and individuated by means of her emotional reactions, whether choleric or phlegmatic, hyperthymic or dysphoric, and there a exists vast tradition of research—from Aristotle's *Rhetoric* to the current theories of affective temperament—that attempts to establish distinct human temperamental types by means of their emotional reactions. On the other hand, our emotions are that which motivates and moves us, and are thus able to perturb our sense of self. I am touched by my emotions and feelings, and I can only be touched by that which is—at least to some extent—other than myself. My emotions can surprise me, frighten me, and make me do inappropriate things in which I do not recognise myself. At times, our emotions make us feel unfamiliar with ourselves, we can be ashamed of our emotions and even condemn them from an ethical point of view. They may also, however, make us discover, or rediscover, aspects of our sensibility that we thought were not there, or had been buried a long time ago. Our emotions, as we have argued throughout the book, do not let our sense of self remain stable and identical to itself.

Hence, our emotions are part of the otherness that represents our inescapable sameness, the implicit stability upon which we conceive, and are recognised to be, the persons that we are. And yet, they can also emerge as an explicit otherness that troubles our implicit sense of sameness and personal stability. In any case, we are all compelled to integrate our emotions into our understanding of who we are during our becoming the person that we are; to become the person that we are, we must, in other words, try to integrate the implicit with the explicit, or otherness with selfhood. My emotions are the vital energy, the existential backbone, which both supports my sense of being a self, and drives the dialectic of selfhood and otherness essential to personal identity. We have to take care of our emotions in order to understand and live with who we are. This means that we have a responsibility, not only to moderate and dominate our emotions, or to control our emotions and avoid being carried away by them, but also to try to understand the multifaceted feelings involved in our emotional life. Our emotions encompass a-rational and rational factors resulting in an ambivalent kind of intelligibility that is both intimate and alienating, personal and anonymous. It is an unpolished, unstable, and a highly fragile intelligibility, which requires a rational effort of interpretation sensitive to the a-rational features of human nature. This interpretation is supposed to try to name what cannot be named, to narrate the inenarrable, to express the inexpressible in the attempt to confer order on our emotional life, and to attribute causes and assign meanings to our ambivalent feelings and conflicting emotions. The ontological ambiguity constitutive of our being personal animals makes this interpretative endeavour an unceasing task. We have to live our life accepting the inescapable emotional ambivalence of our rational effort to understand ourselves.

Our emotional life is central to a therapy of care, since our feelings and emotions are a central part of the concerns, values, and norms that our care is an expression of.[8] Our feelings both constitute and reveal what we care about, and disclose that our care is not limited to what we think or believe that we care about. The cognitively impenetrable character of our emotional life binds us to what we are in our reflective attempt to reappropriate our sense of selfhood, that is, in our constant endeavour to understand who we are and to become who we want to be.[9] We are what we are, but we have to become who we are through a responsible reappropriation of what we are, of what has happened to us, and of what we have said and done. We have developed this narrative approach to personal identity with a particular focus on how our emotions affect our identity as persons.

We have aimed at providing an account of human emotions that includes, and is able to make sense of, the inarticulate moods and feelings. The feelings involved in our moods are often difficult to understand, describe, and live with. Nevertheless, they are fundamental to the emotional life of a person. We suggested a hermeneutical account of the relationship between emotions and personhood that is adequate for articulating these vague and hazy feelings and may thus furnish a language which can help us cope with at least some of the impalpable aspects of our emotional life. We explained how narratives enable us to articulate the complexity of our emotional life, and argued that the narrative structures of our emotional experiences help to bring out the dynamic interplay of the voluntary and involuntary aspects of our emotions and feelings. By focusing on the dialectical development of moods into affects and vice versa, we explained how our identity as persons is always at play in our emotions. The narrative dimension is introduced as *therapy* when a person needs to cope explicitly with the dialectic of selfhood and otherness involved in his or her troubled and troubling experience of being a self.

Our experience and behaviour is brimming with emotions, feelings, and moods that turn the notion of rationality into an open normative question. Often there exists a painful discrepancy between how I feel and what I feel that I should feel. Perhaps I want to feel differently, but no matter how hard I try I am incapable of conjuring up the feelings consistent with the kind of person that I want to be. Also, I know that my

---

[8] The normative problems involved in psychopathology are very delicate. The clinician should, of course, suspend moral judgements and pre-established norms of right and wrong, good or bad, in order to be able to pay close attention to the particular nature of peoples' flaws, and not simply write off thoughts, feelings, behaviour as 'irrational', 'bad', 'wrong' or in any way 'beyond the human pale'—as Blackburn so poignantly puts it. It is in this sense that psychopathology is a descriptive enterprise. Moral judgements would only impair our chances of coming to understand the obscure movements of the disordered mind. And yet, throughout the book we have argued that human personhood is normative in nature: to be a person is a normative task of becoming who and what I am. To be a self is to become a person, and this inescapable relation between selfhood and personhood introduces normative questions at the heart of the descriptive endeavour of psychopathology.

[9] This was what Ricoeur tried to capture with his account of narrative identity: the dialectic of sameness (*idem* or *character*) and selfhood (*ipse* or *keeping one's word*) at the fragile heart of personhood.

feelings tell something about myself, maybe something very important, although I may not want to acknowledge this. Feelings express more powerfully and often in a much less diplomatic manner than reflection the involuntary side of who I am—although they are also much 'dirtier' (to use LeDoux's metaphor) in the sense of being imprecise, inaccurate, and indeterminate. In this sense, feelings *approximate* me to myself. The fact that feelings are able to reveal aspects of myself that I may not be reflectively aware of does not entail, however, that feelings are therefore truer, more correct or more natural expressions of who I am than my reflective conception of who I am. It is simply wrong to ascribe this kind of normative transparency to my emotional life. My feelings can be just as problematic as my thoughts—often they are more so due to the fact that they are nourished by both a-rational and rational factors and therefore do not always tally well with the intentional, rational, or pragmatic structures that characterise my thinking.[10]

Some years ago, the Italian philosopher Umberto Galimberti, who for more than thirty years has worked intensely with the encounter of philosophy and psychopathology, proposed a philosophical approach to mental illness that he named a 'therapy of ideas'. In a recent formulation of this approach, he asks:

> Do our mental sufferings and our existential unease always depend—as psychoanalysis wants us to believe—upon internal conflicts, remote traumas, compulsions [*coazioni*] to repeat past experiences consolidated in us? Or do they sometimes, perhaps in most cases, depend upon our *world view* [*nostra visione del mondo*], which is too narrow [*angusta*], too indurated [*sclerotizzata*], too thoughtless [*irriflessa*] to allow us, on the one hand, to understand the world in which we live and, on the other, to find a meaning for our existence and thus good reasons for living in accordance with ourselves? If the second hypothesis is the correct one, then why not take into consideration *a therapy of ideas*?
>
> (Galimberti 2009, p. 152, our translation)

We believe that Galimberti's idea about a philosophical approach to therapy is on the right track. However, we neither share his suspicion against 'internal conflicts' (although we do not understand such conflicts in a strict psychoanalytical sense, rather as the ubiquitous expression of non-coincidence of the 'wounded Cogito') nor his confidence in our rational capacities to cure the poverty of our 'world view'. We would argue instead for *a therapy of care* that acknowledges the significance of the obscure and cognitively impenetrable aspects of our emotional life without abandoning the importance of our rationality. A therapy of ideas operates with an ontology of human nature that focuses on our particular rational capacities at the cost of the a-rational aspect of our nature. A therapy of care, on the contrary, by acknowledging 'the importance of what

---

[10] The normative questions that my feelings bring about are not simply whether they are right or wrong, true or false, appropriate or inappropriate. Emotional matters are more complicated than the explicit norms by which we judge them—be that rational, biological, ethical, or pragmatic norms. This is perhaps because emotions admit of context-sensitive degrees and are brimming with the subjective features of experience, which 'suggest that they are closer kin to evaluations than to norms' (de Sousa 2006, p. 32). While norms, no matter what their origin, aspire to a kind of objective or even universal measure that is constitutionally deaf to the subjective voice, evaluations carry with them the full force of subjectivity.

we care about' (Frankfurt 1982), understands human nature in terms of an ontology of care that allows us to take seriously the question 'How do you feel?' and articulate it without deciding in advance what is 'rational', 'appropriate', or 'sane' to care about.

The unquestionable fact that there are no straightforward answers to such a question makes evident the vulnerable character of human rationality; or as de Sousa points out, 'while there is a clear rationale for avoiding inconsistent beliefs, there is so far no equally clear rationale for insisting that we ought to avoid feeling inconsistent emotions' (2011, p. 77). We all know that our emotions are not always rational, and neither are always our hopes for the future, our dreams, desires, or actual behaviour. In fact, our feelings often challenge our notion(s) of rationality, because they make us question the normative splendour of rational thinking and behaviour. Is it really a good thing always to behave rationally? Why should I care about the future if that means to deprive myself of the pleasures of what is going on right now? I know that she is bad for me, but I want her! She hurts me again and again, but how can I leave her? Feelings make what we experience matter to us. They make us think about what to say and do. Was it really irrational when it felt good? I also like to sit in a cornfield counting crows while I smoke cigarettes and drink cold beers. Too many beers, and every one of the cigarettes, are bad for me, and I am well aware that it is a stupidly irrational thing to do, if not suicidal. Nonetheless, it makes me happy. I may even value and eventually choose things that I know will make me sad, or are somehow bad for me. The irresistible pleasure of Shakespeare's tragedies, a hopeless love affair or devouring an entire box of chocolate are all examples of the reverse side of rationality that I am. My attraction to, and voluntary enjoyment of, such things makes sense in spite of—or perhaps exactly because of—the fact that it goes against the grain of rational behaviour. I may want to be irrational, love the irrationality of my wife, and be proud of the thoughtless spontaneity of my child. Rational arguments and pragmatic reflection are at times so tedious exactly because they have the tendency to desiccate the a-rational spontaneity that is constitutive of human life. In fact, our existence does not seem particularly rational. Our existence springs from and is constantly affected by a-rational factors that we then try to understand, shape, and develop rationally. We do not need the natural sciences to teach us this. The experiential fact that much of what we feel, from intense joy to devastating sadness, cannot be brought under rational control, should make us leery of attempts to establish strict norms of rational and irrational behaviour.

So instead of following the trajectory of Galimberti's rational therapy of *world views*, we believe that a therapeutic approach to our vulnerability to mental illness would be better off following Remo Bodei's succinct reformulation of the ontological conviction behind Spinoza's philosophical cure of human emotions:

> The philosophy of Spinoza has as its aim the education of human beings who are free both internally and externally, who are neither serfs [*servi*] nor robots [*automi*]. It therefore deals with the passions which are already forms of imaginative understanding [*conoscenza*]. It does not—as a matter of principle—treat those passions as riotous serfs, but as energies and forms of inferior knowledge [*sapere*] which can be guided to their transformation [*metamorforsi*] into affects (and thus to the abandonment of the side of passivity) through a growth of understanding.
>
> (Bodei 1992, p. 184; our translation)

Our rationality is unstable, and the only way to strengthen the use of our rational capacities is to take seriously the a-rational character of our emotional understanding as a *form of knowledge*—though an obscurely ambivalent knowledge—and to transform the inescapable passivity of our inarticulate feelings into a growing understanding of who and what we are. Or to put it differently, understanding the fragile complexity of what we care about helps us make sense of our own vulnerability. To be human is to deal with the fragility of our values and norms by taking upon us the responsibility for articulating, making sense of, and appropriating our ambivalent feelings. A therapy of care may be of help in supporting persons who find it difficult to take this responsibility upon themselves—but such a therapy only works if we start by acknowledging the human fragility that make the life of every person uniquely vulnerable.

References

Agamben, G. (2004). *The Open: Man and Animal.* Translated by Attell, K. Stanford: Stanford University Press; *L'aperto: L'uomo e l'animale.* Torino: Bollati Boringhieri.

Akiskal, H.S. (1994). The Temperamental Borders of Affective Disorders. *Acta Psychiatrica Scandinavica* **89** (379, Suppl.): 32–7.

Akiskal, H.S. (1996). The Temperamental Foundations of Affective Disorders. In: Mundt, C., Hahlweg, K., and Fiedler, P. (eds.) *Interpersonal Factors in the Origin and Course of Affective Disorders.* London: Gaskell, 3–30.

Akiskal, H.S. and Mallya, G. (1987). Criteria for the 'Soft' Bipolar Spectrum: Treatment Implications. *Psychopharmacology Bulletin* **23** (1): 68–73.

Akiskal, K.K. and Akiskal, H.S. (2005). The Theoretical Underpinnings of Affective Temperaments: Implications for Evolutionary Foundations of Bipolarity and Human Nature. *Journal of Affective Disorders* **85** (1–2): 231–9.

Andreasen, N.C. (2001). *Brave New Brain: Conquering Mental Illness in the Era of the Genome.* Oxford: Oxford University Press.

Andreasen, N.C. (2007). DSM and the Death of Phenomenology in America: An Example of Unintended Consequences. *Schizophrenia Bulletin* **33** (1): 108–22.

Baker, L.R. (2000). *Bodies and Persons: A Constitution View.* Cambridge: Cambridge University Press.

Baker, L.R. (2007). *The Metaphysics of Everyday Life: An Essay in Practical Realism.* Cambridge: Cambridge University Press.

Ballerini, A. and Rossi Monti, M. (1990). *La vergogna e il delirio.* Torino: Bollati Boringhieri.

Barcelona, A. (1986). On the Concept of Depression in American English: A Cognitive Approach. *Revista Canaria de Estudios Ingleses* **12**: 7–35.

Baudelaire, C. (1951). *Œuvres complètes.* Paris: Gallimard.

Beedie, C.J., Terry P.C., and Lane A.M. (2005). Distinctions Between Emotion and Mood. *Cognition and Emotion* **19** (6): 847–78.

Bennett, J. (1984). *A Study of Spinoza's Ethics.* Indianapolis: Hackett Publishing Company.

Berner, P. (1991). Delusional Atmosphere. *British Journal of Psychiatry* **159** (Suppl. 14): 88–93.

Berner, P., Gabriel, E., Katsching, H., Kieffer, W., Koehler, K., Lenz, G., Nutzinger, D., Schanda, H., and Simhandl, C. (1992). *Diagnostic Criteria for Functional Psychoses.* Cambridge: Cambridge University Press.

Berner, P., Musalek, M., and Walter, H. (1987). Psychopathological Concepts of Dysphoria. *Psychopathology* **20** (2): 93–100.

Bernstein, R.J. (1995). Whatever Happened to Naturalism? *Proceedings and Addresses of the American Philosophical Association* **69** (2): 57–76.

Berrios, G.E. (1996). *The History of Mental Symptoms: Descriptive Psychopathology since the Nineteenth Century.* Cambridge: Cambridge University Press.

Berze, J. and Guhle, H.W. (1929). *Psychologie der Schizophrenie.* Berlin: Springer Verlag.

Binswanger, L. (1960). *Melancholie und Manie.* Pfullingen: Verlag Günther Neske.

Blackburn, S. (1998). *Ruling Passions: A Theory of Practical Reasoning.* Oxford: Oxford University Press.

Blackburn, S. (2006). Julius Caesar and George Berkeley Play Leapfrog. In: MacDonald, C. and MacDonald, G. (eds.) *McDowell and his Critics.* Oxford: Blackwell Publishing, 203–16.

Blackburn, S. (2010). The Majesty of Reason. *Philosophy* **85** (1): 5–27.

Blankenburg, W. (1971). *Der Verlust der natürlichen Selbstverständlichkeit*. Stuttgart: Enke.

Blankenburg, W. (1980). Phenomenology and Psychopathology. *Journal of Phenomenological Psychology* **11** (2): 52–78.

Blankenburg, W. (1982). A Dialectical Conception of Anthropological Proportions. In: De Koning, A.J.J. and Jenner, F.A. (eds.) *Phenomenology and Psychiatry*. London: Academic Press, 35–50.

Blankenburg, W. (2001/1969). First Steps Toward a Psychopathology of 'Common Sense'. (Translated by Mishara, A.L.) *Philosophy, Psychiatry & Psychology* **8** (4): 303–15.

Bleuler, E. (1911). *Dementia praecox oder Gruppe der Schizophrenien*. Leipzig: Franz Deuticke.

Bodei, R. (1992). *Geometria delle passioni: Paura, speranza e felicità – filosofia e uso politico*. Milano: Feltrinelli.

Bovet, P. and Parnas, J. (1993). Schizophrenic Delusions: A Phenomenological Approach. *Schizophrenia Bulletin* **19** (3): 579–97.

Bruns, G.L. (1992). *Hermeneutics: Ancient and Modern*. New Haven: Yale University Press.

Callieri, B. (1982). *Quando vince l'ombra*. Roma: Città Nuova.

Callieri, B. (1999). Wahnstimmung e perplessità: La sospensione di significato fra gli esordi del delirare schizofrenico. In: Rossi Monti, M. and Stanghellini, G. (eds.) *Psicopatologia della schizofrenia: Prospettive metodologiche e cliniche*. Milano: raffaelo Cortina Editore, 3–12.

Cannon, W.B. (1927). The James-Lange Theory of Emotions: A Critical Examination and an Alternative Theory. *The American Journal of Psychology* **39** (1): 106–24.

Carlson, G.A. and Goodwin, F.K. (1973). The Stages of Mania: A Longitudinal Analysis of the Manic Episode. *Archives of General Psychiatry* **28** (2): 221–8.

Changeux, J.P. and Ricoeur, P. (2000/1998). *What Makes Us Think?* Translated by DeBevoise, M.B. Princeton: Princeton University Press; *La nature et la règle: Ce qui nous fait penser*. Paris: Odile Jacob.

Charland, L.C. (2008). A Moral Line in the Sand: Alexander Crichton and Philippe Pinel on the Psychopathology of the Passions. In: Charland, L.C. and Zachar, P. (eds.) *Fact and Value in Emotion*. Amsterdam: John Benjamins Publishing Company, 15–33.

Charland, L.C. (2010). Science and Morality in the Affective Psychopathology of Philippe Pinel. *History of Psychiatry* **21** (1): 38–53.

Clark, A. (1997). *Being There: Putting Brain, Body, and World Together Again*. Cambridge: The MIT Press.

Coetzee, J.M. (1994). *The Master of Petersburg*. London: Secker & Warburg.

Conrad, K. (1958). *Die beginnende Schizophrenie: Versuch einer Gestaltanalyse des Wahns*. Stuttgart: Georg Thieme Verlag.

Correale, A. (2007). *Area traumatica e campo istituzionale*, seconda edizione. Roma: Borla Edizioni.

Cutting, J. (1989). Gestalt Theory and Psychiatry: Discussion Paper. *Journal of the Royal Society of Medicine* **82** (7): 429–31.

Cutting, J. (1997). *Principles of Psychopathology: Two Minds, Two Worlds, Two Hemispheres*. Oxford: Oxford University Press.

Cutting, J. (1999). *Psychopathology and Modern Philosophy*. West Sussex: The Forest Publishing Co.

Cutting, J. (2002). *The Living, the Dead and the Never-Alive*. West Sussex: The Forest Publishing Co.

Cutting, J. (2009a). Scheler, Phenomenology, and Psychopathology. *Philosophy, Psychiatry & Psychology* **16** (2): 143–59.

Cutting, J. (2009b). Psychopathologists and Philosophers. *Philosophy, Psychiatry & Psychology* **16** (2):175–8.

Cutting, J. (2011). *A Critique of Psychopathology*. West Sussex: The Forest Publishing Company.

Damasio, A.R. (1994). *Descartes' Error: Emotion, Reason, and the Human Brain*. New York: Putnam.

Damasio, A.R. (1999). *The Feeling of What Happens: Body and Emotion in the Making of Consciousness*. New York: Harcourt.

Damasio, A.R. (2000). A Second Chance for Emotions. In: Lane, R.D. and Nadel, L. (eds.) *Cognitive Neuroscience of Emotion*. Oxford: Oxford University Press, 12–23.

Damasio, A.R. (2003). *Looking for Spinoza: Joy, Sorrow, and the Feeling Brain*. New York: Harcourt.

Damasio, A.R. (2004). Emotions and Feelings: A Neurobiological Perspective. In: Manstead, A.S.R., Frijda, N., and Fischer, A. (eds.) *Feelings and Emotions. The Amsterdam Symposium*. Cambridge: Cambridge University Press, 49–57.

Damasio, A.R. (2010). *Self Comes to Mind: Constructing the Conscious Brain*. London: William Heineman.

Davidson, D. (1999). Reply to John McDowell. In: Hahn, L.E. (ed.) *The Philosophy of Donald Davidson*. Chicago: Open Court, 105–9.

de Caro, M. and McArthur, D. (eds.) (2004): *Naturalism in Question*. Cambridge: Harvard University Press.

de Caro, M. and McArthur, D. (eds.) (2010). *Naturalism and Normativity*. New York: Columbia University Press.

de Clérambault, G. (1942). Psychoses à base d'automatisme. Premier article. In: *Oeuvre psychiatrique*, réuni et publié par Fretet, J. Paris: PUF, 528–44.

Deigh, J. (2010). Concepts of Emotions in Modern Philosophy and Psychology. In: Goldie, P. (ed.) *The Oxford Handbook of Philosophy of Emotions*. Oxford: Oxford University Press, 17–40.

Deleuze, G. (1986). *Foucault*. Paris: Les Éditions de Minuit.

Deleuze, G. (2003/2002). *Francis Bacon: The Logic of Sensation*. Translated by Smith, D.W London: Continuum; *Francis Bacon: Logique de la sensation* [1st edition 1981]. Paris: Éditions du Seuil.

Del Pistoia, L. (2008). *Saggi fenomenologici: Psicopatologia, clinica, epistemologia*. Roma: Giovanni Fioriti Editore.

de Martino, E. (1997). *Il mondo magico: Prolegomena a una storia del magismo*. Torino: Bollati Boringhieri.

de Sousa, R. (1987). *The Rationality of Emotions*. Cambridge: The MIT Press.

de Sousa, R. (2006). Restoring Emotion's Bad Rep: The Moral Randomness of Norms. *European Journal of Analytic Philosophy* **2** (1): 27–45.

de Sousa, R. (2007). *Why Think? Evolution and the Rational Mind*. Oxford: Oxford University Press.

de Sousa, R. (2010). The Mind's Bermuda Triangle: Philosophy of Emotions and Empirical Science. In: Goldie, P. (ed.) *The Oxford Handbook of Philosophy of Emotions*. Oxford: Oxford University Press, 93–117.

de Sousa, R. (2011). *Emotional Truth*. Oxford: Oxford University Press.

de Waal, F. (2005). *Our Inner Ape: The Best and Worst of Human Nature*. London: Granata Books.

Dixon, T. (2003). *From Passions to Emotions: The Creation of a Secular Psychological Category*. Cambridge: Cambridge University Press.

Dupré, J. (1993). The *Disorder of Things: The Metaphysical Foundations of the Disunity of Science*. Cambridge: Harvard University Press.

Dupré, J. (2001). *Human Nature and the Limits of Science*. Oxford: Oxford University Press.

Egan, J. (2010). *A Visit from the Goon Squad*. New York: Alfred A. Knopf.

Ekman, P. (1992). An Argument for Basic Emotions. *Cognition and Emotion* **6** (3–4): 169–200.

Ekman, P. (2003). *Emotions Revealed: Understanding Faces and Feelings*. London: Weidenfeld & Nicolson.

Eliot, T.S. (1944). *Four Quartets*. London: Faber and Faber.

Elster, J. (1999). *Alchemies of the Mind*. Cambridge: Cambridge University Press.

Erikson, E. (1968). *Identity: Youth and Crisis*. New York: W.W. Norton & Company.

Evans, J., Akiskal, H.S., Keck Jr, P.E., McElroy, S.L., Sadovnick, A.D., Remick, R.A., and Kelsoe, J.R. (2005). Familiality of Temperament in Bipolar Disorder: Support for a Genetic Spectrum. *Journal of Affective Disorders* **85** (1–2): 153–68.

Ey, H. (1959). Los Delirios. *Revista de psiquiatría del Uruguay* **140**: 3–42.

Faulkner, W. (1930). *As I Lay Dying*. New York: Jonathan Cape–Harrison Smith.

Fergusson, D.M. and Mullen, P.E. (1999). *Childhood Sexual Abuse: An Evidence Based Perspective*. Thousand Oaks: Sage Publications.

Ferreira, B. (2002). *Stimmung bei Heidegger: Das Phänomen der Stimmung im Kontext von Heideggers Existenzialanalyse des Daseins*. Dordrecht: Kluwer Academic Publishers.

Fink, H. (2006). Three Sorts of Naturalism. *European Journal of Philosophy* **14** (2): 202–21.

Fonagy P. and Target M. (1997). Attachment and Reflective Function: Their Role in Self-Organization. *Development and Psychopathology* **9** (4): 679–700.

Foucault, M. (1984). *Histoire de la sexualité 2: L'usage des plaisirs*. Paris: Éditions Gallimard.

Frankfurt, H.G. (1971). Freedom of the Will and the Concept of a Person. *The Journal of Philosophy* **68** (1): 5–20.

Frankfurt, H.G. (1982). The Importance of What We Care About. *Synthese* **53** (2): 257–72.

Freud, S. (1957/1973). Mourning and Melancholia. In: *The Complete Edition of the Psychological Works of Sigmund Freud, Vol. 14*. Edited and translated by Strachey, J. London: Hogarth Press, 243–58; Trauer und Melancholie. In Freud, A. et al. (eds.) *Sigmund Freud. Gesammelte Werke, Band X*. Frankfurt am Main: S. Fischer Verlag, 197–212.

Fuchs, T. (2000). *Leib, Raum, Person. Entwurf einer phänomenologischen Anthropologie*. Stuttgart: Klett-Cotta.

Fuchs, T. (2002). Maske, Selbst, Selbstentfremdung: Zur Anthropologie und Psychopathologie der Person. In: Fuchs, T. *Zeit-Diagnosen: Philosophisch-psychiatrische Essays*. Kusterdingen: Die Graue Edition, 135–63.

Fuchs, T. (2003). The Phenomenology of Shame, Guilt and the Body in Body Dysmorphic Disorder and Depression. *Journal of Phenomenological Psychology* **33** (2): 223–43.

Fuchs, T. (2005). Overcoming Dualism. *Philosophy, Psychiatry & Psychology* **12** (2): 115–17.

Fuchs, T. (2007). Fragmented Selves: Temporality and Identity in Borderline Personality. *Psychopathology* **40** (6): 379–87.

Fuchs, T. (2008). Zur Phänomenologie des Schweigens. In: Fuchs, T. *Leib und Lebenswelt: Neue philosophisch-psychiatrische Essays*. Kusterdingen: Die Graue Edition, 123–47.

Fuchs, T. (2010). Temporality and Psychopathology. *Phenomenology and the Cognitive Sciences*. Available from: http://www.springerlink.com/content/w53g5814n8t49117/.

Fuentenebro, F. and Berrios, G.E. (1995). The Predelusional State: A Conceptual History. *Comprehensive Psychiatry* **36** (4): 251–9.

Fukunishi, I., Nakagawa, T., Nakamura H., and Ogawa, J. (1993). A Comparison of Type A Behaviour Pattern, Hostility and Typus Melancholicus in Japanese and American Students: Effects of Defensiveness. *International Journal of Social Psychiatry* **39** (1): 58–63.

Fulford, K.W.M., Thornton, T., and Graham, G. (2006). *Oxford Textbook of Philosophy and Psychiatry*. Oxford: Oxford University Press.

Gabbani, C. and Stanghellini, G. (2008). What Kind of Objectivity do We Need for Psychiatry? A Commentary to Oulis's Ontological Assumptions in Psychiatric Taxonomy. *Psychopathology* **41** (3): 135–40.

Gabriel, E. (1987). Dysphoric Mood in Paranoid Psychoses. *Psychopathology* **20** (2): 101–6.

Galimberti, U. (2009). *I miti del nostro tempo*. Milano: Feltrinelli.

Gallagher, S. (2004). Hermeneutics and the Cognitive Sciences. *Journal of Consciousness Studies* **11** (10–11): 162–74.

Gallagher, S. (2005). *How the Body Shapes the Mind*. Oxford: Oxford University Press.

Gallagher, S. (2008). How to Undress the Affective Mind: An Interview with Jaak Panksepp. *Journal of Consciousness Studies* **15** (2): 89–119.

Gallagher, S. and Zahavi, D. (2008). *The Phenomenological Mind: An Introduction to Philosophy of Mind and Cognitive Science*. London: Routledge.

Gallese, V. (2010). Embodied Simulation and its Role in Intersubjectivity. In: Fuchs, T., Sattel, H.C., and Henningsen, P. (eds.) *The Embodied Self: Dimensions, Coherence and Disorder*. Stuttgart: Schattauer, 77–92.

Garrett, A.V. (2003). *Meaning in Spinoza's Method*. Cambridge: Cambridge University Press.

Garrett, D. (2002). Spinoza's *Conatus* Argument. In: Koistinen, O. and Biro, J. (eds.) *Spinoza: Metaphysical Themes*. Oxford: Oxford University Press, 127–58.

Gibbard, A. (1990). *Wise Choices, Apt Feelings: A Theory of Normative Judgment*. Oxford: Oxford University Press.

Goldie, P. (2000). *The Emotions: A Philosophical Exploration*. Oxford: Oxford University Press.

Goldie, P. (2002a). Emotion, Personality and Simulation. In: Goldie, P. (ed.) *Understanding Emotions: Mind and Morals*. Aldershot: Ashgate Publishing, 97–109.

Goldie, P. (2002b). Emotions, Feelings and Intentionality. *Phenomenology and the Cognitive Sciences* **1** (3): 235–54.

Goldie, P. (2003a). One's Remembered Past: Narrative Thinking, Emotion, and the External Perspective. *Philosophical Papers* **32** (3): 301–19.

Goldie, P. (2003b). Narrative, Emotion, and Perspective. In: Kieran, M. and Lopes, D. (eds.) *Imagination and the Arts*. London: Routledge, 54–68.

Goldie, P. (2003c). Narrative and Perspective: Values and Appropriate Emotions. In: Hatzimoysis, A. (ed.) *Philosophy and the Emotions*. Cambridge: Cambridge University Press, 201–20.

Goldie, P. (2004). *On Personality*. London: Routledge.

Goldie, P. (2007a). There Are Reasons and Reasons. In: Hutto, D. and Ratcliffe, M.J. (eds.) *Folk Psychology Reassessed*. Dordrecht: Kluwer Academic Press, 103–14.

Goldie, P. (2007b). Dramatic Irony, Narratives, and the External Perspective. In: Hutto, D. (ed.) *Narratives and Understanding Persons*. Cambridge: Cambridge University Press, 69–84.

Goodwin, F.K. and Jamison, K.R. (2007). *Manic-Depressive Illness: Bipolar Disorders and Recurrent Depression*. Second Edition. New York: Oxford University Press.

Gordon, R.M. (1987). *The Structure of Emotions: Investigations in Cognitive Philosophy*. Cambridge: Cambridge University Press.

Graham, G. (2010). *The Disordered Mind: An Introduction to Philosophy of Mind and Mental Illness*. London: Routledge.

Grieg, D. (2001). Introduction. In: Kane, S. *Complete Plays*. London: Methuen, xi–xviii.

Grinberg, L. (1964). On Two Kinds of Guilt: Their Relation with Normal and Pathological Aspects of Mourning. *International Journal of Psychoanalysis* **45** (2–3): 366–71.

Grøn, A. (2004). Self and Identity. In: Zahavi, D., Grünbam, T., and Parnas, J. (eds.) *Structure and Development of Self-Consciousness: Interdisciplinary Perspectives*. Philadelphia: John Benjamins Publishing Company, 123–56.

Grondin, J. (1994/1991). *Introduction to Philosophical Hermeneutics*. Translated by Weinsheimer, J. New Haven: Yale University Press; *Einführung in die philosophische Hermeneutik*. Darmstadt: Wissenschaftliche Buchgesellschaft.

Gunderson, J. and Phillips, K.A. (1991). A Current View of the Interface between Borderline Personality Disorder and Depression. *American Journal of Psychiatry* **148** (8): 967–75.

Handke, P. (1972/1970). *The Goalie's Anxiety at the Penalty Kick*. Translated by Roloff, M. New York: Farrar, Straus and Giroux; *Die Angst des Tormanns beim Elfmeter*. Frankfurt am Main: Suhrkamp Verlag.

Hasker, W. (1999) *The Emergent Self*. Ithaca: Cornell University Press.

Heidegger, M. (1990/1991). *Kant and the Problem of Metaphysics*. Translated by Taft, R. Indiana: Indiana University Press; *Kant und das Problem der Metaphysik*. Gesamtausgabe, Band 3. Frankfurt am Main: Vittorio Klostermann.

Heidegger, M. (1995/1983). *The Fundamental Concepts of Metaphysics: World, Finitude, Solitude*. Translated by McNeil, W. and Walker, N. Indianapolis: Indiana University Press; *Die Grundbegriffe der Metaphysik: Welt – Endlichkeit – Einsamkeit*. Gesamtausgabe, Band 29/30. Frankfurt am Main: Vittorio Klostermann.

Heidegger, M. (2010/1986). *Being and Time*. Translated by Stambaugh, J., revised by Schmidt, D.J. New York: State University of New York Press; *Sein und Zeit*. Tübingen: Max Niemeyer Verlag.

Holland, D. and Kipnis, A. (1995). American Cultural Models of Embarrassment: The Not-So Egocentric Self Laid Bare. In: Russell, J.A., Fernandez-Dols, J.M., Manstead, A.S.R., Wellenkamp, J.C. (eds.) *Everyday Conceptions of Emotions: An Introduction to the Psychology, Anthropology and Linguistics of Emotion.* Dordrecht: Kluwer Academic Press, 181–202.

Hornsby, J. (2000). Personal and Sub-Personal: A Defence of Dennett's Early Distinction. *Philosophical Explorations* **3** (1): 6–24.

Hume, D. (1958). *A Treatise of Human Nature.* Edited by Selby-Bigge, L.A. Oxford: Oxford University Press.

Husserl, E. (1966). *Analysen zur passiven Synthesis. Aus Vorlesungs- und Forschungsmanuskripten 1918–1926.* Den Haag: Martinus Nijhoff.

Husserl. E. (1989/1952). *Ideas Pertaining to a Pure Phenomenology and to a Phenomenological Philosophy, Second Book.* Translated by Rojcewicz, R. and Schuwer, A. Dordrecht: Kluwer Academic Press; *Ideen zu einer reinen Phänomenologie und phänomenologischen Philosophie. Zweites Buch. Phänomenologische Untersuchungen zur Konstitution.* Den Haag: Martinus Nijhoff.

Jacob, F. (1977). Evolution and Tinkering. *Science* **196** (4295): 1161–6.

James, W. (1884). What is an Emotion? *Mind* **9** (34): 188–205.

Jaspers, K. (1978). *Notizen zu Martin Heidegger.* Hrsg. Hans Saner. München: R. Piper & Co. Verlag.

Jaspers, K. (1997/1959). *General Psychopathology.* Translated by Hoenig, J. and Hamilton, M.W. Baltimore: Johns Hopkins University Press; *Allgemeine Psychopathologie,* 7. unveränderte Auflage. Heidelberg: Springer Verlag.

Joyce, J. (1986). *Ulysses.* New York: Random House.

Kane, S. (2001). 4.48 Psychosis. In: Kane, S. *Complete Plays.* London: Methuen, 203–46.

Kant, I. (1996/1911). *Critique of Practical Reason.* Translated by Gregor, M.J. Cambridge: Cambridge University Press; *Kritik der praktischen Vernunft. Kant's gesammelte Schriften,* Band IV. Berlin: Georg Reimer.

Kendler, K. and Parnas, J. (eds.) (2008). *Philosophical Issues in Psychiatry: Explanation, Phenomenology, and Nosology.* Baltimore: The Johns Hopkins University Press.

Kendler, K.S. and Zachar, P. (2008). The Incredible Insecurity of Psychiatric Nosology. In: Kendler, K. and Parnas, J. (eds.) *Philosophical Issues in Psychiatry: Explanation, Phenomenology, and Nosology.* Baltimore: The Johns Hopkins University Press, 368–83.

Kenny, A. (1963). *Action, Emotion and Will.* London: Routledge.

Kepinski, A. (1974). *Schizophrenia.* Warszawa: Państwowy Zaklad Wydawnictw Lekarskich.

Kernberg, O. (1984). *Severe Personality Disorders: Psychotherapeutic Strategies.* New Haven: Yale University Press.

Kim, J. (2003). The American Origins of Naturalism. In: Audi, R. (ed.) *Philosophy in America at the Turn of the Century.* Journal of Philosophical Research (APA Centennial Supplement), 83–98. Charlottesville: Philosophy Documentation Center.

Kimura, B. (1992). *Écrits de psychopathologie phénoménologique.* Trad. Bouderlique, J. Paris: PUF.

Kimura, B. (2000). *L'Entre. Une approche phénoménologique de la schizophrénie.* Trad. Vincent, C. Grenoble: Éditions Jérôme Millon.

Kitcher, P. (1992). The Naturalists Return. *The Philosophical Review* **11** (1): 53–114.

Kitcher, P. (1993). *The Advancement of Science: Science Without Legend, Objectivity Without Illusions.* Oxford: Oxford University Press.

Kitcher, P. (2001). *Science, Truth, and Democracy.* Oxford: Oxford University Press.

Koenigsberg, H.W., Harvey, P.D., Mitropoulou, V., Schmeidler, J., New, A.S., Goodman, M., Silverman, J.M., Serby, M., Schopick, F., and Siever, L.J. (2002). Characterizing Affective Instability in Borderline Personality Disorder. *American Journal of Psychiatry* **159** (5): 784–8.

Kohut, H. (1978). Thoughts on Narcissism and Narcissistic Rage. In: *The Search for the Self, Vol. 2.* Edited by Ornstein, P. New York: International Universities Press, 615–58.

Kövecses, Z. (1986). *Metaphors of Anger, Pride, and Love: A Lexical Approach to the Structure of Concepts.* Amsterdam: John Benjamin.

Kövecses, Z. (1991). Happiness: A Definitional Effort. *Metaphor and Symbolic Activity* **6** (1): 29–46.

Kövecses, Z. (2000a). *Metaphor and Emotion: Language, Culture, and Body in Human Feeling*. Cambridge: Cambridge University Press.

Kövecses, Z. (2000b). The Concept of Anger: Universal or Cultural Specific? *Psychopathology* **33** (4): 159–70.

Kraepelin, E. (1899). *Psychiatrie: Ein Lehrbuch fur Studierende und Aerzte*. 6. Auflage. Leipzig: Barth Verlag.

Kraus, A. (1977). *Sozialverhalten und Psychose Manisch-Depressiver: Eine Existenz- und Rolleanalytische Untersuchung*. Stuttgart: Ferdinand Enke Verlag.

Kretschmer, E. (1966). *Der Sensitive Beziehungswahn: Ein Beitrag zur Paranoiafrage und zur Psychiatrischen Characterlehre*, 4. erweiterte Auflage. Heidelberg: Springer.

Laird, J.D. (2007). *Feelings: The Perception of Self*. Oxford: Oxford University Press.

Laitinen, A. and Ikäheimo, H. (2007). Dimensions of Personhood: Editors' Introduction. In: Laitinen, A. and Ikäheimo, H. (eds.) *Dimensions of Personhood*. Exeter: Imprint Academic, 6–16.

Lakoff, G. and Johnson, M. (1980). *Metaphors We Live By*. Chicago: Chicago University Press.

Lakoff, G. and Kövecses, Z. (1987). The Cognitive Model of Anger Inherent in American English. In: Holland, D. and Quinn, N. (eds.) *Cultural Models in Language and Thought*. Cambridge: Cambridge University Press, 195–221.

Lebuffe, M. (2010). *From Bondage to Freedom: Spinoza on Human Excellence*. Oxford: Oxford University Press.

LeDoux, J.E. (1996). *The Emotional Brain: The Mysterious Underpinnings of Emotional Life*. New York: Simon & Schuster.

Mayer-Gross, W. (1920). Über die Stellungnahme zur abgelaufenen akuten Psychose: Eine Studie über verständliche Zusammenhänge in der Schizophrenie. *Zeitschrift für die gesamte Neurologie und Psychiatrie* **60** (1): 160–212.

Mayr, E. (2004). *What Makes Biology Unique? Consideration on the Autonomy of a Scientific Discipline*. Cambridge: Cambridge University Press.

McDowell, J. (1994). *Mind and World*. Cambridge: Harvard University Press.

McGinn, C. (1989). Can We Solve the Mind-Body Problem? *Mind* **98** (391): 349–66.

Meares, R. (2000). *Intimacy and Alienation: Memory, Trauma and Personal Being*. London: Routledge.

Merleau-Ponty, M. (1945). *Phénoménologie de la perception*. Paris: Gallimard.

Merleau-Ponty, M. (1964). *Le visible et l'Invisible, Suivi de Notes de Travail*. Ed. Lefort, C. Paris: Gallimard.

Minkowski, E. (1927). *La schizophrénie: Psychopathologie des schizoïdes et des schizophrènes*. Paris: Payot.

Minkowski, E. (1933). *Le temps vécu: Études phénoménologiques et psychopathologiques*. Paris: Collection de l'Evolution Psychiatrique.

Minkowski, E. (1997). La notion de perte de contact vital avec la réalité et ses applications en psychopathologie [1st ed. 1926]. In: Minkowski, E. *Au-delà du Rationalisme Morbide*. Paris: L'Harmattan, 35–67.

Monod, J. (1970). *Le hasard et la nécessité: Essai sur la philosophie naturelle de la biologie moderne*. Paris: Éditions du Seuil.

Moyn, S. (2009). The Assumption by Man of His Original Fracturing: Marcel Gauchet, Gladys Swain, and the History of the Self. *Modern Intellectual History* **6** (2): 315–41.

Mundt, C. (1985). *Das Apathiesyndrom der Schizophrenen: Eine psychopathologische und computertomographische Untersuchung*. Heidelberg: Springer.

Mundt, C. (1991). Constituting Reality – Its Decline and Repair in the Long-Term Course of Schizophrenic Psychoses: The Intentionality Model. In: Marneros, A., Andreasen, N.C., and Tsuang, M.T. (eds.) *Negative Versus Positive Schizophrenia*. Heidelberg: Springer, 96–108.

Mundt, C., Backenstrass, M., Kronmiller, K.T., Fiedler, P., Kraus, A., and Stanghellini, G. (1997). Personality and Endogenous/Major Depression: An Empirical Approach to Typus Melancholicus: 2.

Validation of Typus Melancholicus Core-Properties by Personality Inventory Scales. *Psychopathology* **30** (3): 130–9.

Mundt, C., Goldstein, M.J., Halweg, K., and Fiedler, P. (1996). *Interpersonal Factors in the Origin and Course of Affective Disorders*. London: Gaskell.

Murphy, D. (2006). *Psychiatry in the Scientific Image*. Cambridge: The MIT Press.

Musalek, M., Lesch, O.M., and Kieffer, W. (1987). Dysphoric States in the Course of Manic-Depressive Illness. *Psychopathology* **20** (2): 107–114.

Nagel, T. (1974). What It Is Like to Be a Bat. *The Philosophical Review* **83** (4): 435–50.

Nakanishi, T., Isobe, F., and Ogawa, Y. (1993). Chronic Depression of Monopolar, Endogenous Type: With Special Reference to the Premorbid Personality, 'Typus Melancholicus'. *Japanese Journal of Psychiatry & Neurology* **47** (3): 495–504.

Nussbaum, M.C. (2001). *Upheavals of Thought: The Intelligence of Emotions*. Cambridge: Cambridge University Press.

Olson, E.T. (1997). *The Human Animal: Personal Identity without Psychology*. Oxford: Oxford University Press.

Olson, E.T. (1999). There Is No Problem of the Self. In: Gallagher, S. and Shear, J. (eds.) *Models of the Self*. Exeter: Imprint Academic, 49–61.

Olson, E.T. (2007). *What Are We? A Study in Personal Ontology*. Oxford: Oxford University Press.

Panksepp, J. (1998). *Affective Neuroscience: The Foundations of Human and Animal Emotions*. Oxford: Oxford University Press.

Panksepp, J. (2001). On the Subcortical Sources of Basic Human Emotions and the Primacy of Emotional-Affective Action-Perception Processes in Human Consciousness. *Evolution and Cognition* **7** (2): 134–40.

Panksepp, J. (2003). At the Interface of the Affective, Behavioural, and Cognitive Neuroscience: Decoding the Emotional Feelings of the Brain. *Brain and Cognition* **52** (1): 4–14.

Panksepp, J. (2004a). Affective Consciousness and the Origins of Human Mind: A Critical Role of Brain Research on Animal Emotions. *Impuls* **57** (3): 47–60.

Panksepp, J. (2004b). Basic Affects and the Instinctual Systems of the Brain. In: Manstead, A.S.R., Frijda, N., and Fischer, A. (eds.) *Feelings and Emotions. The Amsterdam Symposium*. Cambridge: Cambridge University Press, 175–93.

Panksepp, J. (2004c). Emerging Neuroscience of Fear and Anxiety: Therapeutic Practice and Clinical Implication. In: Panksepp, J. (ed.) *Textbook of Biological Psychiatry*. Hoboken: Wiley-Liss, 489–519.

Panksepp, J. (2005a). Toward a Science of Ultimate Concern (Guest Editorial). *Consciousness and Cognition* **14** (1): 22–9.

Panksepp, J. (2005b). Affective Consciousness: Core Emotional Feelings in Animals and Humans. *Consciousness and Cognition* **14** (1): 30–80.

Panksepp, J. (2005c). On the Embodied Neural Nature of Core Emotional Affects. *Journal of Consciousness Studies* **12** (8–10): 158–84.

Panksepp, J. (2006). Emotional Endophenotypes in Evolutionary Psychiatry. *Progress in Neuro-Psychopharmacology & Biological Psychiatry* **30** (5): 774–84.

Panksepp, J. (2010). Perspectives on Passages Towards an Affective Neurobiology of Mind. In: Koob, G., Le Moal, M., and Thompson, R. (eds.) *Encyclopedia of Behavioral Neuroscience*. New York: Elsevier, xxii–xxix.

Panksepp, J. (2011). Toward a Cross-Species Neuroscientific Understanding of the Affective Mind: Do Animals Have Emotional Feelings? *American Journal of Primatology* **73** (6): 545–61.

Panksepp, J. and Northoff, G. (2009). The Trans-Species Core Self: The Emergence of Active Cultural and Neuro-Ecological Agents through Self-Related Processing within Subcortical Midline Networks. *Consciousness and Cognition* **18** (1): 193–215.

Papineau, D. (1999). Normativity and Judgement. *Supplement to the Proceedings of the Aristotelian Society* **73** (1): 17–43.

Paris, J. (1994). *Borderline Personality Disorder: A Multidimensional Approach*. Washington, DC: American Psychiatric Press.

Paris, J. (2000). *Myths of Childhood*. Philadelphia: Brunner/Mazel.

Parnas, J., Bovet, P., and Zahavi, D. (2002). Schizophrenic Autism: Clinical Phenomenology and Pathogenic Implications. *World Psychiatry* **1** (3): 131–6.

Parnas, J. and Sass, L.A. (2001). Self, Solipsism, and Schizophrenic Delusions. *Philosophy, Psychiatry & Psychology* **8** (2–3): 101–20.

Parnas, J., Zahavi, D., and Sass, L. (2008). Recent Developments in Philosophy of Psychopathology. *Current Opinion in Psychiatry* **21** (6): 578–84.

Pasolini, P.P. (1964). *Poesia in forma rosa*. Milano: Garzanti Editore.

Pazzaglia, A. and Rossi Monti, M. (2000). Dysphoria and Aloneness in Borderline Personality Disorder. *Psychopathology* **33** (4): 220–6.

Pinel, P. (1800). *Traité médico-philosophique sur l'aliénation mentale, ou la manie*. Paris: Richard, Caille et Ravier.

Plantinga, A. (2007). Materialism and Christian Belief. In: Van Inwagen, P. and Zimmerman, D. (eds.) *Persons: Human and Divine*. Oxford: Oxford University Press, 99–141.

Plutchik, R. (1980). *Emotions: A Psychoevolutionary Synthesis*. New York: Harper & Row.

Pocai, R. (1996). *Heideggers Theorie der Befindlichkeit: Sein Denken zwischen 1927 und 1935*. Freiburg/München: Alber.

Preuss, T.M. (2004). What It Is Like to Be a Human. In: Gazzaniga, M.S. (ed.) *The Cognitive Neurosciences III*. Cambridge: The MIT Press, 5–19.

Prinz, J.J. (2004). *Gut Reactions: A Perceptual Theory of Emotion*. New York: Oxford University Press.

Prinz, J.J. (2005). Are Emotions Feelings? *Journal of Consciousness Studies* **12** (8–10): 9–25.

Prinz, J.J. (2007). *The Emotional Construction of Morals*. New York: Oxford University Press.

Pugmire, D. (1998). *Rediscovering Emotion*. Edinburgh: Edinburgh University Press.

Pugmire, D. (2005). *Sound Sentiment: Integrity in the Emotions*. Oxford: Oxford University Press.

Putnam, H. (1999). *The Threefold Cord: Mind, Body, and World*. New York: Columbia University Press.

Putnam, K.M. and Silk, K.R. (2005). Emotion Dysregulation and the Development of Borderline Personality Disorder. *Development and Psychopathology* **17** (4): 899–925.

Radden, J. (ed.) (2004). *The Philosophy of Psychiatry: A Companion*. Oxford: Oxford University Press.

Ratcliffe, M. (2005). The Feeling of Being. *Journal of Consciousness Studies* **12** (8–10): 43–60.

Ratcliffe, M. (2007). *Rethinking Commonsense Psychology: A Critique of Folk Psychology, Theory of Mind and Simulation*. Hampshire: Palgrave Macmillan.

Ratcliffe, M. (2008). *Feelings of Being: Phenomenology, Psychiatry and the Sense of Reality*. Oxford: Oxford University Press.

Ratcliffe, M. (2009). Understanding Existential Changes in Psychiatric Illness: The Indispensability of Phenomenology. In: Broome, M.R. and Bortolotti, L. (eds.) *Psychiatry as Cognitive Neuroscience: Philosophical Perspectives*. Oxford: Oxford University Press, 223–44.

Ratcliffe, M. (2010). The Phenomenology of Mood and the Meaning of Life. In: Goldie, P. (ed.) *The Oxford Handbook of Philosophy of Emotions*. Oxford: Oxford University Press, 349–71.

Ricoeur, P. (1966/1950). *Freedom and Nature: The Voluntary and the Involuntary*. Translated by Kohák, E.V. Evanston: Northwestern University Press; *Philosophie de la volonté I: Le volontaire et l'Involontaire*. Paris: Aubier.

Ricoeur, P. (1977/1965). *Freud and Philosophy: Essay on Interpretation*. Translated by Savage, D. New Haven: Yale University Press; *De l'interprétation: Essai sur Freud*. Paris: Éditions du Seuil.

Ricoeur, P. (1981a/1972). Metaphor and the Central Problem of Hermeneutics. In: Ricoeur, P. *Hermeneutics and the Human Sciences*. Edited and translated by Thompson, J.B. Cambridge: Cambridge University Press, 165–81; La Métaphore et le Problème Centrale de l'Herméneutique. *Revue Philosophique de Louvain* **70** (5): 93–112.

Ricoeur, P. (1981b/1979). The Narrative Function. In: Ricoeur, P. *Hermeneutics and the Human Sciences*. Edited and translated by Thompson, J. B. Cambridge: Cambridge University Press, 165–81; La fonction narrative. *Études théologiques et religieuses* **54**: 209–30.

Ricoeur, P. (1986). Le sentiment. In: Ricoeur, P. *À l'école de la phénoménologie*. Paris: Vrin, 251–65.

Ricoeur, P. (1987/1960). *Fallible Man*. Translated by Kelbley, C.A. New York: Fordham University Press; *Philosophie de la Volonté II: L'homme faillible*. Paris: Aubier.

Ricoeur, P. (1988/1985). *Time and Narrative, III*. Translated by Blamey, K. and Pellauer, D. Chicago: University of Chicago Press; *Temps et récit, tome 3*. Paris: Éditions du Seuil.

Ricoeur, P. (1989). Narrativité, phénoménologie et herméneutique. In: Jacob, A. (ed.) *Encyclopédie Philosophique Universelle I: L'Univers Philosophique*. Paris: PUF, 63–71.

Ricoeur, P. (1991/1986). *From Text to Action: Essays in Hermeneutics, II*. Translated by Blamey, K. and Thompson, J.B. Evanston: Northwestern University Press; *Du texte à l'action: Essais d'herméneutique II*. Paris: Éditions du Seuil.

Ricoeur, P. (1992/1990). *Oneself as Another*. Translated by Blamey, K. Chicago: University of Chicago Press; *Soi-même comme un autre*. Paris: Éditions du Seuil.

Ricoeur, P. (2004/1969). *The Conflict of Interpretations: Essays in Hermeneutics*. Edited by Ihde, D. New York: Continuum; *Le conflit des interprétations: Essais d'herméneutique*. Paris: Éditions du Seuil.

Ricoeur, P. (2005/2004). *The Course of Recognition*. Translated by Pellauer, D. Cambridge: Harvard University Press; *Parcours de la reconnaissance: Trois études*. Paris: Éditions Stock.

Ricoeur, P. (2007a/1986). *Husserl: An Analysis of His Phenomenology*. Translated by Ballard, E.G. and Embree L.E. Evanston: Northwestern University Press; *A l'école de la phénoménologie*. Paris: Vrin.

Ricoeur, P. (2007b/1967). *History and Truth*. Translated by Ch. Kelbley, A. Evanston: Northwestern University Press; *Histoire et vérité*. Paris: Éditions du Seuil.

Rizzolatti, G. and Sinigaglia, C. (2007). *Mirrors in the Brain: How Our Minds Share Actions and Emotions*. Oxford: Oxford University Press.

Roberts, G. (1992). The Origin of Delusions. *The British Journal of Psychiatry* **161** (3): 298–308.

Robinson, J. (2005). *Deeper than Reason: Emotion and Its Role in Literature, Music, and Art*. Oxford: Oxford University Press.

Rosfort, R. and Stanghellini, G. (2009). The Person in between Moods and Affects. *Philosophy, Psychiatry & Psychology* **13** (3): 251–66.

Rossi Monti, M. (2008). *Forme del Delirio e Psicopatologia*. Milano: Cortina.

Russell, B. (1927). *Philosophy*. New York: W.W. Norton & Company, Inc. Publishers.

Russell, J.A. (2003). Core Affect and the Psychological Construction of Emotion. *Psychological Review* **110** (1): 145–72.

Ryle, G. (1949). *The Concept of Mind*. London: Hutchinson's University Library.

Sartre, J.P. (1956/1943). *Being and Nothingness: A Phenomenological Essay on Ontology*. Translated by Barnes, H.E. New York: Philosophical Library; *l'être et le néant: Essai d'ontologie phénoménologique*. Paris: Gallimard.

Sartre, J.P. (1971/1939). *Sketch for a Theory of the Emotions*. Translated by Mairet, P. London: Methuen & Co Ltd; *Esquisse d'une théorie des émotions*. Paris: Hermann.

Sartre, J.P. (1975/1939). *The Wall (Intimacy) and Other Stories*. Translated by Alexander, L. New York: New Directions; *Le mur*. Paris: Gallimard.

Sato, T., Sakado, K., and Sato, S. (1992). Differences between Two Questionnaires for Assessment of Typus Melancholicus, Zerssen's F-list and Kasahara's Scale: The Validity and Relationship to DSM-III-RPersonality Disorders. *Psychiatry and Clinical Neurosciences* **46** (3): 603–8.

Sato, T., Sakado, K., and Sato, S. (1993). Typus Melancholicus Measured by a Questionnaire in Unipolar Depressive Patients: Age- and Sex-Distribution, and Relationship to Clinical Characteristics of Depression. *Psychiatry and Clinical Neurosciences* **47** (1): 1–11.

Sauer, H., Richter, P., and Sass, H. (1989). Zur prämorbiden Persönlichkeit von Patienten mit schizoaffektiven Psychosen. In: Marneros, A. (ed.) *Schizoaffektive Psychosen*. Berlin: Springer, 109–18.

Saunders, G. (2002). *'Love Me or Kill Me': Sarah Kane and the Theatre of the Extremes*. Manchester: Manchester University Press.

Scheler, M. (1966). *Der Formalismus in der Ethik und die materiale Wertethik*. Gesammelte Werke. Band 2. Bern: Francke Verlag.

Scheler, M. (1976). *Die Stellung des Menschen im Kosmos*. Gesammelte Werke. Band 2. Bern: Francke Verlag.

Scheler, M. (2008/1979). My Theory of the Cognitive and Methodological Aspects of Metaphysics. In: Scheler, M. *The Constitution of the Human Being: From the Posthumous Works, Volumes 11 and 12*. Translated by Cutting, J. Milwaukee: Marquette University Press, 77–128; *Gesammelte Werke, Band 11*. Bern: Francke Verlag, 72–117.

Schmidt, G. (1987). A Review of the German Literature on Delusion Between 1914 and 1939. In: Cutting, J. and Shepard, M. (eds.) *The Clinical Roots of the Schizophrenia Concept: Translations of Seminal European Contributions on Schizophrenia*. Cambridge: Cambridge University Press, 104–34.

Schneider, K. (1967). *Klinische Psychopathologie*, 8. ergänzte Auflage. Stuttgart: Georg Thieme Verlag.

Schrank, B., Stanghellini, G., and Slate, H.M. (2008). Hope in Psychiatry: A Review of the Literature. *Acta Psychiatrica Scandinavica* **118** (13): 421–33.

Schrijvers, M. (1999). The Conatus and the Mutual Relationship Between Active and Passive Affects in Spinoza. In: Yovel, Y. (ed.) *Desire and Affect: Spinoza as Psychologist*. New York: Little Room Press, 63–80.

Searle, J. (2000). *Mind, Language and Society*. London: Phoenix, Orion Books Ltd.

Sechehaye, M. (1951/1950). Autobiography of a Schizophrenic Girl. Translated by Rubin-Rabson, G. New York: Grune & Stratton; *Journal d'une schizophrène: Auto-observation d'une schizophrène pendant le traitement psychothérapique*. Paris: PUF.

Sellars, W. (1963a). Philosophy and the Scientific Image of Man. In: *Science, Perception and Reality*. London: Routledge and Kegan Paul, 1–40.

Sellars, W. (1963b). Empiricism and the Philosophy of Mind. In: *Science, Perception and Reality*. London: Routledge and Kegan Paul, 127–96.

Sheets-Johnstone, M. (1999). *The Primacy of Movement*. Amsterdam: John Benjamins.

Siemer, M. (2005). Moods as Multiple-Object Directed and as Objectless Affective States: An Examination of the Dispositional Theory of Moods. *Cognition and Emotion* **19** (6): 815–45.

Siemer, M. (2009). Mood Experience: Implications of a Dispositional Theory of Moods. *Emotion Review* **1** (3): 256–63.

Simpson, G.G. (1966). The Biological Nature of Man. *Science* **152** (3721): 472–8.

Smith, Q. (1986). *The Felt Meanings of the World: A Metaphysics of Feeling*. West Lafayette: Purdue University Press.

Solomon, R.C. (1976). *The Passions*. New York: Anchor Press/Doubleday.

Solomon, R.C. (2003). *Not Passion's Slave: Emotions and Choice*. Oxford: Oxford University Press.

Solomon, R.C. (2007). *True To Our Feelings: What Our Emotions Are Really Telling Us*. Oxford: Oxford University Press.

Spinoza, B. (1985). *The Collected Works of Spinoza, vol. I*. Edited and translated by Curley, E. Princeton: Princeton University Press.

Stanghellini, G. (1997a). *Antropologia della vulnerabilità*. Milano: Feltrinelli.

Stanghellini, G. (1997b). For an Anthropology of Vulnerability. *Psychopathology* **30** (1): 1–11.

Stanghellini, G. (2000). The Doublets of Anger. *Psychopathology* **33** (4): 155–8.

Stanghellini, G. (2004). *Disembodied Spirits and Deanimated Bodies: The Psychopathology of Common Sense*. Oxford: Oxford University Press.

Stanghellini, G. (2007a). The Grammar of Psychiatric Interview: A Plea for a Second-Person Mode of Understanding. *Psychopathology* **40** (2): 69–74.

Stanghellini, G. (2007b). Schizophrenia and the Sixth Sense. In: Chung, M. et al. (eds.) *Reconceiving Schizophrenia*. Oxford: Oxford University Press, 129–49.

Stanghellini, G. (2008). *Psicopatologia del senso comune*. Milano: Raffaello Cortina Editore.

Stanghellini, G. (2009). Embodiment and Schizophrenia. *World Psychiatry* **8** (1): 56–89.

Stanghellini, G. (2010). A Hermeneutic Framework for Psychopathology. *Psychopathology* **43** (5): 319–26.

Stanghellini, G. (2011). Phenomenological Psychopathology, Profundity, and Schizophrenia. *Philosophy, Psychiatry & Psychology* **18** (2): 163–6.

Stanghellini, G. and Ballerini, A. (1992). *Ossessione e rivelazione: Riflessione sui rapporti tra ossessività e delirio*. Torino: Bollati Boringhieri.

Stanghellini, G. and Ballerini, M. (2007a). Criterion B in Persons with Schizophrenia: The Puzzle. *Current Opinion in Psychiatry* **20** (6): 582–7.

Stanghellini, G. and Ballerini, M. (2007b). Values in Persons with Schizophrenia. *Schizophrenia Bulletin* **33** (1): 131–41.

Stanghellini, G. and Ballerini, M. (2008). Qualitative Analysis: Its Place in Psychopathological Research. *Acta Psychiatrica Scandinavica* **117** (3): 161–3.

Stanghellini, G. and Ballerini, M. (2011). What Is It Like to Be a Person with Schizophrenia in the Social World? A First-Person Perspective Study on Schizophrenic Dissociality – Part Two: Methodological Issues and Empirical Findings. *Psychopathology* **44** (3): 183–92.

Stanghellini, G., Ballerini, M., Fusar-Poli, P., and Cutting, J. (2012). Abnormal Bodily Experiences May be a Marker of Early Schizophrenia? *Current Pharmaceutical Design* **18** (4): 392–8.

Stanghellini, G. and Bertelli, M. (2006). Assessing the Social Behaviour of Unipolar Depressives: The Criteria for Typus Melancholicus. *Psychopathology* **39** (4): 179–86.

Stanghellini, G., Bertelli, M., and Raballo, A. (2006). Typus Melancholicus: Personality Structure and the Characteristic of Major Unipolar Depressive Episode. *Journal of Affective Disorders* **93** (1–3): 159–67.

Stanghellini, G. and Mundt, C. (1997). Personality and Endogenous/Major Depression: An Empirical Approach to Typus Melancholicus: 1. Theoretical Issues. *Psychopathology* **30** (3): 119–29.

Stanghellini, G., Quercioli, L., Ricca, V., Strik, W.K., and Cabras, P. (2001). Basic Symptoms and Negative Symptoms in the Light of Language Impairment. *Comprehensive Psychiatry* **32** (2): 141–6.

Stanghellini, G. and Ricca, V. (1995). Alexithymia and Schizophrenia. *Psychopathology* **28** (5): 263–72.

Stanghellini, G. and Rosfort, R. (2010). Affective Temperament and Personal Identity. *Journal of Affective Disorders* **126** (1–2): 317–20.

Stanghellini, G. and Rossi Monti, M. (2009a). *Psicologia del patologico: Una prospettiva fenomenologica-dinamica*. Milano: Raffaello Cortina Editore.

Stanghellini, G. and Rossi Monti, M. (2009b). Explication or Explanation? *Philosophy, Psychiatry & Psychology* **16** (3): 237–9.

Stocker, M. (1996) with Hegeman, E. *Valuing Emotions*. Cambridge: Cambridge University Press.

Stone, M.H. (1988). Toward a Psychobiological Theory of Borderline Personality Disorder: Is Irritability the Red Thread that Runs Through Borderline Conditions? *Dissociation* **1** (2): 2–15.

Störring, G.E. (1939). *Wesen und Bedeutung des Symptoms der Ratlosigkeit bei psychischen Erkrankungen*. Leipzig: Georg Thieme Verlag.

Strasser, S. (1977/1956). *Phenomenology of Feeling: An Essay on the Phenomena of the Heart*. Translated by Wood, R.E. Pittsburgh: Duquesne University Press; *Das Gemüt: Grundgedanken zu einer Phänomenologischen Philosophie und Theorie des Menschlichen Gefühlsleben*. Freiburg: Verlag Herder.

Strauss, J.S. (1969). Hallucinations and Delusions as Points on Continua Function: Rating Scale Evidence. *Archives of General Psychiatry* **21** (5): 581–6.

Strauss, J.S., Hafez, H., Lieberman, P., and Harding, C.M. (1985). The Course of Psychiatric Disorder, III: Longitudinal Principles. *The American Journal of Psychiatry* **142** (3): 289–96.

Strawson, G. (1999). The Self and the SESMET. *Journal of Consciousness Studies* **6** (4): 99–135.

Strawson, G. (2004). Against Narrativity. *Ratio (new series)* **16** (4): 428–52.

Strawson, P.F. (1959). *Individuals: An Essay in Descriptive Metaphysics*. London: Methuen & Co. Ltd.

Strawson, P.F. (1966). *The Bounds of Sense: Essay on Kant's Critique of Pure Reason*. London: Methuen & Co. Ltd.

Swain, G. (1997). *Le sujet de la folie: Naissance de la psychiatrie* [1st ed. 1977]. Précédé de 'De Pinel à Freud' par Marcel Gauchet. Paris: Calmann-Lévy.

Swinburne, R. (2007). From Mental/Physical Identity to Substance Dualism. In: Van Inwagen, P. and Zimmerman, D. (eds.) *Persons: Human and Divine*. Oxford: Oxford University Press, 142–65.

Tappolet, C. (2000). *Émotions et Valeurs*. Paris: PUF.

Tavris, C. (1989). *Anger: The Misunderstood Emotion*. Revised Edition. New York: Simon and Schuster.

Taylor, C. (1985). *Human Agency and Language. Philosophical Papers 1*. Cambridge: Cambridge University Press.

Taylor, C. (1989). *Sources of the Self. The Making of Modern Identity*. Cambridge: Cambridge University Press.

Teichert, D. (2004). Narrative, Identity and the Self. *Journal of Consciousness Studies* **11** (10–11): 175–91.

Tellenbach, H. (1980/1976). *Melancholy. History of the Problem, Endogeneity, Typology, Pathogenesis, Clinical Observation*. Pittsburgh: Duquesne University Press; *Melancholie. Problemgeschichte, Endogenität, Typologie, Pathogenese, Klinik*. Dritte, erweiterte Auflage [1st edition 1961]. Heidelberg: Springer Verlag.

Thagard, P. (2010). *The Brain and the Meaning of Life*. Princeton: Princeton University Press.

Thomas, D. (2003). *The Poems*. Edited by Jones, D. New York: New Directions.

Thompson, E. (2007). *Mind in Life: Biology, Phenomenology, and the Sciences of Mind*. Cambridge: Harvard University Press.

Thornton, T. (2007). *Essential Philosophy of Psychiatry*. Oxford: Oxford University Press.

Tinbergen, N. (1951). *A Study of Instinct*. Oxford: Oxford University Press.

Tölle, R. (1987). Persönlichkeit und Melancholie. *Nervenarzt* **58**: 327–39.

Unger, P. (2006). *All the Power in the World*. Oxford: Oxford University Press.

Urfer, A. (2001). Phenomenology and Psychopathology of Schizophrenia: The Views of Eugene Minkowski. *Philosophy, Psychiatry & Psychology* **8** (4): 279–89.

Varela, F.J., Thompson, E., and Rosch, E. (1991). *The Embodied Mind: Cognitive Science and Human Experience*. Cambridge: The MIT Press.

Vogt, B.A. (2005). Pain and Emotion Interactions in the Subregions of the Cingulate Gyrus. *Nature Review Neuroscience* **6** (7): 533–44.

von Weizsäcker, V. (1940). *Der Gestaltkreis: Theorie und Einheit von Wahrnehmen und Bewegen*. Stuttgart: Georg Thieme Verlag.

von Zerssen, D., Asukai, N., Tsuda, H., Ono, Y., Kizaki, Y., and Cho, Y. (1997). Personality Traits of Japanese Patients in Remission from an Episode of Primary Unipolar Depression. *Journal of Affective Disorders* **44** (2): 145–52.

von Zerssen, D. and Possl, J. (1990). The Premorbid Personality of Patients with Different Subtypes of an Affective Illness. Statistical Analysis of Blind Assignment of Case History Data to Clinical Diagnoses. *Journal of Affective Disorders* **18** (1): 39–50.

von Zerssen, D., Tauscher, R., and Possl, J. (1994). The Relationship of Premorbid Personality to Subtypes of an Affective Illness. A Replication Study by Means of an Operationalized Procedure for the Diagnosis of Personality Structures. *Journal of Affective Disorders* **32** (1): 61–72.

Weiner, D.B. (2008a). The Madman in the Light of Reason. Enlightenment Psychiatry: Part I. Custody, Therapy and the Need for Reform. In Wallace, E.R. and Gach, J. (eds.) *History of Psychiatry and Medical Psychology*. New York: Springer, 255–77.

Weiner, D.B. (2008b). The Madman in the Light of Reason. Enlightenment Psychiatry: Part II. Alienists, Treatises, and the Psychologic Approach in the Era of Pinel. In: Wallace, E.R. and Gach, J. (eds.) *History of Psychiatry and Medical Psychology*. New York: Springer, 281–303.

Wetzel, A. (1922). Das Weltuntergangserlebnis in der Schizophrenie. *Zeitschrift für die gesamte Neurologie und Psychiatrie* **78** (1): 403–28.

Whitman, W. (1993). *Leaves of Grass*. New York: Modern Library.

Wilkinson-Ryan, T. and Westen, D. (2000). Identity Disturbance in Borderline Personality Disorder: An Empirical Investigation. *American Journal of Psychiatry* **157** (4): 528–41.

Williams, B. (1993). *Shame and Necessity*. Berkeley: University of California Press.

Wollheim, R. (1984). *Thread of Life*. Cambridge: Harvard University Press.

Wollheim, R. (1999). *On the Emotions*. New Haven: Yale University Press.

Wood, A.W. (2003). Kant and the Problem of Human Nature. In: Jacobs, B. and Kain, P. (eds.) *Essays on Kant's Anthropology*. Cambridge: Cambridge University Press, 38–59.

Woolf, V. (1941). *To the Lighthouse*. London: The Hogarth Press.

Wyller, T. (2005). The Place of Pain in Life. *Philosophy* **80** (3): 385–93.

Wyrsch, J. (1949). *Die Person des Schizophrenen: Studien zur Klinik, Psychologie, Daseinsweise*. Bern: Verlag Paul Haupt.

Zahavi, D. (1999). *Self-Awareness and Alterity: A Phenomenological Investigation*. Evanston: Northwestern University Press.

Zahavi, D. (2002). Metaphysical Neutrality in the 'Logical Investigations'. In: Zahavi, D. and Stjernfelt, F. (eds.) *One Hundred Years of Phenomenology: Husserl's Logical Investigations Revisited*. Phaenomenologica 164. Dordrecht: Kluwer Academic Publishers, 93–108.

Zahavi, D. (2004). Phenomenology and the Project of Naturalization. *Phenomenology and the Cognitive Sciences* **3** (4): 331–47.

Zahavi, D. (2005). *Subjectivity and Selfhood: Investigating the First-Person Perspective*. Cambridge: The MIT Press.

Zahavi, D. (2010). Naturalized Phenomenology. In: Schmicking, D. and Gallagher, S. (eds.) *Handbook of Phenomenology and Cognitive Science*. Dordrecht: Springer, 3–19.

Zahavi, D. (2011). Unity of Consciousness and the Problem of Self. In: Gallagher, S. (ed.) *The Oxford Handbook of the Self*. Oxford: Oxford University Press, 316–33.

Zanarini, M.C. (2000). Childhood Experiences Associated with the Development of Borderline Personality Disorder. *Psychiatric Clinics of North America* **23** (1): 89–101.

Zanarini, M.C. and Frankenburg, F.R. (1997). Pathways to the Development of Borderline Personality Disorder. *Journal of Personality Disorders* **11** (1): 93–104.

Index

action 76–8, 86–90
 agent 79, 89
 emotional resistance to 174
 motivation for 77–8
 rules and practices 86–7, 89
 versus event 76–8
affections 56
affective instability 265–6
affective neuroscience 121–9
affective values 54–7, 125
affectivity 195, 198
 core affective systems 124–5
 mammalian 126, 128, 195, 197–8
 normative 152, 198, 207–10
 see also emotions; feelings
affect programs 120
affects 163–6, 262
 intentionality 166–8
 temporality 168–70
 see also emotions; feelings
affordances 163, 250–1
Agamben, Giorgio 216
agitation 265–6
aïda 273–4
Akiskal, Hagop S. 169, 266
Akiskal, Kareen K. 169
ambiguity 134–7, 142, 146–8, 181–2, 226–7, 267, 297–9
ambivalence 49–51, 94–5, 119, 181–2, 299–300
 bodily 13, 71, 72–9, 119
 feelings of 157, 162
 personhood 13–14, 133–48, 181–2, 297, 299
analytical philosophy 1–2, 19
Andreasen, Nancy C. 22, 311
anger 261–5, 286–7
 in borderline personality disorder 266, 270, 272, 286–7
 definition 264–5
 metaphors 161–2
anglophone tradition 1–2
anhedonia 270–1
animals 120–1, 191–2
 cross-species research 121–2, 128
 distinction from humans 25, 31–2, 191–2, 198
 human animal 137–40, 142, 188
 mammalian affectivity 116, 118, 195, 197–8
 mammalian brain 121, 123–4
 mammalian selfhood 126–8
 personal animals 137–42, 148, 188
antithetical attitude 259
appropriation 52, 142, 302
a-rationality 36, 47–50, 293, 300
 see also rationality

Aristotle 46
attunement 4–4, 75, 163, 203
 schizophrenia and 246–8
authenticity 38
autism 248

Bacon, Francis 303
bad moods 211, 212–16
 personhood relationship 213–16
 varieties of 264–72
Baker, Lynne R. 137, 140–2
Ballerini, Arnaldo 226, 230, 246, 247, 259, 260
Barcelona, Antonio 161
basic emotions 113, 118–20
Baudelaire, Charles 282–3
Befindlichkeit 163–4, 203
belonging to the world 204–5, 210, 241
Bennett, Jonathan 194
Berner, Peter 228, 231, 232, 265
Bernstein, Richard J. 27
Berrios, Germain E. 229
Bertelli, Marco 269
Berze, Joseph 228
Binswanger, Ludwig 222
biological identity 138–9, 146
biology 189–90
Blackburn, Simon 7, 25, 27, 166, 305
Blankenburg, Wolfgang 11, 223, 257, 259
Bleuler, Eugen 228, 252, 255
Bodei, Remo 316
bodily feelings 86, 102
 neuroscientific investigations 115–29
 see also feelings
body 71, 119–20, 241–2, 250
 abnormal experiences of in schizophrenia 243–6
 ambivalence of 13, 71, 72–9, 119
 body state relation to emotion 105–7
 deanimated 245
 dynamisation 244
 externalisation 244
 see also embodiment
borderline personality disorder 11–12, 217, 261, 303, 307, 309
 delusions 268
 emotions in 261–72, 284–7
 invalidation trauma 275–7
 lived time issues 272–80, 287–90
 otherness and 280–4, 293
 traumatic existence 287–92
 traumatic sequence 290–2
 victim, perpetrator, bystander 293–5
boredom 267

bound of sense 46
Bovet, Pierre 260
brain 123–4
　affective nature of 121–2
　imaging 122
　mammalian brain 121, 123–4

Callieri, Bruno 228–30
Cannon, Walter B. 105
care 92–3, 183–4
　hermeneutics of 95, 180–7
Carlson, Gabrielle A. 270
categorical rationality 304
causality 24–5, 47–8
Changeux, Jean-Pierre 51, 192–3
character 81–2, 175
charismatic delusions 260
choreography of emotions 155–62
Clark, Andy 250–1
clinical phenomenology 224
　schizophrenia 222–8
coenesthopathic flooding 247
Coetzee, J.M. 197–8
cognition 189, 250–1
　emotion relationship 128–9, 159, 192
cognitive theories of emotion 107–10, 114, 185
common sense disorder 221, 223, 224, 227–8
conativity of inner time consciousness 246
conatus 11, 61, 90, 193–8, 242
concerns 299
conflict 44–6, 53–4, 57–63, 88–9
Conrad, Klaus 223, 231–2, 234
conscious emotions 154
consciousness 32, 44, 51, 63
　intentional nature 41
Constitution View 140
continental tradition 1–2, 19
Copernican Revolution 44–5
corporeality 85–6, 250
Correale, Antonello 285, 290, 291
cross-species research 121–2, 128
Cutting, John 101, 230, 232

Damasio, Antonio 105–6, 116–20, 121, 153, 189, 192–3
Davidson, Donald 25
de Clérambault, Gaëtan 252, 255, 258
deep moods 211
Deigh, John 101
Deleuze, Gilles 289, 303
Del Pistoia, Luciano 237
delusional mood 221, 228, 230–5
delusions
　in borderline personality disorder 268
　charismatic 260
　eschatological 260
　philosophical 258
　in schizophrenia 223, 248–9, 257–60
De Martino, Ernesto 239

depersonalisation 224
depressed mood 271–2
depression 270
　in borderline personality disorder 271–2
derealisation 224
Descartes, René 119
desires 57–63, 88–9
desocialisation 224
de Sousa, Ronald 8, 47, 109, 111, 114–15, 130–1, 166, 171–3, 190–2, 254, 299, 304, 315–16
despair 266–7
desperate vitality 262, 285
devitalisation 244–5
de Waal, Frans 136–7, 147–8
dialectical model of psychopathology 252–7, 306–10
　schizophrenia 222, 252–7
Dilthey, Wilhelm 32
disattunement 246–8
disconnectedness 227, 234, 246–8
disembodiment 241–6, 247–52, 257–60
disengagement 227
dispositional theory of moods 167
dispositions 82, 297
disproportion 54
Dixon, Thomas 4, 102–3, 150
dual-aspect monism 122–3, 194–5
Dupré, John 189, 190
dynamisation of bodily construction 244
dysphoria 262–4, 265, 269–70, 272, 284–7
　definition 265
dysphoric emotional complex 266

eclipse of meaning 228
Egan, Jennifer 177
Ekman, Paul 8, 118, 153
Eliot, T.S. 68, 83, 94, 144–5, 186
Elster, Jon 155, 162
embarrassment 156–7
embodiment 180
　borderline personality disorder and 271
　of emotions 9–11, 115–29, 159–60
　melancholia and 271–2
　schizophrenia and 241–6, 247–52
　of subjectivity 50–1, 54
　temporality relationship 245–6
emotional dysregulation 265–6
emotional experience 150, 155, 196, 202
　external perspective 173–4, 176
　narrative identity and 171–80
emotional flooding 247
emotional resistance 174, 176
emotional tonality 168–9
emotions 3–4, 99–100, 101, 150–5, 301–2
　basic emotions 113, 118–20
　body state relation 105–7
　in borderline personality disorder 261–4, 284–7
　choreography of 155–62

cognition relationship 128–9, 159, 192
cognitive theories of 107–10, 114, 185
conscious emotions 154
difficulties 129–32
embodied nature of 9–11, 115–29, 159–60
feeling-sensations of 157–8
feeling theories of 104–7, 113
history of 102–3
metaphors 160–2
narrative theories of 110–15
neuroscientific investigations 115–29
normative character of 113
personal nature of 142
personhood relationship 4–9, 149–50
phenomenological description 155–62
philosophy of 100–7
recognition of 159–60
values and 198–200
versus feelings 118, 126, 150–1
see also affectivity; feelings
enactment 4–5
end-of-the-world experience 229–30
engagement 4–5, 163–4
Erikson, Erik H. 284
eschatological delusions 260
euphoric mood 270
Evans, J. 169
event, versus action 76–8
evolution 25–6, 113–14, 137, 188–92
  of emotions 8–9, 107, 119–28, 189
  intentionality and 189–92
  versus biology 189–90
evolutionary psychology 20–1, 31, 130
evolutionary well-being 198–202
existential feelings 151, 202–12
existential negation 62–3
experience 9–11, 28, 41–3, 54–5
  emotional experience 150, 155
  subjectivity and 44
explication 291
exteriority 274
external perspective 173–4, 176
Ey, Henri 240

fallibility 54
familiarity 228
Faulkner, William 300–1
fear of flying 110
feelings 46, 53, 55–63, 99–102, 150–5, 163–4
  articulating 155–62
  awareness of 159–60
  bodily feelings 86, 102
  difficulties 129–32
  existential feelings 151, 202–12
  fundamental feeling 58–9
  intentional relation 58
  interpretation of 100–7
  reason and 55–6
  tension generated 57–63, 88

values and 214
versus emotions 118, 126, 150–1
  see also affects; emotions; moods
feeling-sensations of emotions 157–8
feeling theory of emotion 104–7, 113
feeling-tonality 158
Fergusson, David M. 290
fiction 67
Fink, Hans 25
flying, fear of 110
Foucault, Michel 289
fragility 198–202, 216–17, 296–302
  heart (*thymos*) 57–63
  identity 178–9, 180–1
  personhood 34, 37, 93–5, 146–8, 183–4, 296, 299
  schizophrenia and 248
Frankenburg, Frances R. 271
Frankfurt, Harry G. 278
Freud, Sigmund 65, 115
Fuchs, Thomas 28, 157, 164, 168, 215, 241, 246, 267, 278–9, 287, 308, 310
functional biology 189–90
fundamental feeling 58–9

Gabbani, Carlo 226
Gadamer, Hans-Georg 33
Galimberti, Umberto 315
Gallagher, Shaun 27, 30, 119, 120, 129, 134, 204
Gallese, Vittorio 247
Gehlen, Arnold 30
Goldie, Peter 102, 109, 111, 114–15, 119–20, 150, 151–4, 166, 168, 173–6, 180
good life, the 88–92
Goodwin, Frederick K. 270
Gordon, Robert M. 108
Graham, George 306
Grinberg, Leon 269
Grøn, Arne 144, 148, 178
Gruhle, Hans W. 228
Guidano, Vittorio 291
guilt 156–7, 268–9
Gunderson, John G. 271

habits 82
hallucinations 223
Handke, Peter 233, 236
happiness metaphors 161
Hasker, William 137
heart (*thymos*) 57, 58, 60
  fragile 57–63
Hegel, Georg Wilhelm Friedrich 65
Heidegger, Martin 5, 20, 32–7, 75, 163–4, 178, 202–3, 206, 209, 215–16, 235, 251
hermeneutics 1–2, 19, 29–30, 32–40
  of care 95, 180–7, 310–17
  clinical 296
  hermeneutical phenomenology 29–32, 65

miscarried 293–6, 310, 311
  of the *I am* 53–4, 292–5
  psychopathology and 227
  Ricoeur's philosophical hermeneutics 34–93, 182–3
  of schizophrenic life-worlds 252–7
  of traumatic existence 290–2
H-instincts 190–1
history 67–70
  personal 83, 192
Holland, Dorothy 162
Hornsby, Jennifer 226
human animal 137–40, 142, 188
humiliation 267–8
Husserl, Edmund 34–5, 40, 44, 50, 51, 66, 164, 237, 249

identity 138–9, 170–80, 239
  ambivalence 142–8
  biological 138–9, 146
  borderline personality disorder and 284
  fragile sense of 178–9, 180–1
  imaginative variations 85–6
  narrative 68–70, 79–86, 170–80
  numerical 80
  qualitative 80, 84
  schizophrenia and 239–40
  temporality and 68–70, 146–7
  uninterrupted continuity 80–1
  voluntary and involuntary aspects 171
Ikäheimo, Heikki 7
imaginative variations of personal identity 85–6
immediateness 273–5
imputability 78
inclinations 56–7
indignation 286
infinite interiority 12, 274–5
instantaneity 273–4
instincts 190–1, 195–6
intellect 194
intelligence 188
intentionality 40–4, 51, 166–8, 189–92, 256, 263
  feelings and 58
  levels of performance 256–7
intention to signify 43
internal agitation 265
interpersonal relationships, borderline personality disorder 277, 279
interpersonal values 38
interpretation 65–6
  of feelings 100–7
intersubjectivity 5
intimacy 275, 282
introspection 55, 155, 160
invalidation trauma 275–7
invasiveness 247
irritability 265
irritable-dysphoric temperament 264, 266

Jacob, François 299
James, William 104–5, 106, 153, 185
James–Lange theory of emotion 104–5, 117
Jamieson, Kay R. 270
Jaspers, Karl 30, 38, 228, 248–9, 258
Joyce, James 144

Kane, Sarah 263, 280–3, 284, 288–9, 293
Kant, Immanuel 35–6, 40, 44–6, 66
keeping one's word 81, 82
Kendler, Kenneth S. 225
Kenny, Anthony 105
Kepinski, Antoni 230
Kim, Jaegwon 31
Kimura, Bin 12, 238–40, 263, 273–5, 277, 285
kinaesthesia 249
kinetic–kinaesthetic experience 156, 160
Kipnis, Andrew 162
Kitcher, Phillip 190
Koenigsberg, Harold W. 265
Kövecses, Zoltán 161–2, 287
Kraepelin, Emil 255
Kraus, Alfred 269
Kretschmer, Ernst 268, 294

Laird, James D. 153
Laitinen, Arto 7
Lakoff, George 161
Lange, Carl G. 104
language 12, 61–4, 159–64, 183–7, 308
  infinite interiority and 274–5
Lebensdrang 11, 242–3
LeDoux, Joseph E. 116, 121, 123, 155
life 76, 88
  the good life 88–92
  personal history of 83, 192
life-drive 242–3
  reduction in schizophrenia 243, 251–2
lived space, changes in schizophrenia 232–5
lived time, in borderline personality disorder 272–80, 287–90
logos 307–10

McDowell, John 23–7
McGinn, Colin 297–8
Mallya, Gopinath 266
mammals
  affectivity 116, 118, 195, 197–8
  brain 121, 123–4
  selfhood 126–8
mania 268, 270
material things, objectualisation of in schizophrenia 235–6
Mayer-Gross, Willy 255–6
Mayr, Ernst 189
meaning 43, 64–5, 250–1
  delusions and 248–9
  eclipse of 228
meaningfulness 249–50
Meares, Russell 275–7, 290

melancholia 268, 271
  versus borderline depression 271–2
memory 143–4
mental alienation theory 253
mental illness *see* psychopathology
mental suffering 311–12
Merleau-Ponty, Maurice 228, 234, 237
metaphorical expression of emotions 160–2
metaphysical enactment 259–60
mind 193–5
  disembodied 245
mind-body problem 297–8
minimal sense of self 43–4, 51–2
Minkowski, Eugene 11, 223, 225, 228, 259
miscarried hermeneutics 293–6, 310, 311
mnemotive factor 228
mood disorders 264–72
moods 8–9, 58, 75, 150, 163–6, 202–3, 212–13, 262–3
  deep moods 211
  delusional 221, 228, 230–5
  depressed 271–2
  dispositional theory of 167
  euphoric 270
  intentionality 167–8
  personhood relationship 213–16
  schizophrenic 230–5, 249–51
  temporality 168–70
  see also bad moods
morbid objectivisation 244–5
motivation 5, 52, 57, 77–8, 153, 190–1
movement 5, 153
  choreography of emotions 155–62
  disorder of 229
Moyn, Samuel 254
Mullen, Paul E. 290
Mundt, Christoph 256, 257, 268–9
Murphy, Dominic 304

narrative configuration 84–6
narrative identity 68–70, 79–86, 170–80
  temporal fragmentation of 277–80
narratives 169–80, 302
  of time 66–70
narrative theories of emotion 110–15
naturalism 20–3, 31, 50–1, 297, 298
  relaxed 23–7, 305
neuroscience 192–8, 297
non-coincidence 60, 65, 68, 73–4, 84, 226, 311
normative affectivity 152, 198, 207–10
normative rationality 304–5
norms 300–1
Northoff, Georg 124, 126–7
numerical identity 80
Nussbaum, Martha 108, 109

objectivity 226
objectualisation of material things 235–6

Olson, Eric T. 137–40, 141, 145–6
ontic tie 260
ontology 260
ontology of care 92–3
originating affirmation 11, 61, 64, 183, 193, 242
otherness 11–12, 37–8, 58, 92
  in borderline personality disorder 280–4, 293
  relations with other persons 88–93
  selfhood and 6, 73–4, 76, 93–5, 184

Panksepp, Jaak 116, 120–9, 189, 192, 194–5, 299
Papineau, David 25–6
paradigm scenarios 171–3
Paris, Joel 266, 290
Parnas, Joseph 22, 259, 260
Pasolini, Pier Paolo 262, 285
passivity 223
pathos 307–10
Pazzagli, Adolfo 262
perception 43, 163, 250
  changes in schizophrenia 230–41, 249–50
perceptual theory of emotions 106–7
perplexity 221, 228–35, 245
persecutory guilt 269–70
personal actions 76–8, 79
  motivation for 77–8
personal animal 137–42, 148, 188
personal history 83, 192
personal identity *see* identity
personality 6
personal level of explanation 226
personal relation to the world 56
personhood 2, 103–4, 133–7, 148, 201, 298
  ambivalence 13–14, 133–48, 181–2, 297, 299
  bad mood relationship 213–16
  being human relationship 6–9
  emotion relationship 4–9, 149–50
  fragile nature of 34, 37, 93–5, 146–8, 183–4, 296, 299
  normative nature 178–9
  ontological basis 136–42
  otherness and 93–5
  see also selfhood
perspectivity 43
pervasiveness of normativity 7
phenomenological approach 1–2, 19, 27–30, 155–62, 206–12
  hermeneutical phenomenology 29–32
  psychopathology 225–7
Philips, Katharine A. 271
philosophical delusions 258
philosophy 21–2
  analytical philosophy tradition 1–2, 19
  of psychiatry 23
  of psychopathology 34, 38
  psychopathology relationship 19–23
Pinel, Philippe 222, 252–3, 306
Plessner, Helmuth 30
Plutchik, Robert 153

position-taking 188, 297
  schizophrenia and 221, 229, 252, 255–6
practices 86–8, 89
pre-reflective awareness 42, 43–4, 51–2
Preuss, Todd M. 72
Prinz, Jesse 106–7, 199–200, 299
profundity 227
protention 273
protentional states 5
psychiatry 22, 31
  philosophy of 23
psychopathology 22–3, 27, 225, 296–7
  dialectical model 252–7, 306–10
  mental alienation theory 253
  philosophy of 34, 38
  philosophy relationship 19–23
  subjectivity 28
  syndromes 225
  therapy of care 310–17
  vulnerability 302–3, 305
  see also borderline personality disorder; schizophrenia
psychotic symptoms 223
see also schizophrenia
Pugmire, David 109, 185–6, 198–9
Putnam, Hilary 25
Putnam, Katherine M. 265

qualitative identity 80, 84
quality of familiarity 228

Ratcliffe, Matthew 102, 113, 151–2, 154, 202–12, 299
rationality 24–7, 36, 46–52, 300, 302–4
  categorical 304
  emotions 107–10
  normative 304–5
  precarious nature of 26–7, 47, 49–50
  sui generis character 24, 25
  types of 48–9
reality, vital contact with 223
reappropriation 52
reason 3–4, 44–6, 53–4
  feelings and 55–6
  tension between reason and sensibility 44–6, 53–4, 57–63
recognition
  absence of 275
  desire for 197
  of emotions 159–60
relaxed naturalism 23–7, 305
resignation 286
responsibility 176–7, 302
retaliation 286–7
retention 273
Ricca, Valdo 259
Ricoeur, Paul 5–6, 30, 34–93, 116, 146–7, 164, 170–1, 182–3, 193–7, 210, 241–2, 277, 279, 298, 310, 314

Roberts, Glenn 231
Robinson, Jenefer 109
Rorty, Richard 33
Rosfort, René 168
Rossi Monti, Mario 252, 253, 262, 289, 291
rules 86–8
Russell, Bertrand 3, 109
Russell, James A. 165
Ryle, Gilbert 212–13

Saas, Louis 233
sadness metaphors 161
Sartre, Jean-Paul 108, 111, 164, 267, 300
Saunders, G. 283
Scheler, Max 11, 30, 164, 235, 236, 242–3, 251–2
schizophrenia 11, 217, 221–2, 302–3, 307–9
  clinical phenomenology 222–8
  delusions 223, 248–9, 257–60
  dialectical model 222, 252–7
  disattunement 246–8
  disembodiment 243–6, 247–52, 257–60
  as disorder of common sense 221, 223, 224, 227–8
  hermeneutical account 252–7
  life-drive reduction 242–3
  metaphysical enactment 259–60
  objectualisation of material things 235–6
  spatial perception changes 230–5, 250
  temporality disintegration 236–41, 250
schizophrenic mood 230–5, 248–51
Schleiermacher, Friedrich 32
Schmidt, Gerhardt 230
Schneider, Kurt 8
Schrank, Beate 290
Searle, John 189
Sechehaye, Marguerite 235–235, 240, 247, 251
seeking 125
self 59–64, 76–9
  borderline personality disorder and 275–7
  life of 76
  minimal sense of 43–4, 51–2
  therapy of 38–9
self awareness 41–4, 51–2, 63–4, 160
  borderline personality disorder 284–5
  feelings and 56, 59–63
self-esteem 91, 176–7
selfhood 35–9, 175, 183, 298
  ambivalence 72–9, 119, 133–48, 181–2
  conflictual nature 35–6
  interpretative recovery of 63–6
  levels of 126–7
  mammalian 126–8
  otherness and 6, 73–4, 76, 93–5
  see also personhood; self
SELF (Simple Ego-type Life Form) 123–7
  proto-SELF 126–7
self-transparency 63
Sellars, Wilfrid 24, 131
sensibility 44–6

tension between sensibility and reason 44–6, 53–4, 57–63
sensitive character 268, 294
shame 156–7, 162, 267–8, 270
  metaphors 162
Sheets-Johnstone, Maxine 153, 250
Siemer, Matthias 167
Silk, Kenneth R. 265
Simpson, George G. 20–1
singular reference 197
slow-motion recollection 290–1
Smith, Quentin 157–9, 164, 267
solicitude 91
see also care
Solomon, Robert C. 108–9, 153–4, 156–7, 185, 189, 265, 299
somatic-marker hypothesis 116–17
spatiality 76
  perceptual changes in schizophrenia 230–5, 250
  temporality relationships 238–41
spatializing-temporalizing vortex 228, 261
Spinoza, Baruch 11, 61, 90, 192–5, 242
spiritual desires 57–63, 88–9
Stanghellini, Giovanni 168, 224, 225, 226, 230, 240, 242, 244, 246, 247, 252, 259, 260, 269, 271, 283, 285, 289, 291
Stocker, Michael 109, 110, 152
Stone, Michael H. 266
Störring, Gustav E. 229, 249
Strasser, Stephan 30, 153, 164, 167, 168, 176, 211, 214
Strauss, John S. 254
Strawson, Galen 179
Strawson, Peter F. 46, 141
sub-apophanic schizophrenia 223, 224, 259
subjectivity 5–6, 19, 28–9, 210, 274
  embodied nature of 50–1, 54
  experiential structures of 44, 59–60
  Ricoeur's hermeneutical theory 34–93, 182–3
substance dualism 137
Swain, Gladys 222, 306
Swinburne, Richard 137
synthesis of inner time consciousness 246

Taylor, Charles 90, 111–13, 178, 252
Teichert, Dieter 175
teleology 190, 196–7
Tellenbach, Hubertus 266, 269, 271
temperament 169
temporality 66–70
  affects and moods 168–70
  anomalies of temporalisation 272–3
  borderline personality disorder 272–80, 287–90
  change with time 146–7, 168
  disintegration of in schizophrenia 236–41, 250

embodiment relationship 245–6
permanence of identity 80–1
spatiality relationships 238–41
see also time
tension between reason and sensibility 44–6, 53–4, 57–63
Thagard, Paul 21
therapy of care 310–17
therapy of the self 38–9
third-time 66–7
Thomas, Dylan 263
Thompson, Evan 9, 27, 153, 213, 250
Thornton, Tim 23, 25, 27, 305
thrownness 75
time 66–70, 79, 143, 146, 169
  change with 146–7, 168
  lived time in borderline personality disorder 272–80
  permanence of identity 80–1
  see also temporality
Tinbergen, Nikolaas 190
T-instincts 190–1
touch 204
transcendental synthesis 44–5, 51
traumatic existence, borderline personality disorder 287–92
  hermeneutics of 290–2
traumatic sequence 290–2
trema 221, 224, 231–2
typus melancholicus (TM) 268–9

understanding 55
  of feelings 100–7
unfathomed flatness of lived space in schizophrenia 230–5
Unger, P. 137
Ur-emotion 11
Urfer, Annick 259

values 64–5, 88–90, 299
  affective 54–7
  emotions and 198–200
  feelings and 214
  interpersonal 38
Varela, Francisco J. 250
Vattimo, Gianni 33
vital contact with reality 223, 259
vital desires 57–63, 88–9
Vogt, Brent A. 311
von Weizsäcker, Viktor 239
vulnerability 11–12, 217, 296–7, 302–6, 310–12, 316–17
  borderline personality disorder 266, 268, 293–5
  schizophrenia 253, 258–9

well-being, fragility of 198–202, 216–17
Westen, Drew 279, 284
West, Rebecca 276

Wetzel, August 229–30
Whitman, Walter 46
Wilkinson-Ryan, Tess 279, 284
Williams, Bernard 269
will to exist 242
Wollheim, Richard 111, 135, 147
Wood, Allan W. 36

Wyller, Truls 311
Wyrsch, Jakob 252, 256, 257

Zachar, Peter 225
Zahavi, Dan 27, 28, 29, 42, 43–4, 127, 134, 204, 234–5, 237
Zanarini, Mary C. 271, 290

Lightning Source UK Ltd.
Milton Keynes UK
UKOW06f0603090216

268009UK00001B/1/P